NURSING RESEARCH
& STATISTICS

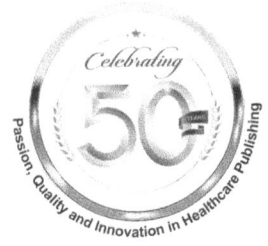

NURSING RESEARCH & STATISTICS

Second Edition

Rajesh Kumar PhD (N) RN RM
Assistant Professor
College of Nursing
All India Institute of Medical Sciences (AIIMS)
Rishikesh, Uttarakhand, India

Foreword
K Reddemma

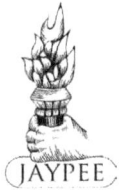

JAYPEE BROTHERS MEDICAL PUBLISHERS
The Health Sciences Publisher
New Delhi | London | Panama

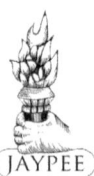 **Jaypee Brothers Medical Publishers (P) Ltd**

Headquarters
Jaypee Brothers Medical Publishers (P) Ltd
4838/24, Ansari Road, Daryaganj
New Delhi 110 002, India
Phone: +91-11-43574357
Fax: +91-11-43574314
Email: jaypee@jaypeebrothers.com

Overseas Offices

J.P. Medical Ltd
83 Victoria Street, London
SW1H 0HW (UK)
Phone: +44 20 3170 8910
Fax: +44 (0)20 3008 6180
Email: info@jpmedpub.com

Jaypee-Highlights Medical Publishers Inc
City of Knowledge, Bld. 235, 2nd Floor
Clayton, Panama City, Panama
Phone: +1 507-301-0496
Fax: +1 507-301-0499
Email: cservice@jphmedical.com

Jaypee Brothers Medical Publishers (P) Ltd
Bhotahity, Kathmandu, Nepal
Phone: +977-9741283608
Email: kathmandu@jaypeebrothers.com

Website: www.jaypeebrothers.com
Website: www.jaypeedigital.com

© 2019, Jaypee Brothers Medical Publishers

The views and opinions expressed in this book are solely those of the original contributor(s)/author(s) and do not necessarily represent those of editor(s) of the book.

All rights reserved. No part of this publication may be reproduced, stored or transmitted in any form or by any means, electronic, mechanical, photocopying, recording or otherwise, without the prior permission in writing of the publishers.

All brand names and product names used in this book are trade names, service marks, trademarks or registered trademarks of their respective owners. The publisher is not associated with any product or vendor mentioned in this book.

Medical knowledge and practice change constantly. This book is designed to provide accurate, authoritative information about the subject matter in question. However, readers are advised to check the most current information available on procedures included and check information from the manufacturer of each product to be administered, to verify the recommended dose, formula, method and duration of administration, adverse effects and contraindications. It is the responsibility of the practitioner to take all appropriate safety precautions. Neither the publisher nor the author(s)/editor(s) assume any liability for any injury and/or damage to persons or property arising from or related to use of material in this book.

This book is sold on the understanding that the publisher is not engaged in providing professional medical services. If such advice or services are required, the services of a competent medical professional should be sought.

Every effort has been made where necessary to contact holders of copyright to obtain permission to reproduce copyright material. If any have been inadvertently overlooked, the publisher will be pleased to make the necessary arrangements at the first opportunity. The **CD/DVD-ROM** (if any) provided in the sealed envelope with this book is complimentary and free of cost. **Not meant for sale.**

Inquiries for bulk sales may be solicited at: jaypee@jaypeebrothers.com

Nursing Research and Statistics

First Edition: 2016

Second Edition: **2019**

ISBN: 978-93-5270-761-4

Printed at

Foreword

It gives me great pleasure to write the Foreword for the book *Nursing Research and Statistics* written by Assistant Professor, Dr Rajesh Kumar, a renowned research scholar. The content is comprehensive, easy and most updated to meet the needs of nursing students. The book is designed as per the nursing curriculum governed by Indian Nursing Council (INC) for graduate and postgraduate nursing students. Each chapter is written in a well-designed manner to meet different needs of nursing students. I must mention that chapters 11 and 12 will sensitize the nursing professionals about research misconduct and statistical analysis for different types of research designs. I am happy to announce that this book will be a landmark in history of nursing research and statistics and enrich the nursing fraternity with updated research knowledge.

I hope this book will be of great help for students of nursing research and will be referred widely. I congratulate the author for his initiative and effort in bringing out this book on nursing research.

K Reddemma
Nodal Officer
National Consortium for PhD in Nursing by
Indian Nursing Council

Formerly, Dean
Behavioral Sciences, and
Senior Professor, Department of Nursing
National Institute of Mental Health and Neurosciences
Bengaluru, Karnataka, India

Preface to the Second Edition

Nursing profession is rapidly changing from conventional nursing to evidence-based nursing. This has created ample of challenges to nursing professionals at every level and also created demand for professionally trained nurse researchers. Consumer awareness, high-tech hospital environment and globalization also augment need of research-trained nursing professionals. Better and efficient quality care with minimum complications became key for success of any organization. The nurse professionals who are passionate in research, dynamic and fully accustomed with research environment can achieve this.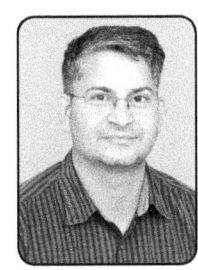

Nursing research can play a wonderful role to achieve high quality care, higher patient satisfaction and efficient use of resources to contribute growth of an organization. To achieve this, nurse professionals are required to be fully equipped with latest and updated knowledge of research and analytic process, especially those which have application at Indian scenarios. A complete and comprehensive knowledge of various basic as well as advanced research strategies will energize them to involve more and more research and research-related activities. Moreover, nursing research and statistics is an integral component of graduate and postgraduate nursing curriculum. A number of nursing students and nursing professionals are involved in research activities at institute and hospital level to explore new facts and evidence.

The present text is the modest attempt to bring the latest and updated material on research tactics, different designs, sampling, research misconduct and publication of the findings. The efforts in this book have been focused to sensitize different category of nursing professionals and to provide a framework for conducting systematic and quality research. The chapters are arranged in a sequence to facilitate reading and learning. The book is a comprehensive package to nursing research and different statistical tests for undergraduate and postgraduate students and practice nurses.

Rajesh Kumar

Preface to the First Edition

Nursing is an evolving profession and is committed to promote health, prevention of illness and restoration of disease. Nursing research plays a significant role to achieve the maxim of nursing profession by finding facts and improving knowledge related to given concept. Nursing research is a scientific inquiry to explore the hidden issues and helps to maintain professional growth and dignity. Research-based knowledge provides scientific basis for developing and refining the professional knowledge and practice. Nursing research helps and gives chance to study population as a whole, i.e. individual, family, and community.

In order to find facts and figures, it is mandatory to have complete and comprehensive knowledge about different steps of research and its relevant concepts; origin of nursing research, progress at different period of interval, scope of nursing research, resources needed to carry research, need and importance of research demanding environment, various problems faced by researcher and opportunities in field.

The book covers all syllabus governed by Indian Nursing Council for graduate and postgraduate nursing students. This book enables nursing faculty, graduate and postgraduate nursing students to learn various notified concepts of nursing research and statistics. Its primary goal is to give simple, realistic and understandable knowledge to nursing fraternity. It covers many relevant and real-life research examples to make the concepts understandable and practical. In addition, this book will help nursing fraternity to learn about various concepts and ways of research publication and enable to publish paper in nursing discipline to improve personal and professional growth.

I hope this book will create a landmark in history of nursing research. It will be my gratification to receive your suggestion and review inputs on *rajeshrak61@gmail.com*.

Rajesh Kumar

Acknowledgments

This textbook is the result of many helping hands and these came in the shape of advisors, colleagues, teachers, family members and many other people. I am thankful to all of them from the core of my heart, for helping me in completing the task within appropriate time limits.

I would like to acknowledge the comments of reviewers, whose feedback greatly influenced me to shape this textbook. Several of the comments triggered my work and motivated me to refine the content from time to time.

I must say thanks to God for giving me such a beautiful and a great human being in the form of my life partner, my wife, **Capt. Kalpana Beniwal**, Assistant Nursing Superintendent (ANS), All India Institute of Medical Sciences (AIIMS), Rishikesh, Uttarakhand. My life was certainly incomplete without her, my sweet daughter, **Rythm R Kataria (Pihoo)** for showing high degree of patience and sacrifices during the work. I owe her time I spent without her while working on this book.

My sincere thanks to Shri Jitendar P Vij (Group Chairman), Mr Ankit Vij (Managing Director) and Mr MS Mani (Group President) of M/s Jaypee Brothers Medical Publishers (P) Ltd, New Delhi, India for giving me an opportunity to share the knowledge with this book.

Above all, I would like to express my deep sense of gratitude to God Almighty for abiding grace and blessing, which gave me the strength for completing this book successfully.

Contents

Chapter 1 — Introduction to Nursing Research — 1
- Introduction 1
- Problem-solving 1
- Scientific Methods and Research 3
- Methods of Acquiring Knowledge in Nursing 5
- Research and Nursing Research 6
- Characteristics of Good Research 8
- Purposes of Research 8
- History of Nursing Research 9
- Types of Research 13
- Scope and Areas of Nursing Research 17
- Significance of Research in Nursing 19
- Evidence-based Practice 20
- Review Questions and Answer 25

Chapter 2 — Research Problem, Research Question and Hypothesis — 29
- Introduction 29
- Research Problem 29
- Sources of Research Problem 30
- Steps of Identifying a Research Problem 32
- Components of a Problem Statement 32
- Research Question 33
- Evaluation Criteria for a Research Problem 34
- Variables 36
- Operational Definitions 37
- Research Objectives 39
- Assumptions 40
- Hypothesis 42
- Delimitations 46
- Limitations 48
- Review Questions and Answer 48

Chapter 3 — The Research Process: An Overview — 52
- Introduction 52
- Fundamental Research Terms 52
- Quantitative Research Process: Overview 53
- Steps in Qualitative Study 56
- Review Questions and Answer 59

Chapter 4 | Ethical Issues in Research — 61
- Introduction *61*
- Code of Ethics *61*
- Importance of Ethics in Research *63*
- Ethical Principles for Protecting Human Rights *63*
- Measures to Protect the Rights of Study Participants *65*
- Ethical Issues in Animal Research *68*
- Review Questions and Answer *68*

Chapter 5 | Review of Literature — 71
- Introduction *71*
- Definitions *71*
- Characteristics of a Quality Review *72*
- Factors Affecting Literature Review *72*
- Purposes of Literature Review *73*
- Importance of Literature Review *73*
- Types of Literature Review *74*
- Sources of Literature Review *75*
- Steps of Literature Review *80*
- Organization of Literature Review *82*
- Tips for Writing Literature Review *82*
- Critical Appraisal of Review *83*
- Review Questions and Answer *84*

Chapter 6 | Theories and Conceptual Models in Research — 86
- Introduction *86*
- Theory *86*
- Terminology of Theory *87*
- Importance of Theory in Nursing *87*
- Model *87*
- Conceptual Framework *88*
- Theoretical Framework *91*
- Types of Theories *92*
- Importance of Theory, Models and Framework in Research *93*
- Use of Theory in Research *94*
- Relationship between Theory, Research and Practice *97*
- Process of Conceptual Framework Development *97*
- Review Questions and Answer *98*

Chapter 7 | Research Designs — 101
- Introduction *101*
- Definitions *101*

- Characteristics of a Good Research Design   102
- Factors Affecting Selection of Study Design   102
- Quantitative Research   103
- Experimental Research   106
- True Experimental Research   106
- Quasi-experimental Research   114
- Pre-experimental Research   117
- Non-experimental Designs   119
- Descriptive Research   120
- Epidemiological Research   122
- Analytical Studies   123
- Developmental Research   124
- Survey Research   126
- Additional Types of Quantitative Research   128
- Qualitative Research Design   130
- Phenomenology   132
- Ethnography   134
- Grounded Theory   136
- Historical Research   137
- Case Study   139
- Action Research   140
- Delphi Technique   143
- Review Questions and Answer   145

Chapter 8 | Sample and Sampling Techniques   151
- Introduction   151
- Sampling Terms   151
- Sampling Criteria   153
- Importance of Sampling in Research   154
- Characteristics of a Good Sample   154
- Types of Sampling Techniques   155
- Probability Sampling Techniques   155
- Non-probability Sampling   160
- Factors Affecting Sampling/Sample Size   164
- Sampling Process in Quantitative Research   165
- Problems in Sampling   166
- Sample Size Calculation   166
- Power Analysis   169
- Sample Size for Animal Studies   169
- Review Questions and Answer   170

Chapter 9 | Data Collection Methods in Research   173
- Introduction   173
- Purposes of Data Collection   173

- Types of Data 174
- Sources of Data 174
- Data Collection Plan 175
- Data Collection Methods 176
- Questionnaire 178
- Rating Scale 184
- Checklist 188
- Interview Method 190
- Observation Method 195
- Biophysiological Methods 198
- Record Analysis 200
- Q-sort 201
- Vignettes 202
- Projective Techniques 204
- Validity and Reliability 205
- Cultural Equivalence of an Instrument 213
- Pilot Study/Feasibility Study 214
- Review Questions and Answer 215

Chapter 10 Data Analysis and Interpretation 219
- Introduction 219
- Statistical Procedures 219
- Descriptive Statistics 219
- Levels of Measurement 220
- Frequency Distribution 221
- Normal Distribution Curve 221
- Measures of Central Tendency 221
- Measures of Dispersion/Variability 222
- Data Processing 223
- Data Presentation 225
- Inferential Statistics 239
- Qualitative Data Analysis 241
- Ethnographic Analysis 248
- Grounded Theory Analysis 249
- Phenomenological Analysis 250
- Review Questions and Answer 253

Chapter 11 Communication and Dissemination of Research Findings 257
- Introduction 257
- Communication of Research Findings 257
- Research Report 260
- References and Bibliography 263
- Critical Appraisal of Research Report 264

- Research Proposal 266
- Research and Publication Misconduct 269
- Research Utilization 271
- Evidence-based Practice 271
- Facilitating Research Utilization 273
- Review Questions and Answer 274

Chapter 12: Introduction to Statistics 277

- Introduction 277
- Meaning and Definition 277
- Characteristics of Statistics 278
- Functions of Statistics 278
- Common Statistical Terms 279
- Levels of Measurement 279
- Descriptive Statistics 281
- Methods of Data Presentation 281
- Measures of Central Tendency 290
- Measure of Dispersion/Variability 297
- Coefficient of Correlation 305
- Spearman's Rank Correlation Coefficient 308
- Normal Distribution Curve 309
- Inferential Statistics 312
- Parametric and Nonparametric Tests 314
- Tests of Significance 315
- Statistical Packages and Analysis 323
- Review Questions and Answer 324

Appendices 327
Glossary 343
Index 361

Chapter 1

Introduction to Nursing Research

INTRODUCTION

Nursing is noble profession which needs a continuous growing and expanding body of knowledge. Knowledge can be developed through many ways and research is one of them. Nurses are increasingly expected to understand and conduct research to develop a scientific basis for improving knowledge. Research is a systematic way of exploring the hidden issues and helps to maintain professional growth and dignity. Research-based knowledge provides scientific basis for developing and refining the professional knowledge and practice.

Because nursing is a practice profession, it is important that clinical practice should be based on scientific knowledge. Evidences generated through nursing research provide support for quality and cost effectiveness of nursing intervention. Thus, recipient of health care and particularly nursing care–reap benefits when nurses attend to research evidence and introduce change based on that evidence into nursing practice. The result of research provides foundation on which practice, decision and behavior are based.

PROBLEM-SOLVING

A problem is a situation that can be quantitative or qualitative, confront an individual or groups of individual, and require solution. Problem-solving is a powerful human activity; it is a process, an activity, whereby the best solution is selected from available solutions. The ability to solve a problem comes from doing it. Many things must put together to solve a problem. Researchers have proposed many different models of problem-solving. The basic model of problem-solving is discussed in Figure 1.1.

Problem-solving Process

Problem solving process is a series of logical steps which progress to a solution for a selected problem. Problem solving process consist six steps easy approach to resolve a issue or problem faced by the students and clinician at their work place. It is simple and systematic way to approach a problem with clearly defined steps to answer, 'WHAT DO WE DO NEXT?'. The problem-solving model follows a series of six steps. The steps are explained here:

1. *Problem identification:* The first step, identifying the problem is a broad view. In this first stage, researcher needs to write down about the problem in details. Writing about the problem in detail will help to comprehend the problem.
2. *Problem analysis:* Once you have defined the problem, you can begin with analyzing the problem from different angles such as magnitude of problem, factors affects problem,

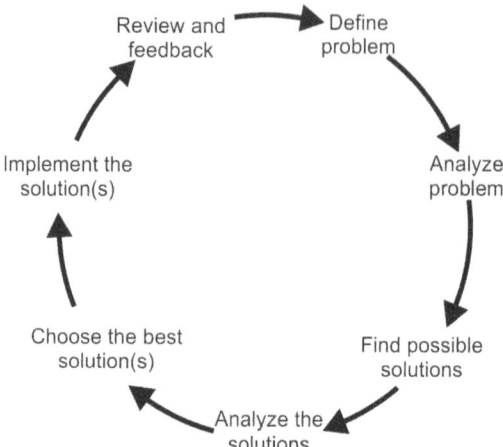

Fig. 1.1: Problem-solving model.

how problem affect researcher and heath care cost and many such issues. Furthermore, Problem analysis develop insight into a researcher about the problem and its relative impacts on different spheres such as in clinical, research and education. Overall, problem analysis develop deeper understanding of gravity of the problem and factors contributing to the problem.

3. *Search best available evidence(s):* Once you explore the root cause of the problem, you may move to find the possible solutions. This is a creative and practical step where every possible solution is identified. However, a creative problem-solving requires use of brain storming and other cognitive processes (i.e. intuition) to explore a full range of possible solutions. Assemble all possible alternative solutions and move to next step.
4. *Analyze evidence(s) for its strengths and weaknesses:* At this step, now you may have a variety of solution to fix the problem given the circumstances, resources, and other considerations. Here, the individual trying to choose the best possible solution in given situation. There are always a number of things that can affect a solution; money, time, people, procedure, policies and so on. All of these factors must be taken in consideration. An effective solution should be technically feasible and sound. The solution should be acceptable to those who will have to implement it.
5. *Select best evidence for clinical practice:* This seems to be an easy step but it really requires a scientific approach to observing specifically what is going on with the implemented solution. Choosing the solution does not immediately solve the problem. Implementing a solution into action may help to solve the problem.
6. *Evaluate outcomes and revise, if necessary:* This is the final stage of problem-solving process. In this step, evaluation is made to judge the effectiveness of the solution to resolve the problem. This will helps to evaluate change in practice. This step enables an researcher to ask, 'Did the solution work? If not, why not? What went right, and what went wrong?'. Answer of all these questions enable the individual to act on finding best solution again. In case of failure, redefine and revise the problem and start the process again.

Table 1.1: Research process and problem-solving: A comparison.

Research process	Problem-solving
Research focus on multiple problems of an individual or organization	Target on single problem of individual or organization
Research contribute to professional growth by replication or generalization of findings	Solution derived from problem-solving cannot be replicated on others, as others may have different cause for same problem
Research process need to stick with certain ethical issues	No ethical issues come across in problem-solving process
Research subject to undergone external and peer review process to determine validity and reliability	A problem of an particular individual or organization is an isolated problem and only need solution

Both, problem-solving and research process use abstract critical thinking and complex reasoning to solve a problem. However, research process should be distinguished from problem-solving on following criteria as given in Table 1.1.

SCIENTIFIC METHODS AND RESEARCH

Scientific method is a systematic and objective method of investigation. Scientific method is the basis of scientific investigation. In scientific method, the investigator poses a research question and formulates hypotheses to answer research question. The hypotheses states a potential explanation or answer to question. Research is also systematic and based on empirical evidences to explore the issue under investigation.

Characteristics of Scientific Method

A scientific method should reflect following characteristics:
- *Systematic process:* Scientific method is an orderly process. Investigator proceeds logically through a series of steps according to specified plan of action.
- *Control:* Researcher imposes certain conditions on the research situation to minimize biases and maximize precision and validity of result.
- *Empirical (Objective) evidences:* Researcher collect empirical evidence through the objective method like observation, sense, touch, smell, hear or taste.
- *Quantitative information:* Usually, collected information in scientific method is numerical in nature. Numeric information is collected through use of valid and reliable measurement tools like questionnaire, rating scale or biophysiological report, etc.
- *Generalizability:* Findings of the scientific method can be generalized over other population.

Limitations of Scientific Method

The scientific method has enjoyed considerable stature as a method of inquiry and has been used productively by nurse researchers studying a range of nursing problems. However, scientific method imposed certain limitations.
- *Moral-ethical problem:* The scientific method cannot be used to answer certain moral or ethical issues. For example, legalization of female feticides, legalization of Euthanasia, etc.

- *Measurement related problem:* The traditional research approach study a phenomena by measuring a construct. Sometimes, researcher do not have sound measurement device to measure a specific construct like assessment of moral status, hope, motivation, etc.
- *Human behavior complexity:* Human are inherently complex and diverse in nature. Scientific method can only study a handful of human characteristics, i.e. height, weight, anxiety, depression, etc. Scientific method fails to study the variation of one parameter among different human being. For example, why some people show quick reaction to something not others?, why some people get easily annoyed not others?, etc.
- *Control problem:* The rigorous control is the core of scientific method. Hence, a specific problem is studied in a systematic and objective ways by keeping rigorous control and holding condition constant which permits only variation to phenomena comes under study. Sometime, researcher fails to control over external and internal environmental condition that can influence the phenomena under study.

Steps of Scientific Methods

Scientific methods follow a series of systematic steps. These steps may vary in different research designs. However, the main steps remain same in a scientific method. These steps are explained here:

- *Selection of area and research problem:* Researcher choose the area of interest and explore it for possible research problems. Selection of research problem and defining a specific research question enable researcher to progress the research study.
- *List down the objectives for the study:* A well-framed, specific and measurable objective help to focus on the study. A research may have varied number of objectives.
- *Review the literature:* Researcher explore the possible sources of information to develop insight about related issues of the research problem under study.
- *Define the variables under study:* Variables are defined in terms of their outcomes to conclude the results of the study.
- *State hypothesis:* Hypothesis helps to find out the association and relationship between different variables and concepts under study. Hypothesis helps to reach on a significant conclusion of the study.
- *Ethical consideration:* Researcher should seek ethical permission after clarifying all ethical principles before ethical board or ethical committee. Ethical permission helps a researcher to get rid out from any unethical claims in future (if any).
- *Describe research methodology:* A well-defined research methodology is the heart of a research study. A methodology should consist population, setting, sample size, sampling techniques and details of methods of data collection.
- *Collect data from subjects:* This is the implementation phase of a research study where the intervention is being delivered to population. Researcher collect information with the help of standardized measures/tools.
- *Analysis and interpretation of data:* Data will be analyzed as per stating objective and hypothesis.
- *Dissemination of findings:* The researcher should disseminate the findings by using any ways of dissemination such as oral presentation or publication in a journal, etc.

METHODS OF ACQUIRING KNOWLEDGE IN NURSING

Knowledge is essential information acquired in a variety of ways, expected to be an accurate reflection of reality and incorporated and used to direct a person's life. The quality of nursing practice has direct relation with the quality of knowledge that a nurse acquired. Knowledge may be acquired through many ways. The quality of nursing care depends on the selection of the source of knowledge of a health care workers. Nurses have relied on several sources of knowledge to guide nursing practice. These source are broadly classified in following two ways.

Unstructured Methods

These sources of information considered more informal and based on personal opinions of self or seniors in a profession. These methods have very little scientific rationale for the information you acquired. Knowledge from traditional things, higher authority and intuition are few examples of unstructured sources.

- *Authority:* An authority is a person with much knowledge and experience and who is capable to influence the others. Nurses who are frequently involved in research work and publication are considered authority. Knowledge acquired from higher authority does not have any scientific basis for truth. But, it is a great source of acquiring knowledge to novice researchers either from higher authority or from their published work.
- *Brainstorming:* It is another cost effective and efficient means of acquiring knowledge. In brainstorming, a group of experts will sit together and discuss the problem from different point of views to reach on a common consensus. Brainstorming helps to take ideas from different background and specialized experts for an issue.
- *Intuition:* Intuition is a part of thinking, including intuition in critical thinking helps to expand the person's ability to know about something. Intuition described as gut feeling or 'hunch' for something. It is an insight or understanding for a particular phenomenon. Some people do not believe in intuition. Nurses may have feeling of intuition while they provide care, for example, 'I just have this feeling that Mr Ram is heading for problem'. It is hard to explain what it is but it happens.
- *Subjective experience and clinical field work:* Gaining knowledge by being personally involved in an event, situation or circumstance is called subjective experience. Nurse's everyday experience is a rich source of acquiring knowledge. Personal experience in clinical setting is a provocative source of knowledge. A nurse can acquire knowledge from day-to-day routine in clinical area. Learning from experience enabled the nurses to gather ideas in a meaningful way. For example, you may read about mouth care procedure in book but in reality you do not know how to give mouth care until you either assist or do the procedure on a patient in clinical area.
- *Trial and error:* Since the existence of human being on earth, trial and error method are used to acquire and expand the knowledge. Likewise, nurses may use trial and error method while providing care. However, trial and error method does not have any scientific steps to follow, but it will help to improve the knowledge.
- *Tradition:* Many question and problem are solved in the preview of traditional views or belief that is based on customs and traditional trends. Nursing tradition from past to present generation is transferred through oral or written communication. However, in the

scenario of evidence-based practice (EBP), nursing knowledge must be based on scientific facts rather than traditional views to have a powerful impact on patient outcomes.

Structured Methods

Knowledge acquired from highly structured sources believe to deliver better quality of care. Logical reasoning, scientific methods or research and problem-solving are few examples of structured sources of knowledge.

- *Borrowing:* Borrowing in nursing involves the appropriation and use of knowledge from other fields or disciplines to guide nursing practice. Knowledge can be borrowed from other health and other disciplines like medicine, sociology, psychology and physical sciences to improve nursing knowledge.
- *Scientific research:* Scientific research is a most objective and reliable source of nursing knowledge. The knowledge needed for practice should be specific and outcomes focused. Thus, a variety of research methods are needed to generate nursing knowledge. Quantitative, qualitative and many other types of research are used to generate nursing knowledge.
- *Literature review:* Reading literature is a good source to acquire knowledge about certain topics in nursing. Novice researchers can profit from regularly reading published and unpublished work on nursing and its related issues. Reviewing literature need experience and multidimensional skills like critical appraisal, reasoning, and analytic skills.

RESEARCH AND NURSING RESEARCH

Research

The word *Research* is derived from *'French'* word and it literal meaning is *'to investigate thoroughly'*. Research is to search again or examine carefully. The term *Research* in *'Latin'* means *'to know'.* So, research is a careful, systematic patient study and investigation in some field of knowledge, undertaken to establish facts or principles. Given the complex nature of research, finding one definition that achieves consensus is difficult. Most research textbooks will contain a variation on this theme as a definition of research. Some important definitions are given below:

'Systematic inquiry that use disciplined method to answer questions or solve problem'.
(Polit and Beck, 2008)

'Research is an attempt to increase the sum of what is known, usually referred to as a 'body of knowledge' by the discovery of new facts or relationship through a process of systematic enquiry, the research process'. *(Hockey, 1984)*

'The attempt to derive generalization new knowledge by addressing clearly defined questions with systematic and rigorous method'. *(DOH, 2005)*

'A methodological examination that uses regimented techniques to resolve questions or decipher dilemmas'. *(Boswal and Cannon, 2007)*

'A careful investigation or inquiry especially through search for new facts in any branch of knowledge'. *(The Advanced Learner's Dictionary)*

'Research is a systematized effort to gain new knowledge'. *(Redman and Mory, 1933)*

'The manipulation of things, concepts or symbols for the purpose of generalizing to extend, correct or verify knowledge, whether that knowledge aids in construction of theory or in the practice of an art'. *(Encyclopedia of Social Sciences)*

'It is search for knowledge through objective and systematic method of findings solution to a problem.'

'Research is a structural inquiry that utilizes acceptable scientific methodology to solve problem and create new knowledge that is generally applicable.'

'A systematic approach concerning generalization and the formulation of theory.'

'Research comprises defining and redefining problem, formulating hypothesis or suggested solution; collecting, organizing and evaluating data; making deductions and reaching conclusions; and it last carefully testing the conclusions to determine whether they fit the following hypothesis.'

'Systematic method consisting of enunciating the problem, formulating a hypothesis, collecting the facts or data, analyzing the facts and reaching certain conclusion either in the form of solution(s) towards the concerned problem or in certain generalization for some theoretical formulation.'

Nursing Research

The purpose of nursing research is to build knowledge in a discipline through the generation and/or testing theory. Research is conducted to describe, explain, and predict the outcomes. Nursing research concerned with the study of individual, its interaction with environment and discovering intervention that promotes optimal functioning and wellness across the lifespan. Nursing research is systematic, objective process of analyzing phenomena of importance to nursing. It includes studies concerning nursing practice, nursing education, nursing administration and nurses themselves. Clinical nursing research is research that has potential for affecting the care of clients.

'Scientific process that validates and refines existing knowledge and generate new knowledge that directly or indirectly influence nursing practice.'

'Systematic inquiry designed to develop knowledge about issues of importance to the nursing profession including nursing practice, education, administration and informatics.'
(Polit and Beck, 2004)

'A systematic approach to gathering information for the purpose of answering questions and solving problems in the pursuit of creating new knowledge about nursing practice, education and policy.' *(Moule and Hek, 2011)*

'Nursing research refers to use of systematic, controlled, empirical and critical investigation in attempting to discover or conform facts that relate to specific problem or question about the practice of nursing.' *(Waltz and Bausell, 1981)*

'Nursing research is a way to identify new knowledge, improve professional education and practices and use of resources effectively.' *(ICN, 1986)*

'Nursing research is a systematic enquiry that seeks to add new nursing knowledge to benefits patients, families and communities. It encompasses all aspects of health that are interest to nursing, including promotion of health, prevention of illness, care of people of all ages during illness and recovery towards a peaceful and dignified death.' *(ICN, 2009)*

Research is directed towards understanding the nursing care of individuals and groups and the biological, physiological, social, behavioral and environmental mechanism influencing health and disease that are relevant to nursing care.

CHARACTERISTICS OF GOOD RESEARCH

Research is a systematic, controlled and orderly process. A good research should have following features in it:
- *Systematic and orderly process:* A well-designed research is based on scientific process and follow a standard process from selection of research problem to dissemination of findings. Therefore, a quality research conducted in systematic and orderly manner.
- *Strive to find solution of the problem:* Findings solution of the professional problems is the primary purpose of scientific research. Research always focused on findings alternative and efficient solution for refining and upgrading professional practice.
- *Focus on improvement of existing professional practice:* A well-planned and controlled research significantly contribute in refinement and improvement of existing outdated professional practice. Therefore, a good research should be always focus to improve professional practices.
- *Based on current issues of the profession:* A good research always focused on resolution of the current issues of a profession. Therefore, research based on current professional issue helps to upgrade the profession.
- *Focused to improve body of knowledge:* A good research always strive to build up new empirical evidences to refine the existing knowledge in a profession. It is considered as a primary objective of a research to improve body of professional knowledge.
- *Always focus on empirical evidences:* An orderly and systematic designed research focus on empirical information, which can be used to improve the professional practice. Therefore, a good research always relies on empirical information.
- *Use of appropriate methods and measures*: Selection of appropriate research methods and measures is key to collect empirical information and generate evidences. Therefore, a sound research based on selection of appropriate methodology and measures.
- *Geared towards evidences development*: A research can only be considered good if it helps to build up high quality evidences. High quality evidences helps to refine the outdated professional practices. Therefore, a good research should focus on generation of high quality of evidences.
- *Adequate reporting and recording:* A research is considered incomplete until and unless it is not recorded and reported to anyone. A well-recorded research information work as source of information and helps in generation of quality evidence in professional practice.
- *Timely communicated:* A research is not complete if it is not communicated to others. Therefore, research findings should be timely communicated to its target users.

PURPOSES OF RESEARCH

The main purpose of the research is to answer the research question through the application of scientific procedure. Through, each research study has its own specific purpose. The specific purpose of nursing research includes identification, description, exploration, prediction and control of phenomena. However, nursing research serve following purposes:
- Describe a particular individual or group of individual or organization
- Test the hypothesis of a casual relationship between two variables
- Determine the frequency with which something occurs or with which it is associated with something else

- Enhance the body of professional knowledge to improve patient care and outcomes
- Improve personal and professional growth
- Enhance the professional identity
- Improve consumer (patient and their relative) satisfaction
- Formulate and test nursing theories for possible refinement and change
- Gain familiarity with a phenomenon or to achieve new insight into it
- Help in prediction and control of certain phenomena in nursing practice
- Explore areas where little is known or to investigate the problem in depth
- Discover or establish the existence of relationship between two or more than two phenomena
- Explain why and how the relation between two or more than two phenomena exists.

HISTORY OF NURSING RESEARCH

Nursing research was slow to develop in India as well as in the rest of the world. Slow growth of nursing research was related to lack of higher cadre nursing education. Nursing research was able to develop and expand only as nurses received advanced educational preparation. The growth of nursing research seems to be directly related to the educational level of nurses. In the early era of nursing, nursing leaders were more concerned about increasing the number of nurses and establishing hospital affiliated nursing school than with establishing university programs. Because nurses were not prepared to conduct research, many of the early nursing studies were conducted by member of other disciplines.

As nurses received advanced educational preparation and became qualified to conduct research, many of the studies they carried out were in nursing education because most of nurses before 1950 received their advanced degree in education. However, even during the early half century, the need for clinical nursing research was evident. Although, Florence Nightingale recommended clinical nursing research in the mid-1800s, her advice was ignored by nurses until over 100 years later. She emphasized some of the studies like environmental health hazards, are being conducted today.

There are many noteworthy events reported in the historical development of nursing research. Some of important milestones in history of nursing research at national and international level are given here:

Major Milestone of Nursing Research at International Level

In the 19th century, Florence Nightingale, founder of modern nursing, was first nurse to do research in connection with nursing, when she used statistics in the analysis of her data. She was the first biostatician in nursing. Nightingale did her work alone and not until after world war II there an organized, continuing effort to conduct further nursing research. The following are some the major hallmarks in the history of nursing research.

1920: Josephine Goldmark, under the direction of Haven Emerson, conducted a comprehensive survey that identified the inadequacies of housing and instructional facilities for nursing students.

1924: The first nursing doctoral program was established at Teacher's College, Columbia University.

1935: ANA published some facts about nursing: A handbook for speakers and others, which contained yearly compilation of statistical data about registered nurses.

1943: The *National Organization of Public Health Nursing* surveyed needs and resources for home care in the 16 communities. The work was reported in public health nursing care of the sick.

1949: ANA conducted its first national inventory of professional registered nurses in the United States and Puerto Rico.

1950: The *National Nursing Accrediting Services* established a system for accrediting Nursing Schools.

1952: The *Journal of Nursing Research* was published in June 1952. It was the ANA's first official journal for reporting nursing and health research.

1954: ANA established a committee on research and studies to plan, to promote, and to guide relating to the functions of the ANA (1968 published) *ANA Guidelines in Ethical Values*.

1955: ANA established the *American Nurse's Foundation*, a center for research to receive and administer funds and grants for nursing research.

1956: The study on patient care and patient satisfaction in 60 hospitals was published.

1957: The department of Nursing established at *Walter Reed Army Institute of Research*, provided opportunities for growth of *Military Nursing Services*.

1959: *The National League for Nursing (NLN) Research* studies was established to conduct research.

1960: Faye Abdellah developed the first federally tested coronary care unit and published patient centered approach to nursing, which altered nursing theory and practice.

1965: ANA Nursing Research Conferences (1965-1980s) provided a forum for critiquing nursing research.

1966: *The International Nursing Index* was published. One of the first textbook of nursing research was published by Abdellah and Levine: *Better Patient Care through Nursing Research*.

1970: ANA Commission on Nursing Research was established.

1970: The Western Council for Higher Education for Nursing (WCHEN) and Conduct and Utilization Research in Nursing (CURN) project implemented for utilization of research in nursing.

1971: ANA *Council of Nurses Research* was established.

1974: ANA Commission published Guidelines on Human rights for nurses in clinical and others research.

1976: The Stetller Model of Research Utilization (RU) was implemented

1977: *Nursing Research* became first Nursing Journal to be included in MEDLINE.

1980: ANA published a social policy statement which defined the nature and scope of nursing practice and characteristics of specialization in nursing.

1983: *The Volume of Annual Review of Nursing Research Survives* was published *by Springer Publishing Company*.

1983: *The Institute of Medicine* recommended that nursing research be included in the mainstream of bio-medical behavioral sciences.

1984: NIH task force study found that nursing research activities are relevant to NIH mission.

1985: The National Center for Nursing Research (NINR) was established in US Public Health Service (USPHS).

1993: The NINR launched Cochrane collaboration for funding of nursing research.

1994: *The Journal of Qualitative Research* started being published.

1998: Sigma Theta Tau sponsored the first *International Research Utilization Conference* in Toronto.

2003: The NINR supported clinical and basic research to establish a scientific basis for *the care of individual across the lifespan.*

2004: *The Journal Worldviews on Evidence-based Nursing* started.

Major Milestone of Nursing Research at National Level

Nursing research in India has its roots in the Philosophy of Florence Nightingale, which stated that profession is committed to the task of enlarging professional body of knowledge through systematic approach to solve problems. The statistics on the unsanitary conditions in the Indian army prepared by Florence Nightingale may be starting point of nursing research in India. Afterwards, many developments have taken place in India. Some of the major landmarks in history of Nursing Research in India are as follows:

1946: Bhore Committee (1943) submitted a report in which recommendation were made for the improvement of various aspects of nursing profession, nursing education, nursing research, working condition, nursing services in both hospital and community, sending nurses for higher education to abroad, etc.

1953: Ms. Edith Buchanan, Vice Principal, Rajkumari Amrit Kaur (RAK) College of Nursing, New Delhi, was the first nurse from India who was sent to Columbia University to earn Doctorate in Education (DEd) under World Health Organization (WHO) fellowship program.

1955: Ms. Margaretta Craig, Principal, College of Nursing, New Delhi, attended International Council of Nurses (ICN) meet at France to present a paper on the need for nursing research.

1960: First two years' master degree program in nursing was started at RAK College of Nursing, New Delhi, which included nursing research as a full subject with a thesis work on nursing topics. Nursing research recommended on all India basis along with a master's degree program in nursing in an intensive manner, although nurse leaders had been already participating in research at various levels. Clinical studies were even being carried on short-term basis by the beginning-level postgraduate nursing students.

1963: A study of health services was carried out in connection with the revision of syllabus of General Nursing and Midwifery (GNM) by the Indian Nursing Council in 1963. The study provided valuable insights into trends in the health services and implications for nursing.

1964: Dr Marie Ferguson, a public health nurse who joined RAK College of Nursing, New Delhi, was able to create greater appreciation and understanding and value of the research in nursing for nursing practice, administration and education. With senior nursing leaders of the country, she conducted a research study titled *'Activity Study to define Nursing and Non-Nursing Functions of Nurses in Selected Health Institutions of India'*.

1966: Trained Nurses Association of India (TNAI) established a research section under the guidance of chairwomen Ms Margareta Craig. TNAI conducted Nurses *'time utilization study'* with assistance from Ms Anna Gupta, Principal RAK College of Nursing, New Delhi under supervision of Dr Sulochana Krishnan.

1971: TNAI conducted a study on socioeconomic status of Nurses in India.

1976: Dr Marie Farrell and Dr Aparna Bhaduri of RAK College of Nursing, New Delhi conducted seminars on nursing research for educationists at Delhi, Mussoorie (Uttarakhand) and Yercaud (Tamil Nadu) to strengthen the nursing research in India.

1981: Dr Farrell and Dr Bhaduri's book *Health Research: A Community-Based Approach* was published by the WHO.

1984: A nursing research workshop was launched titled *Teaching Nursing Research to Nursing College Teachers* at Bengaluru, which was sponsored by University Grant Commission (UGC). This workshop was open all the teachers of all the nursing colleges in India. A workshop was conducted on 'Nursing Process' by Dr Marie Farrell at Leelabai Thackersey College of Nursing, SNDT Women University Mumbai, which was sponsored by the WHO.

1986: The Nursing Research Society of India (NRSI) was established to promote research within and related to nursing. Dr (Mrs) Inderjit Walia was founder president, and Mrs Uma Handa was its first secretary. The association continues to organize conference every year.

1986: M Phil Program started at RAK College of Nursing, University of Delhi, New Delhi.

1986: Introduction of nursing research process was introduced in BSc Nursing syllabus by Indian Nursing Council (INC).

1986: PhD in Nursing started in College of Nursing, PGIMER Chandigarh and some private colleges such as Manipal College of Nursing, Manipal and Shri Ramchandran College of Nursing, Chennai.

1998: Nursing Research Interest Section was organized under the chairmanship of Mr R Raj Arathnam (A senior nursing tutor, NIMHANS, Bengaluru).

2002: INC revised syllabus of GNM and Post Basic BSc Nursing (revised 2005) and included nursing research as individual subject.

2004: Publication of Nightingale Nursing Times was started by Jain and Co. Noida, Uttar Pradesh.

2005: Nursing and Midwifery Research Journal was started at National Institute of Nursing Education (NINE), PGIMER under the editorship of Dr Inderjit Walia. Principal NINE, PGIMER, Chandigarh.

2005: National Consortium PhD nursing has been started by INC under the leadership of Shri T. Dileep Kumar, President, INC, New Delhi to promote research activities in various fields of nursing collaboration with Rajiv Gandhi University of Health Sciences (RGUHS) Bengaluru in support of WHO. Initially 6 centers established with web-conferencing facility and later on 2 more centers were added on. These centers are; NIMHANS, Bengaluru, RAK College of Nursing, New Delhi; Christian Medical College (CMC), Vellore; Christian Medical College (CMC), Ludhiana; Seth Sukhlal Karnani Memorial (SSKM) Hospital, Kolkata; Government College of Nursing, Thiruvananthapuram; Government College of Nursing, Hyderabad; and Institute of Nursing Education (INE), Mumbai.

2009: Central Institute of Nursing and Research (CIN) was brought in existence under control of TNAI, New Delhi.

2009: Indira Gandhi National Open University (IGNOU) started PhD in Nursing.

2010: Faculty of Nursing Sciences, Baba Farid University of Health Sciences Faridkot, Punjab started PhD in Nursing.

2017: Faculty of Nursing Sciences, All India Institute of Medical Sciences (AIIMS), Rishikesh, Uttrakhand started PhD in Nursing.

TYPES OF RESEARCH

Research process provides a general strategy for gathering, analyzing and interpreting data to answer a research question or test hypothesis. Broadly, research is classified on the basis of purpose of the study and approach of studying a phenomenon. The basic types of research are as follows:

1. Basic and Applied Research
2. Quantitative and Qualitative Research

Basic and Applied Research (Table 1.2)

Basic Research

Basic Research is often referred as a *pure or fundamental research*. The major purpose of basic research is to gain knowledge to improve body of knowledge. It helps to obtain empirical information that can be used to develop, refine, or test a theory for direct application to clinical practice. For example, work of laboratory technician or scientist in a laboratory. A research conducted on adolescents towards their attitude about sex practices. So, the prime purpose of the investigator to know more about sex practices of adolescents. Sometimes, these findings

Table 1.2: Basic and applied research: A comparison.

Basic research	Applied research
It is pure or fundamental research	It is used in the field of practice to solve a problem
It is conducted to study a general phenomenon or a process	It is targeted to solve a practical problem for utilization purpose
It is abstract or theoretical in nature	A theory or part of theory is tested to find the utility
It is conducted to enhance body of professional knowledge	It generate quality evidence to solve clinical problems

do not have any direct benefits to others and have no commercial value as their primary purpose is to expand body of knowledge about the concept under study. So, the basic research conducted to serve following purposes:
1. To gain more understanding about the phenomena.
2. To enhance body of professional knowledge.
3. To develop, test and refine theories by supplementing new knowledge.

> **Box 1.1:** Example of Basic Research.
>
> A researcher carries out a study on impact of leadership styles adopted by nurse administrators on interpersonal relationship, quality care and work performance of nursing officers in an organization.
> Here, researcher observed that nursing officers' performance improved with democratic leadership style. Further, it is observed that nursing officers shows better harmonious relationship to nurse administrators who used democratic leadership styles.

Applied Research

Applied Research is conducted to gain knowledge that can be used in practical settings to improve the quality care. This type of research is conducted in actual practical conditions. Most of clinical research falls in category of applied research. Although, many times applied research serve the purpose of basic research by enhancing the body of professional knowledge. Many studied provide clinical application as well as new knowledge that contribute to theoretical understanding of basic behavior. Here, applied research helps to provide information that can be used to solve problems or make important decision in clinical, education and administrative areas.

> **Box 1.2:** Example of Applied Research.
>
> A researcher has planned to conducted a study to see the effect of blood pH value on mortality risk among brain trauma patients.
> Here, researcher interested to solve the problem of high-risk mortality among brain injury patients with the help of assessing pH value and decide to maintain pH in this category of patients at the time of admission to emergency department.

Quantitative and Qualitative Research (Table 1.3)

Quantitative Research

Quantitative research is a systematic collection of numerical information, often under conditions of considerable control to test a hypothesis or refine a theory. The collected information are analyzed with the help of statistical procedure. Experimental, quasi-experimental and non-experimental design are main quantitative research approaches.

> **Box 1.3:** Example of Quantitative Research.
>
> A descriptive study to assess stress and coping strategies among nursing students at a selected private nursing college, Punjab.
> In this study, researcher collect numerical information from the subjects to determine the study variables.

Qualitative Research

Qualitative research deals with the systematic collection of subjective and narrative information to develop in depth understanding about the topic. Qualitative research is important

Table 1.3: Quantitative and qualitative research.

Characteristics	Quantitative research	Qualitative research
Philosophical origin	Logical positivism	Naturalistic, interpretive and humanistic
General nature	Objective approach to seek precise measurement in numerical form and also known as 'hard science'	Subjective approach to study a phenomena in depth and also known as 'soft science'
Aims	To test hypothesis or to refine theory	To develop theory, and assumptions
Focus	Concise and narrow	Broad and complete
Knowledge of Variable	Study variable are operationally defined and well understood	Researcher may have only rough ideas of study variables
Research design selection	Study is planned properly and a rigorous methodology is selected before preceding the study. It is reductionist in nature	Research methodology is flexible and design emerges in between the study and called 'emergent design'. It is holistic in nature
Origin of research problem	Researcher have to use deductive approach to formulate problem	Inductive approach is helpful to reason out problem
Sample size	Quantitative studies based on large sample size in order to generalize the findings	Usually, a small sample size is obtained
Data types	Numerical data	Narrative or descriptive data
Duration of data collection	It takes long time to collect data in case of large sample size	Usually, it is short but time consuming to explore the minute details
Study instruments	Usually questionnaire, rating scale and checklist are used to collect numerical information	Interview (structured, unstructured, focus group) and observation are common method used to collect information
Duration of data analysis	Usually, it takes very short time to analysis data with the help of many statistical software like SPSS, Minitab and SYSTAT	It takes very long time in indexing, coding the data. Scope for statistical software application is negligent
Use of statistics	Researcher use descriptive and inferential statistic to analyze data	Scope of descriptive and inferential statistics is narrow. Researcher analyze the data through words, pictures, indexing, and thematic analysis, etc.
Role of researcher	Researcher is passive in quantitative study	Researcher has to participate actively to explore the given construct

when quantitative research is not feasible to study some aspects of human behavior like studying hope, and motivation level in a dying patient is easy to explore through qualitative study. Here, data are analyzed with the help of coding, indexing and narrations for the purpose of discovering meaning and pattern of relationship in underlying construct. The major qualitative research designs are phenomenology, grounded theory, ethnography, case study and historical research.

> **Box 1.4:** Example of Qualitative Research.
> - A phenomenology on life experience of HIV/AIDS patients admitted in a palliative care center, New Delhi, India.
> - A phenomenology on life experiences of victims of Bhopal gas tragedy at Bhopal, Madhya Pradesh.
>
> In these studies researcher collect narrative information from the study subjects to understand the phenomenon in depth.

Characteristics of Qualitative Research

Many attempts have been made to characterize qualities that distinguish qualitative work from others research approaches. The following are some salient features of qualitative study:

- *Natural setting:* Qualitative study conducted in natural setting to explore the phenomena in depth. In qualitative work, the intent is to explore human behaviors within the contexts of their natural settings.
- *Subjectivity:* Qualitative researcher is interested in inner states of human activity. Because these inner states are not directly observable. Qualitative researcher must rely on subjective judgment to bring them to light. Most qualitative researcher would deny the possibility of pure objectivity in any scientific endeavors.
- *Participant perspective:* Qualitative research seeks to understand the world from the perspective of research participants. Qualitative studies try to capture the perspective that human use as basis for their action in special social setting.
- *Researcher a data gathering instrument:* Traditional quantitative methods generate information through the use of instruments such as questionnaire, scale, checklist, test and other measurement device, while the principal data for qualitative research are gathered directly by the researcher themselves. The logic behind research as instrument approach is that the human capacities necessary to participate in social life are the same capacities that enables researcher to make sense of the actions, intentions and understanding of those being studied.
- *Wholeness and complexity:* Qualitative work starts with the assumptions that social settings are unique, dynamic and complex. Qualitative method provide means whereby social contexts can be systematically examined as whole, without breaking down in to isolated, incomplete and disconnected variable. Qualitative report are usually complete, detailed and narrative that included the voice of participants being studied.
- *Emergent design:* It is characteristic of qualitative study that study change as they are being placed into operation. The goal of qualitative study is to get into a social phenomenon in deep inside in a special social setting, therefore, it is impossible to construct and choose a design before actual conduction of the study. So, design will be emerged during study process and so called '*emergent design*'.
- *Inductive data analysis:* Qualitative researchers do not start with null hypothesis to retain or reject. They collect as many details information necessary from the research setting as possible, then establish pattern of relationship among the phenomena.
- *Reflexivity:* This is another important characteristic of a qualitative study. Reflexivity can be broadly described as qualitative researcher's engagement for continuous examination and explanation about how they have influenced research project. Reflexivity involves an awareness that the researcher and the object of the study affect each others mutually and

continually in the research process. However, the extent to which researchers engage in reflexivity depends on the methodological approach they have adopted for the study.

SCOPE AND AREAS OF NURSING RESEARCH

The research findings can be utilized to solve problems in government, business, society and health care. Nursing research has wide scope in nursing practice, education and management/administration. The research findings are utilized in different areas of nursing in order to expand and improve knowledge for improving quality education and practice. The scope of research may be classified under following headings:

- Research in nursing education
- Research in clinical nursing practice
- Research in nursing administration.

Research in Nursing Education

Nursing education is an important area to build up theoretical knowledge about nursing and its related issues. Nursing education research centers on developing and testing more efficient educational processes, identifying new ways to incorporate technology in order to enhance learning and discovering more efficient approaches to promoting lifelong learning. To achieve these goals, the use of rigorous research strategies in the assessment of teaching and learning process and outcomes at all level of nursing education is essential. The expectation and competencies of graduate at each level of nursing education in regards to research are described below. Areas of research as per National League for Nursing, (NLN, 2008) in Nursing eduction are given here:

- Curriculum design and evaluation, including community driven model for curriculum development
- New pedagogies
- Innovation in teaching and learning
- Use of instructional technology, including new approaches to simulated learning
- Student/teacher learning partnership
- Client teaching model
- Assessment of students learning in classroom settings and practice
- New model for teacher preparation and faculty development
- Quality improvement processes
- Educational system and infrastructures.

Research in Clinical Nursing Practice

High quality and cost effective care is the demand of consumers nowadays. In the scenario of EBP, the scope of research is widely recognized in clinical nursing practice. Nursing's expanded view of health emphasizes health promotion, restoration, and rehabilitation as well commitment to caring and comfort. The scope of research in practice ranges from acute to chronic care, promotion, prevention and rehabilitation of individual, family and community.

Research areas as per International Council of Nurses (ICN, 2009 and NINR, 2007, 2010) for clinical nursing practice are as follows.

- Health promotion, prevention of illness and control of symptoms
- Quality and cost effectiveness of care
- Impact of nursing intervention on client outcomes
- Evidence-based nursing practice
- Community and primary health care
- Living with chronic condition and quality of life
- Caring for clients experiencing change in their health and illness
- Assessing and monitoring client problems
- Providing and testing nursing care intervention
- Symptom management, self management and care giving
- End of life research.

In practice, many other subareas maybe possible. However, researcher may select the topic of interest and area of specialization for research.

Research in Nursing Administration

This is extremely important area of nursing practice as well as hospital management. Research may also be used to explore problems related to nursing management and administration in order to improve staff satisfaction, decrease turn over and augment work satisfaction.

Many international and national bodies and organization like World Health Organization (WHO), Ministry of Health and Family Welfare (MoHFW), Indian Nursing Council (INC) and Trained Nurses Association of India (TNAI) and many other agencies also given certain sub-areas where research may be conducted to explore the hidden and buried issues

Research areas as per International Council of Nurses (ICN, 2009) for Nursing administration are given below:
- Nursing manpower including quality nurses, work life, retention, turn over, satisfaction with work
- Nursing research in delivery of care services
- Impact of health care reform on health policy, programme planning and evaluation (impact studies)
- Financing health sector.
- Impact of equity and access to nursing care and its effect on nursing (outcome research).

Apart from above mention areas, many other sub-areas may be possible in nursing management and administration which need investigation.

Indian Nursing Council (INC) also proposed following research areas for nursing management:
- Clinical intervention studies
- Practice standards in various nursing specialties
- Nursing education measurement, evaluation competencies, innovation in teaching strategies
- Manpower planning
- Cost benefit analysis
- Quality assurance in education and practice
- Development of tools
- Testing nursing theories and model and theory development

- Impact studies that have policy implications for nursing education and practice
- Independent nursing practice related research.

Survey by nurse executives from Magnet Hospital (2007) also proposed research areas for nursing administration:
- Clinical outcomes
- Practice environment issues satisfaction
- Human resources issues.

Research areas proposed by Sigma Theta Tau International Honor Society for nursing administration are given below:
- Promotion of healthy community through health promotion and disease prevention
- Implementation of evidence-based practice
- Targeting the needs of vulnerable populations (chronically ill)
- Capacity development for research by nurses.

SIGNIFICANCE OF RESEARCH IN NURSING

Nursing research has an important place in nursing science and is becoming increasingly recognized. Research is a vital aspect of the health services and essential to the provision of effective and safe health and social care. It is believed that patients and the public have the right to expect their care to be based on the best available research evidence. As nurses play a pivotal role in delivering health and social care, research on nursing practice and key nursing issues is essential to ensure continuous improvement and safe, effective and evidence-based health and social care for people seeking health care services. Some facts that justify the importance of conducting research are as follows:

- *Research promotes evidenced based nursing care:* The nursing profession exists to provide services to individual, community or society as whole. The provided services based on scientific knowledge. Research has been determined to be the most reliable method of obtaining knowledge. Nursing research is essential for the development of empirical knowledge that enable nurses to provide evidence-based nursing care. Evidence-based nursing practice means that nurses make clinical decision based on best available research evidences, their clinical practice and the health care preferences of their patient/clients.
- *Provide accountability of nursing practice:* Independent role of nurse brought a greater need of accountability in practice. To be accountable for their practice, nurses should have sound scientific research based knowledge.
- *Develop model and framework for nursing practice:* Nursing research helps to formulate models and framework for variety of nursing settings. It provides a scientific basis for development of nursing models and theory. Nursing models helps to provide nursing care systematically. Models are useful as they allow the concepts in nursing theory to be successfully applied to nursing practice.
- *Ensure credibility of nursing profession:* Nurses must demonstrate to the general public that nursing makes difference in the health status. In the past nursing was thought of a vocation than profession. Research builds a body of professional knowledge that made nursing distinct from other disciplines.
- *Improve cost effectiveness in nursing practice:* The goal of nursing services is to help people to achieve or maintain health, regardless of cost. The reality of the health care picture has

forced nurses to think in monetary terms. Consumers have become more aware of the cost of health care and asking for explanation of service they receive. Nursing services consumes a large percentage of a hospital's budget. Quality patient care and reduction in cost through careful management of resources are the function of well designed research. By encouraging ongoing improvement to practice and exploring new approaches, research can improve the productivity and efficiency of the health and social organization.

- *Miscellaneous:*
    - Research helps to understand the practice environment and therefore help to design treatment in different environment.
    - Research helps to understand the nurses to deliver best possible care.
    - It develop new insight about the process involved in receiving and giving care.
    - A research intensive environment is essential in order to generate the science base for nursing and interpersonal practice and to educate future generations of nurse scientists.
    - Nurses' frontline role puts them in a unique position to reflect the needs and concern of patients and the public. Encouraging nurses to lead and contribute to research keeps research activity focused on patient care and the needs of our health services.
    - Fully resourced nursing research in priority areas of practice improves the quality of care given to patients and thereby increases public confidence in health and social care services.
    - Nursing research and evidence implementation are essential parts of the education and training of India's existing and future nursing workforce.

EVIDENCE-BASED PRACTICE

Over the past several years, the concept of evidence-based practice (EBP) has appeared with increasing frequency in the nursing literature. EBP is similar to research-based practice and has been called an approach to problem-solving in clinical practice that conscientiously uses the current 'best' evidence in the patient care. It involves identifying a clinical problem, searching in literature, critically evaluating the research evidence, and determining appropriate interventions. EBP will help to fill the gap between research, theory and practice.

History of Evidence-based Practice

The concept of EBP originated in the late 1980s. EBP was built on the premises that health professionals should not center practice on tradition and belief but on sound research based information. EBP and research are not synonymous. They are both scholarly process but focus on different phases of knowledge development. EBP refers to the integration of individual clinical expertise with the best available external clinical evidence from systematic search.

Definitions

In medicine, EBP has been defined as conscientious, explicit and judicious use of the current best evidence in making decision about the care of individual patient. To distinguish nursing from medicine regarding EBP, a number of different definitions are given by many scholars. Some important definitions are as follows.

'EBP is the conscientious, explicit, and judicious use of theory derived research base information in making decision about care delivery of individual or group of patients and in the consideration of individual needs and preferences.' *(Ingersoll, 2000)*

'EBP is the using of best available evidence available to guide clinical decision making.' *(Benefield, 2002)*

'EBP is the use of evidence to support decision-making in health care.' *(Greenberg and Pyle, 2004)*

'EBP is an integration of the best evidence available, nursing expertise, and the values and preferences of the individual, families and communities who are served.' *(Sigma Theta Tau, 2005)*

'EBP is an integration of the best research evidence with clinical expertise and patient value to facilitate clinical decision making.' *(Di Censo, et al. 2005)*

So, all above definitions indicates that EBP is a problem-solving approach using current best evidence to answer a clinical question incorporating one's own clinical expertise, and patient values and preferences.

Components of Evidence-based Practice

Nurse play a pivotal role in implementation of evidence-based practice on clinical unit at hospital setting. EBP is an approach that requires the decisions about health care should be based on the best available, current, valid and relevant evidence. In addition, evidence-based decisions should be made by those receiving care, informed by the tacit and explicit knowledge of those providing care, within the context of available resources.

- *Best research evidence:* The research evidence are ranked and described here. Researcher has to select the best available evidence according to clinical research questions (Fig. 1.2). Level 1 is the best resource to use when looking for evidence-based practice.
- *Clinical expertise:* The knowledge and experience of the clinician (physician, nurse and other health professionals).
- *Patient value and preferences:* These are individual's own concern, preferences, expectation and social and financial resources that impact the health and health care.

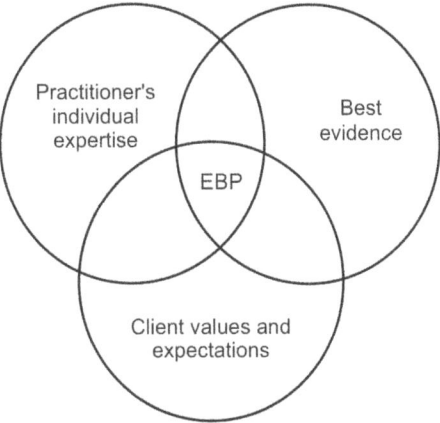

Fig. 1.2: The evidence-based practice model.

- *Clinical data (assessment) and history:* A patient's assessment includes important evidences that should be considered in treatment decision.

Box 1.5: Levels of Evidences.

Level I	Evidence collected from systematic review or meta-analysis of all similar randomized control trails (RCTs)
Level II	Evidence come from single good quality RCT
Level III	Evidence obtained from RCT completed without randomization
Level IV	Evidence collected from case control or cohort studies
Level V	Evidence collected from systematic review of descriptive or qualitative studies
Level VI	Evidence generated from a single descriptive or qualitative study
Level VII	Evidence collected based on expert opinion or expert committee decision

Source: http://www.cebm.net.

Salient Features of Evidence-based Practice

Evidence-based practice (EBP) has several critical features. Some of the important features are given below:
- It is problem-based approach and considered the context of the practioner's current experience.
- EBP bring together the best available evidence and current practice by combining research with tacit knowledge and theory.
- EBP is a systematic and objective process.
- EBP facilitates the application of research findings by incorporating first and second hand knowledge.

A comparison of nursing research and evidence-based practice is discussed in Table 1.5.

Steps of Evidence-Based Practice (Fig. 1.3)

Melnyk and Fineout-Overhott (2011) suggest that EBP involve five critical steps:

Select a Clinical Research Question

The first step of EBP is to select a research question from clinical area. The selection of clinical research problem can be result of following triggers:
- *Knowledge focused triggers:* These triggers come from advancement of knowledge of health care professionals through reading literature or attending professional conferences. For example, implementation of revised guidelines or standard to improve the health care practices.

Table 1.5: Nursing research and evidence-based practice: A comparison.

Nursing research	Evidence-based practice
Problem identification	Clinical problem identification
Conducting research	Using research already conducted
Following steps of research process	Synthesizing all of the evidence and integrating with expert opinion and patient input
Findings usually not immediately applicable and need to be translated to practice through research or EBNP	Findings usually applied at bed side and tailored to individual patient

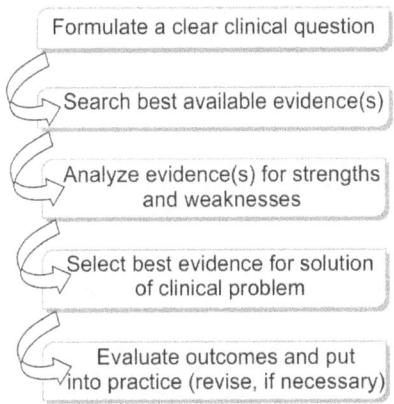

Fig. 1.3: Steps of evidence-based practice.

- *Problem focused triggers:* These triggers are identified by the health care professionals in response to clinical problem, barriers or any others constrained face in day-to-day life in clinical areas. Problem focused triggers may arise in the course of clinical practice or in the context of quality assessment of quality improvement efforts. For example, problem of high sepsis or relapse rate in ICUs or high fall rate of patients, etc. The clinician should appropriately frame clinical research question by using following acronym called PICO. PICO should be part of every search for evidence to improve practice.

Box 1.6: PICO(T) Format.

P– Population-Patient-Problem: Group of people undergoing research
I– Intervention or Underlying Issue: Intervention planned to test
C– Comparison Group or Intervention: Comparison of groups or interventions
O– Outcomes or Expected Results: Expected outcomes or results
(T)– Time Frame or Time Leg: Time frame in which change or effect is expected to occurs

(T) – t = Time frame is an optional alternative or constituents in evidence based practice

Search Best Available Evidence(s)

Once the clinical question selected, the researcher should explore the relevant literature review through clinical studies, meta-analysis findings, expert opinions or existing EBP guidelines. Before concluding the literature, it is also a good strategy to read and understands the literature in whole.

For example, 'are self-management strategies are more effective than medical care alone for improving health status, quality of life and occupational functioning among adult with coronary artery disease?'

Box 1.7: Use of PICO Approach.

P	I	C	O
Client with coronary artery disease	Self-management strategy (ies)	Medical care (drugs and supplement)	• Subjective well-being • Morbidity • Occupational functioning

Analyze Evidence(s) for its Weaknesses and Strength

The available evidences should be critically evaluated for strengthen and weaknesses. Critical appraisal should be focused for evaluation of their feasibility like in term of cost, duration, need of manpower, and other resources, etc.

Select the Best Evidence for Clinical Problem

After critical appraisal of the evidence, the researchers should decide to implement the best available evidence in clinical setting. Following review and analysis of the systematic data, the nurse must determine what the research demonstrate and decide the level of evidence in order to make recommendations to promote EBP. The best evidence should be integrated with patient preferences, values, clinical experts, and patients' assessment information before actual implementation in clinical practice.

Evaluate Outcomes and put into Practice (revise, if necessary)

Finally, the researcher must evaluate the evidence for efficacy, pitfalls and performance for clinical practice to determine the expected change in practice and level of evidence in order to make recommendations to promote evidence-based practice.

Box 1.8: 5 A's of Evidence-based Practice.

1. **Ask:** Formulate the question
2. **Acquire:** Evidence search for answers
3. **Appraise:** The evidence for quality and relevance
4. **Apply:** The results
5. **Assess:** The outcome

Significance of EBP in Nursing

Nursing is a practice profession; it is important that clinical practice to be based on research-based evidence rather than intuition and other traditional belief. EBP help to improve the nursing care by providing evidence-based nursing care. Importance of EBP in nursing are given below:
- EBP improve patient care
- Incorporating research findings in practice helps in decision-making
- It improves nurses and other health care professional's job satisfaction and reduce employees turnover in a organization
- Providing evidence-based care develop confidence in health professionals
- EBP improve the consumer (patient and their family members) satisfaction in health care services
- EBP support for quality and cost effectiveness of nursing intervention.

Barriers to EBP in Nursing

The concept of EBP is relatively new in nursing, still somewhat sophisticated because many nursing practices are based on tradition, belief, experience, common sense and untested theories. Although, there is significant support for increasing emphasis on EBP in nursing still,

Introduction to Nursing Research

there are many barriers to implement EBP in nursing. Some of the common barriers to EBP in nursing are as follows (For more details refer Chapter 11):

- *Barriers related to nurses:* These are individual barriers related to nurses includes lack of knowledge bout the scientific research process, lack of interest of higher authority to change and adopt new practices, lack of supportive colleagues, lack of knowledge of technical language of research process published in scientific work, overwhelming patient load, and lack of time to do quality research, etc.
- *Barriers related to organization:* Organizational qualities that may negatively influence evidence-based practice includes lack of recognition in organization in terms of salary, incentive and promotion, lack of resources, apathy of nurse administrator towards novel ideas and lack of decentralization and formalization in an organization.

REVIEW QUESTIONS AND ANSWER

Long and Short Answer Questions

1. What are the methods of acquiring knowledge in nursing? *(PGI, MSc N-2006)*
2. What is the need of nursing research? *(RGUHS, MSc N-2014)*
3. Explain problem solving and scientific methods in details along with its differences. *(AIIMS, MSc N-2003)*
4. Elaborate the need, scope, purpose of nursing research. *(AIIMS, MSc N-2009)*
5. Briefly explain the history of nursing research. *(KUHAS, MSc N-2013)*
6. Define nursing reach along with its types. *(TNMGRMU, MSc N-2007)*
7. Explain nursing research along with its characteristics. *(BFUHS, MSc N-2011)*

Multiple Choice Questions

1. The process of developing generalizations from a specific observation is known as:
   a. Deductive reasoning
   b. Inductive reasoning
   c. Disciplined reasoning
   d. Intuitive reasoning

2. Which of the following type of research focused on finding a solution to an immediate practical problem?
   a. Basic research
   b. Applied research
   c. Conceptual research
   d. Empirical research

3. Florence Nightingale's landmark publication in early Nursing Research *"Notes on Nursing"* was published in the year:
   a. 1759
   b. 1769
   c. 1859
   d. 1869

4. "An in-depth study to describe the coping mechanisms of women with breast cancer in the period between diagnosis and surgery", is an example of following research:
   a. Quantitative research
   b. Qualitative research
   c. Mixed Method research
   d. Historical research

5. Which one of the following is the best source of knowledge in nursing research?
   a. Tradition
   b. Trial and error
   c. Scientific research
   d. Clinical experience

6. Which one of the following is the highest level of evidence by which one can change the nursing practice?
   a. Systematic review of RCT's
   b. A single RCT
   c. Correlation study
   d. Descriptive study

7. If a researcher is studying the effect of using laptops in his classroom to ascertain their merit and worth, he is likely go for which of following types of research?
   a. Basic research
   b. Applied research
   c. Evaluative research
   d. Experimental research

8. The initial and one of the most significant step in conducting the research process is:
   a. Defining the research variable
   b. Identifying the research problem
   c. Stating the research purposes
   d. Determining the feasibility of the study

9. National Consortium for PhD in Nursing to promote research activities in various field of nursing was started in year:
   a. 2001
   b. 2003
   c. 2005
   d. 2007

10. It is a systematic collection of numerical information under controlled condition to test hypothesis or develop theory.
    a. Basic research
    b. Applied research
    c. Qualitative research
    d. Evidence-based practice

11. In Reference to evidence-based practice (EBP), in PICO approach; P stand for
    a. Population
    b. Person
    c. Pool of data
    d. Problems in EBP

12. In terms of rigor of research evidence, which of the following is considered best research evidence in evidence hierarchy?
    a. Randomized control trails
    b. Meta-analysis
    c. Quasi-experimental study and personal opinions
    d. Single correlational and observational research

13. The process of drawing a specific conclusion from a set of ideas is called as:
    a. Deductive reasoning
    b. Inductive reasoning
    c. Pragmatism
    d. Logical reasoning

14. Which of the following is the most objective source of nursing knowledge?
    a. Textbooks
    b. Higher authority/experts
    c. Experience
    d. Scientific research

15. PICO in evidence-based practice stand for:
    a. Polio, influenza, chicken pox, ovulation
    b. Prevalence, incidence, cohort, observation
    c. Population, intervention, comparison, outcome
    d. Patient, injection, catheterization, operation

Answer Key

1.	2.	3.	4.	5.	6.	7.	8.	9.	10.	11.	12.	13.	14.	15.
b.	b.	c.	b.	c.	a.	c.	b.	d.	c.	a.	b.	a.	d.	c.

SUGGESTED READING

1. Benefield LE. Evidence-based practice: Basic strategies for success, home health care nurse. Home Healthc Nurse. 2002; 20(12): 803-7.
2. Boswall C, Canon S. Introduction to nursing research: Incorporating evidence-based practice. Sunbury, MA: Jones and Bartlett; 2007.
3. Burn N, Grove S K. Understanding nursing research: building an evidence-based practice, 4th edition. St Louis: Saunders Elsevier; 2002
4. Burn N, Grove S K. Understanding nursing research: building an evidence-based practice, 4th edition. St Louis: Saunders Elsevier; 2007.
5. Cartabellotta A, Martin J, Hopayian K, Porzsolt F, Burls A, Osborne J. Second international conference of evidence-based health care teachers and developers. Sicily statement on evidence-based practice. BMC Med Educ. 2005;5:1.
6. Chinn PL, Kramer MK. Theory and Nursing: Integrated knowledge development, 5th edition. St. Louis: Mosby; 1999.
7. Chrastina J. PICO(T) and PCD format of clinically relevant questions in the conceptualization of special education. Journal of exceptional people. 2016;1(8):31-9.
8. Clamp C, Gough S, Land L. Resources for nursing research: An annotated bibliography, 4th edition. London: SAGE; 2004.
9. Department of Health (DOH). Research Governance framework for health and social care, 2nd edition. London: DOH; 2005.
10. DiCenso A, Guyatt G, Ciliska D. Introduction to evidence-based nursing. In: DiCenso A, Guyatt G, Ciliska D (Eds). Evidence-based nursing: A guide to clinical practice. St Louis: Mosby. 2006; pp. 3-19.
11. Finkelman A, Kenner C. Professional nursing concepts: competency for quality leadership. James and Bartlett Publishers; 2010.
12. Fitzaptrick JJ. Making a commitment to go public (editorial). Applied Nursing Research. 2004;17:223.
13. Gerrish K, Lacey A. The research process in Nursing, 6th edition. United Kingdom: John Wiley and sons;2013.
14. Greenberg M, Pyle B. Achieving evidence-based nursing practice in ambulatory care, viewpoint. 2004;26(1):8-12.

15. Hockey L. The nature and purpose of research. In: Cormack DFs (ed). The research process in nursing, 1st edition. London: Blackwell sciences; 1984; pp. 1-10.
16. Ingersoll GL. Evidence-based nursing: What it is and what it isn't. Nursing Outlook. 2000; 48(4): 151-2.
17. James FA. Reading, understand and applying nursing research (Google e-book): E.A. Davis. 2013.
18. Kedar P. Nursing research: Principles, process and issues. New York: Palgrave Macmillan; 1997.
19. Melnyk BM, Fineout-Overhott E, Stone P, Ackerman M. Evidence-based practice, the post treatment and recommendation for new millennium. Pediatric Nursing. 2006; 26(1): 77-80.
20. Moule P, Hek G. Making sense of research: an instruction for health and social care. London: Sage publication; 2011.
21. Nightingale F. Noyes on nursing: What it is not? New York : Dover publications; 1969.
22. Nursing Research Society of India. Nursing research and statistics, India: Pearson education.
23. Polit D, Beck C. Essential of Nursing Research: Methods, Appraisal and Utilization, 6th edition. Philadelphia: Lippincott William Wilkins; 2008.
24. Polit D F, Beck CT. Nursing Research- principle and methods, 7th edition. Philadelphia: Lippincott William Wilkins; 2004.
25. Redman LL, Mory AVH. The romance of research. (1st ed). Baltimore: William and Wilkins, 1933.
26. Sackett D, Straus S, Richardson W, Rosenberg W, Haynes R. In: Dawes M, Summerskill W, Glasziou P (Eds). Evidence based medicine: How to practice and teach EBM. Edinburgh: Churchill Livingstone; 2000.
27. Sackett DL, Straus SE, Richardson WS, Rosenberg W, Haynes RB. Evidence-based practice medicine: How practice and teach EBM, 2nd edition, London: Churchill Livingstone; 2000.
28. Salomnd S. Advancing evidence-based practice: a primer. Orthopedic Nursing. 2007;26(2): 114-23.
29. Sigma Theta Tau international. Position statement of evidence-based practice. 2005. Available at http://www.nursingsociety.org/aboutus/positionpapers/pages/EBN_positionpaper.aspx [Accessed Nov. 2014].
30. Stokke K, Olsen NR, Espehaug B, Nortvedt MW. Evidence based practice beliefs and implementation among nurses: a cross-sectional study. BMC Nursing.2014;13(1):8.
31. Treece E W, Treece JW. Elements of research in nursing, 4th edition. St. Louis: Mosby; 1986.
32. Waltz CF, Bausell RB. Nursing research: Design, statistics and computer analysis. Philadelphia: F.A. Davis; 1981.
33. Whittemore R. Combining evidence in nursing research: Methods and implications. Nursing research. 2005;54(1):56-62.

Chapter 2

Research Problem, Research Question and Hypothesis

INTRODUCTION

Every research study begins with a problem the researcher would like to solve. For such a problem to be researchable, it must be one that can be studied through collecting and analyzing the data. Some problem, although interesting for researcher but not an appropriate research problem as they are not researchable. Developing and identifying research problem is a creative process.

Researcher often begin with interest in a broad area, and then develop a more specific researchable problem. A good researcher jot down all the areas of interest as they come to his mind. Selection of research problem depend on many factors like interest, knowledge of researcher, significance of problem to nursing profession, implications, feasibility of turning research problem into a study and availability and cooperation of research subjects and other colleagues. Many nurses may wonder what there is to be studied, while others may have a variety of ideas and difficulty choosing among them. The problem statement may arise from a difficult situation encountered in practice or from the nurse's particular area of interest.

Defining the Research Problem

Defining the research problem is frequently the most difficult part of doing research. This step of research process maybe most difficult of all and may take a great deal of time. A research problem is a broad topic of interest that has perplexing or troubling aspects which can be 'solved' by the gathering of relevant information and evidences. For example, a nurse is concerned about the healing of wound in patients with burns, this is a problem faced by nursing and can be taken for research purpose.

RESEARCH PROBLEM

In practice, research problem and problem statement are used interchangeably, but these two aspects are distinct to each others. A research problem is merely stating the troubling condition in declarative sentence, but a problem statement in quantitative studies often have following six components:
1. *Problem identification:* What is wrong with the present situation?
2. *Background:* Nature and context of the problem
3. *Scope of the problem:* Magnitude of problem, i.e. how big the problem is it or how many people affected or going to affect, etc.
4. *Consequences of the problem:* What is the cost of not solving the problem?

5. *Knowledge gap:* What is lacking about the problem?
6. *Proposed solution:* How the new study findings help to solve the current problem?

Problem statement for qualitative study express nature of the problem, its context, scope and information needed to solve it.

Box 2.1: Problem Statement.

Example 1: 'A study on factors associated with 2009 pandemic influenza A (H1N1) vaccination acceptance among university students from India during the post-pandemic phase'. *(Suresh PS, et al. 2011)*
- **Problem identification:** Personal witness of H1N1 outbreaks and deaths in clinical practice
- **Background:** A highly contagious and communicable disease that can lead to fatal results
- **Scope of the problem:** A large number of death, burden on health care sector, and huge impact on socioeconomic reforms of country
- **Consequences of the problem:** A large number of death and loss of health care resources
- **Knowledge gap:** Management and prevention of H1N1
- **Proposed solution:** Vaccination is the one of the intervention strategy used to mitigate H1N1.

Example 2: 'A descriptive study on self-esteem and depression among nursing students studying at a private College of Nursing Amritsar, Punjab'. *(Kumar R, 2016)*
- **Problem identification:** Personal experience of symptoms of low self-esteem and depression among nursing students, and by reading increase number of attempted suicide cases in nursing students.
- **Background:** Low self-esteem and depression are common in adolescents as many physiological and psychological changes take place.
- **Scope of the problem:** Decrease academic performance, and use of more negative coping strategies among nursing students
- **Consequences of the problem:** Increase number of suicidal death among nursing students, poor grade and emergence of more indiscipline related problems
- **Knowledge gap:** Measure to improve self-esteem and depression
- **Proposed solution:** Counseling, planned intervention program and consultation with psychologist and psychiatrist

---

SOURCES OF RESEARCH PROBLEM (FIG. 2.1)

Where do you look for research topic? Findings a research problem is not as hard as it first seems. When you develop the ability to look for researchable topic, they appear everywhere. Experienced researchers become so good at spotting research problem as they usually have at least a dozen of ideas waiting to be implemented, but finding topic can be intimidating at first. The most fruitful area for research problem is your own interest, observation and experiences. Because research is a time consuming process, curiosity and interest in a topic is essential. A variety of explicit sources can help the researcher to choose a topic, including following:

- *Clinical experience:* Personal experience, whether health care professional or as a consumer of health care is a rich source of ideas for research topic. A nurse may get ideas from knowledge focused and problem focused triggers in practice and education. For example, why the infection rate is higher in ICU and surgical wards? (*problem focused trigger*), what are the new guidelines for conducing CPR? (*knowledge focused triggers*).
- *The nursing literature:* The nursing literature can also be a valuable source for research problem; particularly for novice researcher. Researcher might identify a topic of interest and

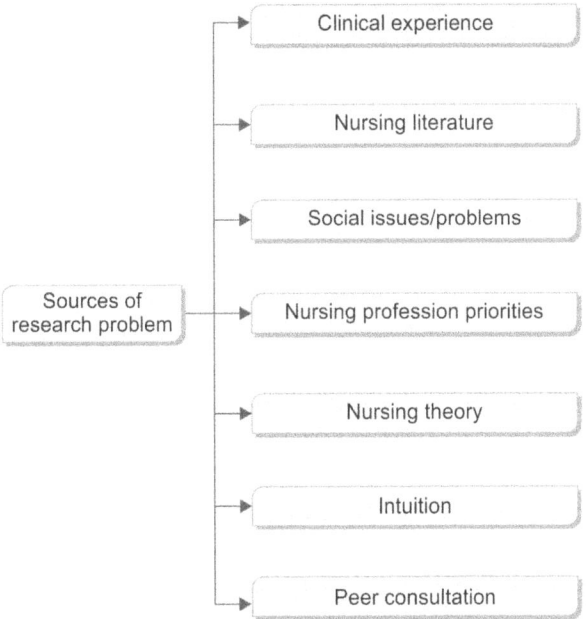

Fig. 2.1: Sources of research problem.

then review the nursing literature to determine which kind of studies already conducted and what can be possible now. The nursing literature, including unpublished thesis and dissertation as well as published research articles may provide direct assistance for further research in the area.

- *Social issues/problems:* Social issue often give rise the topics relevant to health care research. For example, problem of domestic violence, substance abuse, gender discrimination, problems of vulnerable population and other related issues can give ideas for research in nursing.
- *The research priorities of the profession:* Sometimes, hospital management, funding agencies (i.e. WHO, UNICEF) and nursing bodies (i.e. INC, TNAI) might be interested to get information on certain contemporary and innovative topics to generate information to take further step accordingly. For example, a hospital management might be interested to explore the factors related to high bed occupancy in hospital. INC Consortium also defined certain areas for INC PhD students to take for research study, i.e. manpower planning, testing theories, developing/refining standards, etc.
- *Nursing theory:* Nursing and non-nursing theories are also an important source of research problem. Quantitative research conducted either to test or refine existing theories or a part of theory, while qualitative research conducted to develop theory.
- *Intuition:* Intuition is a good source of knowledge as well research ideas and problems. It is believe that reflective mind is a good source for generating research problem.
- *Peer consultation:* Sometimes, sharing ideas with other experts and peer give rise a research problem. In addition, experts may suggest some areas or topic for research study.

STEPS OF IDENTIFYING A RESEARCH PROBLEM (FIG. 2.2)

Although, it is very difficult to step down the exact process of identifying and selection of research process, but some of the common steps maybe followed to identify a research problem, including followings:

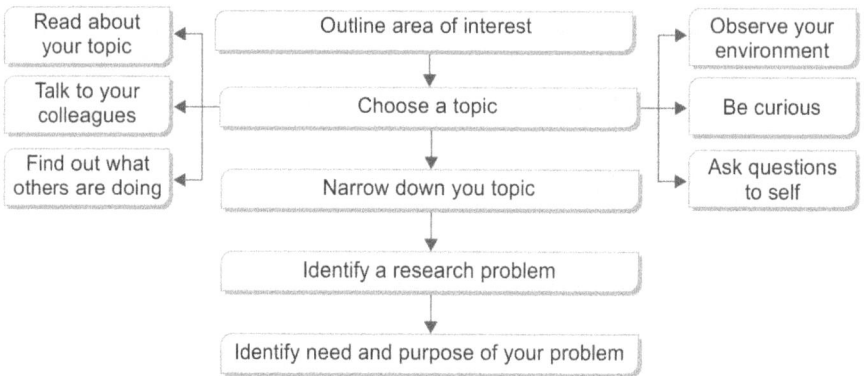

Fig. 2.2: Steps of identifying research problem.

COMPONENTS OF A PROBLEM STATEMENT

A well-framed problem statement for quantitative study, whether written as declarative statement or a question, has at a minimum; two components:
1. The population of concern
2. The variables to be studied

However, PICOT approach has the advantage of clarifying more clearly the population as well as intervention, comparison and expected outcomes

For example, a researcher might be interested in investigating 'the effect of play therapy on reduction of anxiety level among preschool age children at pediatric ward'.

Box 2.2: PICOT Format.		
P	Population	Preschool age children
I	Intervention	Play therapy
C	Comparison	Would be no play therapy group
O	Outcome	Reduction of anxiety level
T	Time frame	Duration of hospitalization

However, some scholars suggest that a well-framed research problem should consist following components
- Research study design
- Variable of interest
- Population under investigation
- Research setting.

> **Box 2.3:** Example of Research Statement.
>
> **Example 1:** 'A descriptive study on self-esteem, stress and depression among nursing students studying at SGRD College of Nursing, Amritsar, Punjab'. *(Kumar R, 2016)*
> - **Research study design:** Descriptive study
> - **Variable of interest:** Self-esteem, stress and depression
> - **Population under investigation:** Nursing students
> - **Research setting:** SGRD College of Nursing, Amritsar, Punjab.
>
> **Example 2:** 'A descriptive study on academic climate, academic stress and self-esteem among baccalaureate nursing students at AIIMS Rishikesh, Uttarakhand'. *(Kumar R, 2018)*
> - **Research study design:** Descriptive design
> - **Variables of interest:** Academic climate, academic stress and self-esteem
> - **Population under investigation:** Nursing students
> - **Research setting:** AIIMS, Rishikesh, Uttarakhand.

RESEARCH QUESTION

Although, the term *research question* and *problem statement* are sometimes used interchangeably, but in practical both are distinct to each others. The problem statement is a general view of why a particular research study is necessary; it is neither prescriptive enough to give specific guidance to design and methodology of the study. For this purpose, a focused research question is necessary.

A research question is a clear and concise interrogative statement that is worded in the present tense includes one or more variables and is expressed to guide the implementation of study. The research question is a final step prior to beginning research design, and it outlines the primary components that will be studied. A clear, simple and straightforward question provides direction for subsequent methodological decisions and enables the researcher to focus on research process. Research question can be used to guide both quantitative and qualitative studies. Quantitative studies are often initiated to answer several research question derived from the problem of interest, each focus on a specific variable to be studied in the population.

Need of a Research Question

- It enable the researcher to select appropriate design and methodology for the study
- It helps the researcher to take decision of certain practical constraints of the study, i.e. feasibility and time frame
- It provide foundation for decision that must be made about the research process
- It helps to guide the research process in planned direction and therefore, make the research process systematic.

Elements of a Good Research Question

Two approaches are helpful in developing a good research question in quantitative studies, one of them known as PICO approach (for formulating research question) and other is FINER (for appraisal of a question) approach.

For example, 'Using preoperative education for short stays patients undergoing cardiac catheterization on quality of life'.

Box 2.4: PICO Approach (for selection of research problem).

P	**P**opulation	Patients admitted for cardiac catheterization
I	**I**ntervention	Preoperative teaching
C	**C**omparison	Compared to standard preoperative teaching
O	Expected **O**utcomes	Lead to better quality of life as measured by quality of life scale

However, PICO approach mostly useful to frame research questions for experimental studies only.

Box 2.5: FINER Approach (for appraisal of research question).

F	**F**easibility	In terms of time, money, and availability of subjects, etc.
I	**I**nteresting	Researcher's interest in the study
N	**N**ovel	Study is new or can provide some new information
E	**E**thical	Ethical consideration and protection of rights of the study subjects
R	**R**elevant	Implications for education, practice and administration

Types of Research Question

Most research question can be classified in one of the following three ways:
1. *Descriptive question:* Question that seek to describe a phenomenon, concept, variable or population. For example, what is the level of burden in caregivers of stroke survivors?
2. *Relationship question:* Question that seek to quantify the nature of relationship between variables or between subjects. For example, what is the relationship between caregiver burden and quality of life in caregiver of stroke survivors?
3. *Cause-effect question:* Question that seek to investigate cause-effect relationship of one thing on another. For example, do smoking cause lung cancer?

Box 2.6: Example of a Research Question.

'A cross-sectional study on needs, burden and quality of life among caregivers of stroke survivors'.
(Kumar R, 2015)

Research questions
1. What are the needs of caregivers of stroke survivors?
2. Do the caregiving task put burden on caregivers of stroke survivors?
3. Do the level of burden affects the quality of life of caregivers of stroke survivors?

■ EVALUATION CRITERIA FOR A RESEARCH PROBLEM

Once the research problem has been identified, the researcher must determine the significance of the problem, to nursing as well as feasibility and researchability of studying the problem. A good research problem should answer all the following questions; is the problem significant to nursing? Is there access to enough subjects? Is the cooperation of others is needed? Will the study get cooperation of subjects? Do the sufficient resources available to conduct the study?
- *Determine the significance of the problem:* A research problem should reflect significance to nursing profession. Significance refers to that the research problem contributes to nursing knowledge and practice. A significant nursing study must answer following questions:

1. Is the problem important to nursing?
2. Will patient care benefits from the research study?
3. Will the findings extends or support current theory or generate new theory?
4. Will the findings applicable to nursing practice, education and administration?

If the answer of above questions is 'yes', then the problem should be taken for further consideration.

- *Determine feasibility of research problem:* (*Use of FINER Approach*) Feasibility refers to whether study can be carried out or not. It includes consideration such as cost, time frame, availability of subjects, cooperation of colleagues and others members, interest and experience of the researcher, etc.
  - *Cost:* All research studies cost money to some degree. It is researcher's task to obtain sufficient money from funding agencies, both within institution itself and outside agencies. A research study maybe self-financed. So, the cost related problem must be considered before initiating a research study.
  - *Time frame:* Research studies done to pursue academic degree (i.e. BSc Nursing, MSc nursing or PhD, etc.) are time bounded. For academic degree, a research study that can be completed in given time period is considered feasible. For a study to be considered time feasibility, it must have possibility of being completed within the applicable time frame.
  - *Availability of subjects:* The type and number of subjects vary depending on the purpose and design of the study. A researcher may believe that study subjects may available while data collection, a sufficient number of subjects must be available for the study to be feasible. For example, a researcher is interested to conduct a study on 8–10th class students in the month of December. Here, researcher should make sure the availability of the students during given time frame as most of the schools usually close in month of December due to extreme winter or Christmas holiday.
  - *Availability of facilities and equipment:* All research projects need help of numerous resources like vehicle, recording device, printing, fax, xerox facilities, stationary, etc. Both, the cost and availability of above given resources must be decided when determining the feasibility of the study.
- *Interest of researcher:* Usually, a researcher will take more interest in the study in which he is actually interested. The study that is not of interest to the researcher can take very long time to complete and sometime left incomplete.
- *Experience of the researcher:* Usually, it would have been better if the researcher already have previous experience in the area of study. It is believed that forthcoming difficulties and problems in research project can be dealt with the help of previous experience.
- *Cooperation of colleagues and others:* Research study cannot be done alone, it need cooperation and expertise of others from selection of research problem to analysis and communication the findings. So, a researcher may need assistance and cooperation of other in order to accomplish research project.
- *Ethical consideration:* A researcher should make it sure that research study will get ethical approval without any further hurdle. In case of ethical disapproval, it is impossible to carry-out a research project.
- *Researchability of the problem:* The selected research problem should be researchable. Usually, it is very difficult the topic which is vague and vary from person to person. For example, study related to moral ethical values, i.e. legalization of euthanasia process, DNR order, legalization of female feticides, etc.

VARIABLES

Variables are properties, characteristics and qualities attached to any element, object, situation or an individual that vary or change. Variables are vary from one situation to another. A fixed or stable feature attached to a situation is not a variable. In quantitative research, variables under research study are defined in measurable way.

'A variable is a characteristic, events or responses that represent the elements of the research question in a detectable way'. *(Creswal, 2008)*

Classification of Variables

There are several types of variables represent the intent of a research question. Following are common types of variables studied in a research study.

Dependent Variables

A dependent variable is outcome of interest. In an experimental research, it is expected that an independent variable will have an effect on dependent variable. The dependent variable is a response or outcome to a researcher interested to know or predict.

Independent Variables

An independent variable is one that is applied to the experimental situation to measure its effects. The independent variable is in the hand of researcher and can be manipulated purposefully to see effect on dependent variable. Independent variable is a factor that is artificially introduced into a study explicitly to measure an expected outcome. It is also called as 'cause', 'question' or 'input variable'. In terms of PICO, the dependent variable corresponds to the 'O' (outcome) and independent variable correspond to the 'I' (intervention).

Box 2.7: Example of Dependent and Independent Variables.

Example 1: 'A pre-experimental study to see the effect of assertiveness education on communication skills given to nursing students in Eastern Turkey'. *(Gultekin A, et al. 2018)*
- **Independent variable:** Assertive education
- **Dependent variable:** Communication skills

Example 2: 'An experimental study to see the effect of reminiscence therapy on cognition, depression, and activities of daily living for patients with Alzheimer disease'. *(Dura AG, et al. 2016)*
- **Independent variable:** Reminiscence therapy
- **Dependent variable:** Cognition, depression, and activities of daily living
---

Research Variables

In non-experimental research (descriptive, exploratory, comparative, correlational) and qualitative studies, variables are observed in natural setting without undue manipulation or change. These variables are observed to describe or explore a particular phenomenon called research variables.

Box 2.8: Example of Research Variables.

'A descriptive study on burden and coping strategies among caregivers of mentally ill patients at IHBAS hospital, Delhi'. *(Kumar R, Saini R, 2012)*
Research variables: Burden and coping strategies

Extraneous Variables

Goal of a high quality research is to have control on external influences to minimize biases in order to get accurate findings. External influences may exert an effect on outcome but actually not being a part of the planned experiments called as extraneous variables. Realistically, extraneous variables exist in each and every study but they are most problematic in experiments. Extraneous variables can be controlled if they are expected and recognized when they occur.

Box 2.9: Example of Extraneous Variables.

'A quasi-experimental study to see the effect of self-care education program on reducing HbA1c levels in patients with type 2 diabetes in Zahedan city'. *(Zareban I, et al. 2014)*
- **Independent variable:** Self-care education program
- **Dependent variable:** HbA1c level
- **Extraneous variables:** Reading newspaper, watching a diabetes awareness program on television or radio and abstinence or change in habit of alcohol intake, etc.

Confounding Variables

Confounding variable is a specific type of extraneous variable. Confounding variables are those variables that can influence the outcome of a study in a ways that are not intended by the investigator. These variables are not a part of primary investigation but exist as a part of the investigation.

Since the majority of nursing studies take place in the real world with human subjects, it is impossible to eliminate confounding variables. In literature, confounding and extraneous variables are used interchangeably.

Box 2.10: Example of Confounding Variables.

'An experimental study on exercise and weight loss reduce blood pressure in men and women with mild hypertension at Duke University Medical Center, Durham, North Carolina'. *(Blumenthal JA, et al. 2000)*
Confounding variables: Age, gender, and other sociodemographic characteristics, etc.

Use of random sampling technique, matching subjects and statistical analysis of covariance are the most common way to control confounders.

For example, a researcher might be interested to investigate 'the effect of individual exercise intervention on physical activity compliance on male adults'. Here, a researcher must choose a homogeneous group to control over confounding variables such as taking only men of a specific age group. However, this kind of control is impossible in a study.

Sociodemographic Variables

In most of the non-experimental studies, a researcher make an attempt to study the personal characteristics of the study subjects. Sometimes, researcher also try to establish association and relationship of these sociodemographic variables with research variables. Age, gender, education level, marital status, habitat, occupational status, income, and religion are common sociodemographic variables used in a research study.

OPERATIONAL DEFINITIONS

Operational definition is definition of a variable in terms of the operation (process or activities) a researcher used to measure or manipulates. Research process is a set of procedures (i.e.

instruments, laboratory protocol, sampling and setting, etc.) that will be performed in a systematic way to assign a value for the concept.

It is a procedure to measure and defining a construct under study. It specifies a measurement procedure (a set of operation) proceeding to fulfill the need of a researcher. Operational definitions describe the procedure in accordance to your plan, i.e. what are you going to do in this procedure, how, when and who will carry the procedure, etc. A quality research always based on operationally defined variables and concepts.

Box 2.11: Examples of Operational Definitions.

Example 1: 'Quality of life among caregivers of patients with schizophrenia: a cross-cultural comparison of Chilean and French families'. *(Boyer L, et al. 2012)*
Theoretical and operational definition of quality of life
- **Theoretical definition:** A complex, multidimensional concept in which a person's sense of well-being stems from satisfaction or dissatisfaction with the areas of life that are most important to him/her.
- **Operational definition:** A complex, multidimensional concept in which a person's sense of well-being stems from satisfaction or dissatisfaction with the areas of life that are most important to him/her as measured by World Health Organization Quality of Life-BREF scale.

Example 2: 'A descriptive study on self-esteem and coping among nursing students at AIIMS, Rishikesh, Uttarakhand'. (Hypothetical statement).
Theoretical definition and operational definitions of self-esteem, and coping.
- **Theoretical definition:**
  - *Self-esteem:* A person's sense of self-worth or value
  - *Coping:* Cognitive and behavioral efforts to manage specific external and/or internal demands that are appraised as taxing and exceeding the resources of the person.
- **Operational definition:**
  - *Self-esteem:* A person is self-worth or value as measured by Rosenberg self-esteem scale
  - *Coping:* Cognitive and behavioral efforts to manage specific external and/or internal demands that are appraised as taxing and exceeding the resources of the person as measured by Coping checklist. *(CCL, Kiran R, et al. 1989)*

Significance of Operational Definitions

It is an integral and essential part of research to define the variable operationally. It will ensure that the particular variables under study are measured, or manipulated consistently throughout the research study. It will also help to communicate the ideas to audience explicitly.

The process of developing operational definitions involves deleting all aspects of the variables except in which researcher is interested. In simple, your operational definition says what you study and how will you study. This whole process called *operationalizing of variables*.

Operational definitions of the variables under study helps a researcher in following ways:
1. Operational definitions give precise indications of the fundamental attributes of a concept/variable under study.
2. It helps in precise measurement of the concept and its characteristics in whole.
3. Operational definition sensitize researcher about measurement to observe or record the attributes the way researcher want to observe or record it.
4. An operational definition is useful tool which energize the researcher to focus on observation or measurement of variable of interest and avoid attention on measurement of other similar but irrelevant phenomenon.

RESEARCH OBJECTIVES

Once the research question is explicit, it is possible to begin to specify the objectives. Research objectives describe the individual task that need to be carried out in order to meet the study aims. The research objectives are clear, concise and declarative statement expressed in the present tense to specify the study purposes. Objectives are more specific and measurable explanation of aims. They enable the researcher to determine whether the problem has been solved or not. The objectives of a research study summaries what is to be achieved by the study. Objectives are closely related to the statement of problem.

Characteristics of Research Objectives (Clement, 2012)

- Research objective is a concrete statement describing what the research trying to achieve
- A well worded objective will be **SMART**, i.e. **S**pecific, **M**easurable, **A**ttainable, **R**elevant, and **T**ime bound.
- Research objective should be feasible, logical, observable, unequivocal and measurable
- The objectives of a research study summarize what is to be achieved by the study
- The research objectives are specific accomplishments the researcher hope to achieve by the study
- Objectives included obtaining answer to research question or testing the hypothesis.

Types of Research Objectives

Broadly, research objectives are classified in following two ways:
1. *General objectives:* These are the main objectives of the research study. These objectives focused on broad outcomes a researcher has to achieve at the end of the study.
2. *Specific objectives:* Specific objectives prepared on the basis of general objectives and usually short term goal oriented. All specific objectives merge together to make a general objective. Usually, specific objectives are more in number and focus on different aspects of a problem. Specific objectives are the one which reply to what, where, when and why of a research study.

Box 2.12: Example of General and Specific Objectives.

'A quasi-experimental study to see the effect of laughter therapy on anxiety and blood pressure among elderly residing at old age home, Rishikesh, Uttrakhand'. (Hypothetical statement).

General objective:
- To assess the effect of laughter therapy on anxiety and blood pressure among elderly

Specific objectives:
- To assess the level of anxiety and blood pressure among elderly
- To compare the effect of laughter therapy on anxiety and blood pressure among elderly
- To find out the association of post-test anxiety and blood pressure with selected sociodemographic variables of elderly

---

Significance of Research Objectives

The formulation of research objectives will help the researcher in following ways:
- *Focus:* A well clear and specific objectives enable the researcher to focus on the study steps. If a researcher knows what they have to achieve ultimately, they will concentrate on the ways to achieve it. It also helps to define the study and avoid the unnecessary findings.

- *Avoid:* The research objective helps the researcher to collect the necessary information for the study and avoid collecting unnecessary and irrelevant trivial information.
- *Organize the study:* The formulation of specific objectives will help to organize the study in well manner. For example, a researcher is interested in conducting 'a study on stress and burnout among critical care nurses', where objectives are formulated as:
    - To assess stress level among critical care nurses
    - To assess burnout among critical care nurses.

  Here, objectives will helps to organize and limit the study results in two sections only.
- *Direction:* A well-framed specific objective will give direction to research study. It enables the researcher to choose appropriate methodology, analysis and interpretation of the results.

Tips for Writing Research Objectives

Writing research objective is not as simple as you think. It needs lot of expertise, knowledge of action verbs and experience. A researcher should keep in mind certain points while writing objectives, including following:
- The objective should be clear, concise and written in declarative format
- The objective should be written in present tense
- Use of appropriate action verb makes the objectives realistic and achievable
- A well written objective should be specific to a variable
- The objective should be written in sequence for variables as given in the problem statement
- Researcher should try to omit the words that are repetitively used in objective statement, i.e. of, an, is, among, etc.
- It should be written in measurable format.

Box 2.13: Example of Research Objectives.

'A cross-sectional observational survey on hand hygiene compliance, attitude and barriers faced by health care workers at a tertiary care teaching hospital, Uttarakhand'. *(Kumar R, et al. 2017)*

Objectives:
The study objective are to:
1. Determine hand hygiene compliance among health care workers
2. Assess attitude of health care workers towards hand hygiene practices
3. Identify the barriers to hand hygiene practices

ASSUMPTIONS

An assumption is an idea or blind guess of a researcher that is taken to be true. It is realistic expectation, i.e. something that we believe to be true. However, there is no enough evidence to support this belief. Assumptions do not have empirical evidence to justify it. Assumptions play an important role in the development of research methodology and instrument and therefore influence the development of research process.

Definitions

'Assumptions defined as the statement that are taken granted or are considered true without any empirical evidences or any scientific testing.'

'Assumptions are those principles which are accepted to be true but without empirical evidence or proof.'

'These are statement taken for granted or considered true without any scientific base or background'.

Researchers have doubt about use of assumption in varied types of research study. Some researcher agree to the fact that assumptions should be only used in survey types of studies and other strongly recommend its use in experimental studies. In fact, there is no such kind of evidence for use of assumption related to types of research design. Besides, use of assumption should be irrespective to the types of research methodology.

Assumptions and Research Hypotheses

Generally, in health sciences research, experts feel confuse regarding use of hypotheses and assumptions. Hypotheses and assumption both are different to each other and serve different purpose in a research study. Some of the distinct features of hypothesis and assumptions are given in Table 2.1.

Table 2.1: Features of Assumptions and hypotheses.

Assumptions	Hypotheses
It is personal belief or ideas that we hold to be true	Predictions made by researcher
Little or no evidence for statistical testing	Usually, tested by statistical test and accepted or rejected
It does not show relationship between variables, only indicate belief about research methodology	It predict relationship between two or more than two variables
Researcher attempts to find out/verify the authenticity of belied made in the beginning of the study	Statistically tested to conclude the study

Types of Assumptions

A researcher can make following types of assumptions. Formulation of research assumption based on research study and it methodological aspects. Common types of assumption are as follows:

- *Universal assumptions:* These are belief that assumed to be true by a large part of society or universe. Testing of such assumption is not always possible. For example, some of the Divine power controlling the universe.
- *Assumptions based on theories:* The basic purpose of research is to either refine the existing theories or developing new theories. In theory-based research, assumptions of underlying theory become the assumptions of your research study. For example, Study based on Betty Neuman System model follows the assumptions of Betty Neuman System model in the study.
- *Methodological assumptions:* Researcher has to formulate some of the methodological assumption to conduct a research study. For example:
  - The self-structured knowledge questionnaire can assess the knowledge regarding universal precautions among staff nurses
  - Participate will willingly participate in the study and respond o research tools honestly.
- *Warranted assumptions:* These types of assumptions stated along with the proof or evidences to support. For example, regular practice of art of living bring biochemical changes in the brain.

- *Unwarranted assumptions:* These assumptions do not have supportive evidence or proof. Sometimes, it will be difficult to fulfill theses kind of assumptions. For example: God is existing everywhere in this universe.

Importance of Assumptions in Research

The followings are common importance of use of assumptions in the research:
- Assumptions works as a foundation or base for researcher. A researcher should have something to discover or search out
- Selection of research topic can be based on written assumption or assumptions of the previous studies
- Assumptions helps in research process and conclude the research study
- Verified and tested assumptions expand the body of knowledge.

HYPOTHESIS

A hypothesis is used when you wish to test the relationship between two or more than two variables. Hypothesis is a tentative statement of the expected relationship(s) between two or more than two variables in a specified population. In scientific research, hypotheses are intelligent guess that assist the researcher in seeking the solution to a problem. A hypothesis translates the research question and purpose into a clear explanation or prediction of the expected results or outcomes of the selected study.

Definitions

'Hypothesis is a conjectural statement of the relations between two or more variables.'
(Kerlinger, 1986)
'Hypothesis is a tentative statement about the relationship, if any between two or more variables.'
(Parahoo, 1997)
'Hypothesis is a statement of the relationship between two or more variables.'
(Polit and Beck, 2004)

Hypothesis should always be written before the study and should not be changed after the study results are examined.

Purposes of Hypothesis in Research

Hypothesis serves several purposes in research studies, including followings:
- They provide objectivity to scientific investigation by pinpointing a specific part of theory to be tested
- They help to advance the knowledge by supporting or rejecting the tested theory
- Hypothesis provides direction and guide to a research study
- It guides research design and dictate the type of statistical analysis to be used with the data
- It provide bridge between theory and practice
- It serves as a framework for drawing conclusion of a research study
- Hypothesis provides the reader an understandings of the researcher's expectations about the study before collection begins.

Sources of Hypothesis

Hypotheses are not wild guess or shots in the dark. The researcher should be able to state the sources or rational for each hypothesis. The hypothesis may generate from personal experience, previous research studies, nursing theories, or reviewing the literature, etc.

- *Personal experiences:* A nurse may have a hunch or guess that comes from day-to-day personal experiences. For example, a nurse may have noticed that a psychiatric patient seems to become more anxious as the time for discharges approach. Observations continue to be made. Patient charts are examined to determine the behavioral reports by other staff nurses. The behavioral records on the charts seem to agree with your observation. Here is a possible hypothesis, 'as the time for discharge draw near, the anxiety level of psychiatric patients increase.
- *Nursing literature:* Hypotheses for nursing studies can also be generated by reading nursing literature or from findings of the other studies. The research may test the assumption of another study or test a hypothesis based on findings of the others.
- *Theoretical/conceptual framework:* This is most important source for generating hypotheses. This process of hypotheses development involves deducting reasoning. A propositional statement is isolated from the study framework and empirically tested. For example, using Maslow's theory of Human needs, you might decide to test the proposition that safety needs take precedence over self-esteem needs.

Classification of Hypotheses

Hypotheses maybe categorized as simple hypotheses, and complex hypotheses. They may also be classified as research hypotheses and statistical or null hypotheses. Research hypotheses maybe further divided into non-directional and directional hypotheses.

Simple Hypothesis

A simple hypothesis concern the relationships between one independent and one dependent variable. It is also known as *bivariate.*

> **Box 2.14:** Example of Simple Hypothesis.
> - 'Birth weight is lower among infants of alcoholic mother than among infants of non-alcoholic mother'
> - 'The greater the degree of sleep deprivation, the higher the anxiety level in ICU patients'
> - 'The greater the amount of use of benzodiazepines, higher the level of psychosis in ICU patients'

Complex Hypothesis

A complex hypothesis shows a relationship of two or more independent variables, two or more dependent variables or both. It is also considered as *multivariate.*

> **Box 2.15:** Example of Complex Hypothesis.
> - 'The greater the amount of use of benzodiazepines and higher $PaCO_2$ level, higher the level of psychosis in ICU patients'
> - 'Daily weight loss is greater for adult who follow a reduced calorie diet and exercise than for those who do not follow a reduced calorie diet and do not exercise daily'
> - 'More postpartum depression and feelings of inadequacy are reported by women who give birth by cesarean section than those who deliver vaginally'

Null Hypothesis (H_0)

Null hypothesis or statistical hypothesis states no relationship between variables. A null hypothesis is subjects to statistical analysis therefore called *statistical hypotheses*.

> **Box 2.16:** Example of Null Hypothesis.
> - 'There is no relationship between internet addiction and depression among engineering students'
> - 'There is no relationship between knowledge and practice of staff nurses on universal precautions'

Research Hypotheses (H_1)

Research hypothesis or alternate hypothesis state the existence of relationship between variables. It is also called *scientific, substantive or theoretical hypothesis*.

> **Box 2.17:** Example of Research Hypothesis.
> - 'There is a positive relationship between depression and suicide'
> - 'There is a positive relationship between stress and use of negative coping strategies among adolescents'

Directional Hypothesis

Research hypotheses maybe presented as being directional or nondirectional hypotheses. In the directional hypotheses, the expected relationship and direction of relationship between variables is presented. Directional hypotheses have several advantages like they may clear the researcher's expectation, and allow more precise testing of theoretical propositions and allow the use of one tailed tests.

> **Box 2.18:** Example of Directional Hypothesis.
> - 'There is a positive relationship between increasing age and osteoporosis'
> - 'There is a positive relationship between increasing age and depression'

Non-directional Hypothesis

Non-directional hypotheses state the relationship between variables, but does not specify the directions of relationship between variables.

> **Box 2.19:** Example of Non-directional Hypothesis.
> - 'There is a relationship between age and depression'
> - 'There is a relationship between organizational commitment and job satisfaction'

Associative Hypothesis

Associate hypotheses state the relationship between two or more than two variables that occur in natural setting, so that when one variable change, another variable also change. These hypotheses only identify the relationship but do not indicate that one cause or effect on another.

> **Box 2.20:** Example of Associative Hypothesis.
> 'High level of job satisfaction would be associated with less frequent reported adverse events in staff nurses'

Casual Hypotheses

Casual hypotheses state the cause and effect relationship between two variables, referred to as independent and dependent variables.

Research Problem, Research Question and Hypothesis

Box 2.21: Example of Casual Hypothesis.

- 'Effect of instillation of 0.5 mm normal saline during suctioning on change in blood pressure and heart rate'
- 'Smoking causes lung cancer'

Characteristics of a Good Hypothesis

A good hypothesis must be written in declarative sentence, using present tense. A hypothesis must be well worded and clear to understand. The main characteristics of a good hypothesis are as follows:

- *Should be written in declarative sentence:* A hypothesis must be written in declarative sentence as it presents an answer or tentative solution to the problem. It is possible to transpose only two words in some problem statement and change them into non-directional research hypothesis.
  For example, 'there is a change in the anxiety level of preoperative patients after listening to music'.
- *Written in present tense:* Hypotheses found in literature are frequently written in the future tense. However, hypotheses are tested in present tense and should be written in present tense only.

Box 2.22: Example of Hypothesis.

Future tense: 'There will be a positive relationship between length of ventilator stay and ICU psychosis among ICU patients'
Present tense: 'There is a positive relationship between length of ventilator stay and ICU psychosis among ICU patients'

- *Should contains the population:* A complete and well framed hypothesis should identified the population, just as it is in the problem statement.
- *Contain the variables:* A scientific hypothesis contains at least two variables. The hypothesis may links two or more variables together. The variables in the hypothesis should be same as those in the corresponding research statement.
- *Contains the instrument(s) or tool(s):* Frequently, the hypotheses contain the instruments or tools that will be used to measure the dependent variables.
- *Reflect the level of significance:* A hypothesis should be mentioned with the desired level of significance. The level of significance should be fixed before writing the hypotheses and it should not be changed. Usually nursing studies choose 0.05 level of significance for hypotheses testing.

Box 2.23: Example of Hypothesis.

'There is a significant relationship between increasing age and depression as measured by Beck Depression Inventory (BDI) at 0.05 level of significance'

- *Empirically tested:* A hypothesis that cannot be empirically tested has no scientific merit. Ethical and moral values related issues are two areas that are inappropriate for hypothesis testing because data cannot be obtained that can be empirically tested.

Components of Hypotheses

A well written and complete hypothesis must contain variables, population under study, and should be stated in accordance to objectives and problem statement. The main elements of a hypothesis are followings:
1. *Population:* Group of subjects under study
2. *Variables:* Concept under investigation
3. *Instruments(s) or tool(s):* Instruments used to measure dependent variables
4. *Level of significance:* The desired level of significance for testing of hypotheses
5. *Anticipated relationship:* Positive, negative or no relationship between variables.

Box 2.24: Hypothesis and its Elements.

'A study on relationship between depression and internet addiction among University students in Jordan'
(Rabdi L, et al. 2017)

H_o: There is a significant positive relationship between internet addiction and depression among university students as measured by Young's Internet Addiction Scale & The online cognition scale (OCS) at 0.05 level of significance.
- **Population:** University of science and technology students
- **Variables:** Internet addiction and depression
- **Instruments(s) or tool(s):** Young's Internet Addiction Scale and the online cognition scale (OCS)
- **Level of significance:** 0.05 level of significance
- **Anticipated relationship:** Positive relationship

Stating the Hypotheses

A hypothesis can be written in different ways and its vary from one person to another. The language of writing hypothesis could be different but it should conclude similar meaning. Some of the common ways of writing hypothesis are exemplified.

In above example, the hypotheses state the population (older patient), the independent variable (age), the dependent variable (falling) and an anticipated relationship.

Box 2.25: Styles of Writing Hypothesis.

For example,' Prevalence of falls in elderly women'. *(Vitor VR, et al. 2015)*
Hypothesis:
- The risk of falling increase with the age of the patients
- Younger patients are at lower risk of falling than older patients
- There is a relationship between patient's age and the likelihood of falling
- The older the patient, the greater the likelihood that he or she will fall
- Older patient differ from younger ones with respect to their risk of falling
- Older patient more likely falling than younger patients

DELIMITATIONS

Delimitations are the boundaries a researcher follows for a study. These boundaries are defined by the researcher to guide the research process in planned way. Delimitations helps researcher to plan the study in a systematic way. Delimitation works as skeleton for the researcher and research process.

Purposes of Delimitations in Research

The following are the important delimitations in the research process:
- It aides as guide to researcher
- It helps to copy out the study in a systematic way
- It will show path to researcher and research process
- It has economic advantages lies in terms of expenses and other expenditure in research process
- It helps researcher to concentrate on the work by defining the boundaries.

Delimitations are the choices made by the researcher to confine the scope of research. They describes the boundaries that a researcher has taken in the study to study a concept more clearly. Following are common research parameters which are defined and addressed in delimitations.

- *Settings of the study:* Confinement of geographical boundaries for the study. For example, the present study delimited to high school students studying in government schools only.
- *Population:* Population which is under study. For example, the study will be delimited to population age group more than 18 years and male only.
- *Research tools/instruments:* Use of particular tool in the study to explore a concept under study. For example, study will use Zarit burden interview schedule (ZBIS) for assessing burden among caregivers of stroke patients.
- *Use of sampling techniques/size:* Use of sample size and sampling technique in the study. For example, use of simple random sampling technique and number of participants in the study.

Characteristics of a Well-framed Delimitation

While writing delimitations, following points should be kept in mind.
- Delimitation should be written in concise term and should be written specifically.
- It should be reasonable to the research study.
- Mention the reason for taking a particular delimitation in the research study.
- A researcher should justify why for a particular research parameter, delimitation is not framed.

Box 2.26: Example of Delimitations.

Example 1: 'A study on pattern of burden and quality of life among caregivers of stroke survivors'.
(Kumar R, et al. 2015)

Delimitations:
- Unpaid primary family caregivers/relatives of stroke patients caring since one month at home
- Perceived burden, and Health related quality of life (HRQoL) of caregivers of stroke patients
- Perceived burden, and health related quality of life are measurable by using Zarit burden interview Schedule, and WHOQoL-BREF.
- Assessment of perceived burden, and Health related quality of life (HRQoL) of caregivers of stroke patients once only
- Caregivers who will be willing to participate and write consent for the study.

Example 2: 'A study on high school students' perception of nursing as a career at selected high schools at Uttarakhand state'.
(Sharma SK, Kumar R, et al. 2017)

Delimitations:
- Students who are studying in 12th class
- Students belong to high schools of district Rishikesh, Uttarakhand
- Students studying at government schools only

LIMITATIONS

Limitation and delimitations are used in research interchangeably but are distinct to each others. Limitations are the weakness or restrictions of the study in terms of theoretical or methodological aspects. Limitations decrease the credibility of research study. Use of rigorous theoretical framework and sound methodological assets will help to overcome certain limitations and subsequently make the generalization possible.

Usually, a researcher or primary investigator is aware about the study limitations and use rigorous ways to improve upon the limitations. A credible research concludes with minimum limitations.

Types of Limitations

A research study can have following types of limitations.
- *Theoretical limitations:* The prime purpose of research is to either test existing theories or to develop new theories. Research based on certain theoretical concept. Inappropriate operationalization of theses theoretical concepts limit the generalization of findings.

  For example: "Stress and coping among caregivers of mentally ill patients". The conceptual framework for this study was based on Betty Neuman System Model. According to this model the caregivers should be defined as client system (as given in Betty Neuman System model). Improper operation definition of client system (caregivers) will limit the study and decrease the credibility and generalization of the findings.

- *Methodological limitations:* A sound research methodology is foremost important for a quality research. It is backbone of the research study. A research study could have many limitations from methodological perspective, i.e. research design, sample, size, sampling technique, methods of data collection, their validity and reliability, control on extraneous variables, maintaining group homogeneity, etc. Every study, no matter how well designed, has certain limitations. An experienced and trained researcher will identify these limitations and take appropriate measures to improve the credibility of the study.

  For example: "Perception of high school students towards nursing as future job perspective". The said research study use systematic random sampling techniques. Now, researcher should adequately defined the process of systematic random sampling in terms of how, when, where and who, etc. Incomplete and inappropriate explanation of sampling technique could limit the generalization of the study.

REVIEW QUESTIONS AND ANSWER

Long and Short Answer Questions

1. Define reach problems and enlist the steps in selection of reach problem. *(KUHAS, MSc N-2002)*
2. How to frame a good research problem? *(RGUHS, MSc N-2017)*
3. Define hypothesis and explain its need in research. *(PGI, MSc N-2013)*
4. Differentiate between statistical hypotheses and research hypotheses. *(KUHAS, MSc N-2016)*
5. What are type-I and type-II errors? *(KUHAS, MSc N-2001)*
6. List done the criteria to frame a research problem. *(PGI, MSc N-2009)*
7. Differentiate between dependent and independent variable. *(KUHAS, MSc N-2008)*
8. List done the sources of research problem. *(TNMGRMU, MSc N-2012)*

9. Define operational definition and explain in detail. (RGUHS, MSc N-2016)
10. Differentiate between assumptions and hypotheses. (BFUHS, MSc N-2005)

Multiple Choice Questions

1. A variable in experimental study that can interfere with an intervention but cannot be controlled is called as:
   a. Independent variables
   b. Dependent variables
   c. Extraneous variables
   d. Confounding variables

2. A variable in experimental study that is presumed to cause a change in another variable is called a(n):
   a. Research variables
   b. Independent variables
   c. Dependent variables
   d. Confounding variables

3. Which of the following is an example of categorical variables?
   a. Age
   b. Gender
   c. Religion
   d. Annual income

4. A formal statement state relationship between two or more than two variables in a specified population. The formal statement is called as:
   a. Assumption
   b. Hypotheses
   c. Research question
   d. Research objectives

5. Which of the following types of design is most suitable for testing cause and effect relationships?
   a. Descriptive design
   b. Exploratory design
   c. Experimental design
   d. Grounded theory

6. A condition or characteristic that can take on different values or categories is called as:
   a. Hypotheses
   b. Variable
   c. Assumption
   d. Objective

7. Which of the following is not an element of a well framed research statement?
   a. Variables
   b. Population
   c. Setting
   d. Tools of the study

8. Problem identification in the research process would be equivalent to which step in the nursing process?
   a. Goal identification
   b. Data collection
   c. Identifying solution
   d. Nursing diagnosis

9. Which of the following is not an element of a well-framed hypothesis?
   a. Variables
   b. Level of significance
   c. Setting of the study
   d. Research instruments

10. Which of the following hypothesis undergone statistical testing in research?
    a. Null hypothesis
    b. Research hypothesis
    c. Casual hypothesis
    d. Directional hypothesis

11. This is the hypothesis state no relationship between dependent and independent variables in an experimental study:
    a. Research hypothesis
    b. Null hypothesis
    c. Casual hypothesis
    d. Directional hypothesis

12. A hypothesis which state relationship between one dependent and independent variable is called:
    a. Simple hypothesis
    b. Research hypothesis
    c. Casual hypothesis
    d. Directional hypothesis

13. Basic principles that are accepted as being true on the basis of logic or reason, without proof or verification is called as:
    a. Assumption
    b. Hypothesis
    c. Propositions
    d. Concepts

14. Which of the following term describe the boundaries that a researcher has set for the study?
    a. Limitations
    b. Delimitations
    c. Hypothesis
    d. Operational definitions

Answer Key

1.	2.	3.	4.	5.	6.	7.	8.	9.	10.	11.	12.	13.	14.
c.	b.	c.	b.	c.	b.	d.	d.	c.	a.	b.	a.	a.	b.

SUGGESTED READING

1. Blumenthal JA, Sherwood A, Gullette ECD, et al. Exercise and weight loss reduce blood pressure in men and women with mild hypertension effects on cardiovascular, metabolic, and hemodynamic functioning. Arch Intern Med. 2000;160(13):1947-58.
2. Boyer L, Caqueo-Urízar A, Richieri R, Lancon C, Gutiérrez-Maldonado J, Auquier P. Quality of life among caregivers of patients with schizophrenia: a cross-cultural comparison of Chilean and French families. BMC Family Practice. 2012;13: 42. doi:10.1186/1471-2296-13-42.
3. Carolyni W, Ora LS, Elizabeth L. Measurement in nursing and health research, 4th edition. Springer Publishing Company; 2010.
4. Clement I. Nursing solved question paper for BSc Nursing IV year (2012–1999), 2nd edition. India: Jaypee; 2012.
5. Creswell J. Research design: qualitative, quantitative and mixed methods approaches, 3rd edition. SAGE Publications; 2008.
6. Duru Aşiret G, Kapucu S. The effect of reminiscence therapy on cognition, depression, and activities of daily living for patients with Alzheimer Disease. Journal of Geriatric Psychiatry and Neurology. 2016;29(1): 31-7.
7. Fain E. Reading, understanding and applying nursing research, Philadelphia: FA. Davis; 2008.
8. Gultekin A, Ozdemir AA, Budak F. The effects of assertiveness education on communication skills given to nursing students. International Journal of Caring Sciences. 2018;11(1):395-401.
9. Harting D, Touchette D. Overview of the clinical research design. American Journal of Health System Pharmacy. 2009; 66(15), 398-407.
10. Houser J. Nursing research, 2nd edition, Jones and Bartlett publishers; 2011.

11. Kerliner F. Foundation of behavioral research, 3rd edition, New York: Halt, Rinehart and Winston; 1986.
12. Kumar R, Gupta PK, Sharma P, et al. Hand hygiene, attitude and barriers among health care workers at a tertiary care teaching hospital, Uttarakhand. Int J Health Sci Res. 2017; 7(9):159-65.
13. Kumar R, Kaur S, Reddemma K. Pattern of burden and quality of life among caregivers of stroke survivors. Int J Health Sci Res. 2015; 5(4):208-14.
14. Kumar R. Academic climate, academic stress and self esteem among baccalaureate nursing students. Nursing and Midwifery Research Journal. 2018;14(2):53-61.
15. Kumar R. Need, burden, coping and quality of life in stroke caregivers: a pilot survey. Nursing and Midwifery Research Journal. 2015;11(2):57-67.
16. Kumar R, Saini R. Extent of burden and coping strategies among caregivers of mentally-ill patients. Nursing and Midwifery Research Journal. 2012;8(4):74-84.
17. Kumar R. Self esteem, stress and depression on nursing students. Indian Journal of Continuing Nursing Education. 2016;17(1):30-6.
18. Macnee CL, Susan MC. Understanding nursing research: Using research in evidence based practice. Lippincott William and Wilkins; 2008.
19. McEwan M, Wills EM. Theoretical basis for nursing. Philadelphia: Lippincott Williams and Wilkins; 2007.
20. Mc-Grath JP, Polit DF, Beck CT. Canadian essential of nursing. Philadelphia: Lippincott William and Wilkins; 2010.
21. Meleis A. Theoretical nursing: developmental progress, 3rd edition, Philadelphia: JB Lippincott company; 2007.
22. Moule P, Goodman M. Nursing research: An introduction: SAGE Publications; 2013.
23. Munhall P. Nursing research: a qualitative perspective, 4th edition. Sudbury MA: Jones and Bartlett; 2006.
24. Nieswiadomy RM. Foundation of nursing research. India: Person Education; 2008.
25. Parahoo K. Nursing research: principle, process and issues. London: Macmillan; 1997.
26. Polit DF, Beck CT. Essential of nursing research: apprising evidence for nursing practice, 8th edition. Philadelphia: Lippincott William and Wilkins; 2013.
27. Polit DF, Beck CT. Nursing research: principles and methods, 7th edition. Philadelphia: Lippincott William and Wilkins; 2004.
28. Potter AP, Perry AG, Stockert P, Hall A. Fundamental of nursing, 8th edition. Elsevier health sciences; 2013.
29. Rabadi L, Ajlouni M, Masannat S, Bataineh S, Batarseh G, et al. The Relationship between Depression and Internet Addiction among University Students in Jordan. J Addict Res Ther. 2017;8: 349.
30. Sharma SK, Kumar R, Singh B. High school students perception of nursing as a career-a pilot survey. Indian Journal of Advanced Nursing. 2017;III(I):15-23.
31. Suresh PS, Thejaswini V, Rajan T. Factors associated with 2009 pandemic influenza A (H1N1) vaccination acceptance among university students from India during the post-pandemic phase. BMC Infectious Diseases. 2011; 11:205.
32. Vitor PR, de Oliveira AC, Kohler R, Winter GR, Rodacki C, Krause MP. Prevalence of falls in elderly women. Acta Ortopedica Brasileira. 2015; 23(3):158-61.
33. Wood M, Janet CK. Basic steps in planning nursing research: From question to proposal. Jones and Bartlett Learning; 2010.
34. Zareban I, Karimy M, Niknami S, Haidarnia A, Rakhshani F. The effect of self-care education program on reducing HbA1c levels in patients with type 2 diabetes. Journal of Education and Health Promotion. 2014;3:123.

Chapter 3

The Research Process: An Overview

INTRODUCTION

The research process encompasses planning and conducting the research study. The manner in which thought and ideas about the research are put into operation and become reality will decide the success of the research study. There are number of sequential stage in the research process that customarily, but not invariably, follows each other. These stages found in each research and in written report. Furthermore, steps in quantitative and qualitative study are not similar. However, there maybe variation in the steps of research process in quantitative and qualitative research study.

FUNDAMENTAL RESEARCH TERMS

- *Abstract:* A brief and concise description of the proposed study. Abstract usually placed in the beginning of the study. It should not be more than 1 00-200 words.
- *Variables:* An attribute that varies and can have more than one value such as height, weight, temperature, etc. Common used variables in research are:
    - *Independent variables:* The variable that is purposely manipulated by researcher to see influence on dependent variable. For example, in experimental studies, the treatment is independent variable. It is also known as stimulus, cause, question, input variable.
    - *Dependent variables:* The variable that is hypothesized depends on independent variable for change or outcome. It is also known as response, answer, effect or outcome variable, etc.
    - *Research variables:* These are qualities, properties and characteristics related to an individual, or organization which are directly measured in natural setting.
    - *Extraneous variables:* The variables which is not a part of study but may confound the study outcomes and need to be controlled by researcher.
    - *Continuous variables:* A variable have an infinite value along a continuum. For example, height, weight and other physical parameters. The number of value for 1 kg and 2 kg is limitless between two points: 1.05, 1.06, 1.07, 1.09 and so on.
    - *Discrete variables:* A variable has fixed or finite number of value between any two points. For example, male and female, number of children, etc.
    - *Categorical variables:* A variable represent some categories but do not represent quantity. For example, blood types, male and female. When categorical variables take only two values, they are called *dichotomous variables.*
- *Subject/key informant:* An individual who participate and provide information in a study. In qualitative study, term 'key informant' word is used in place of subject.

- *Sample:* A part or segment of population selected to participate in the study.
- *Sampling:* The process used to draw sample from a define population is called sampling.
- *Researcher/investigator:* A person who conducts the study is called researcher or investigator.
- *Peer-review:* A researcher who review and critique of a research proposal or report of another person to find out strengths and weakness.
- *Concept:* A mental image inferred from observation of phenomena, behavior, situation, or characteristics (e.g. pain, anxiety).
- *Operational definition:* The definition of a concept or variable in terms of the procedure by which it is to be measured. It is researcher's own definition for concept and variable under investigation.
- *Pilot study:* It is a small scale try-out of main study on similar sample at different setting. It is also called as feasibility study.

QUANTITATIVE RESEARCH PROCESS: OVERVIEW

Quantitative research is a systematic and objective approach for generating information about a particular variable. Quantitative research studies are conducted to describe, explain and explore a phenomenon under investigation. Researcher follow a systematic process from selection of research problem or question to design methodology and end with generation and communicating the research finding to the audience. However, following stages are common in quantitative research (Fig. 3.1):

- The conceptual phase
- The design and planning phase
- The empirical phase
- The analytic phase
- The dissemination phase

The Conceptual Phase

The quantitative research is a result of strong conceptual and intellectual elements. These concept or ideas are result of reading books, journals, literature and of discussion with the colleagues. A sound research concept makes the research rigorous and credible. The conceptual phase includes following sub steps:

Formulating Research Problem

It is suggested here that first part of the research process is the *"research idea".* In fact, a good research begins with a good idea. The research process begins in the mind of the researcher before actually implantation of these ideas into action. The identification of research problem and question determine the significance of the research study.

Searching the Relevant Literature Review

Research never been conducted in vacuum. A good research is based on sound and relevant literature review. A thorough and relevant literature review provides foundation for selection of adequate size of sample, design, research instrument and analysis and interpretation of the findings.

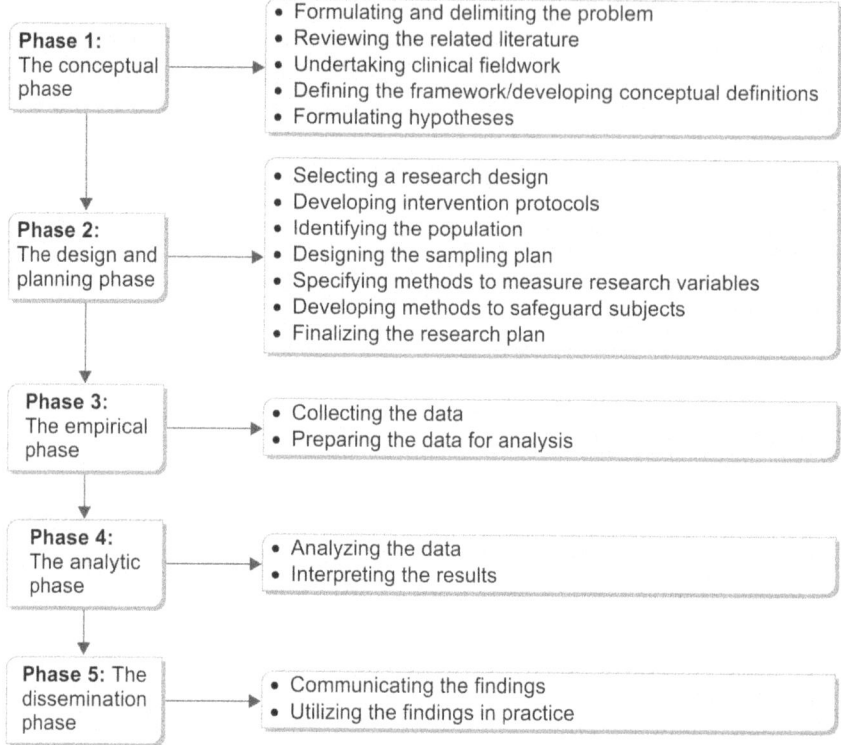

Fig. 3.1: Steps of quantitative research process.

Developing Conceptual Framework

The aim of the quantitative study is to test or refine the existing theory. Researcher may choose or develop his/her own conceptual framework for research study.

Formulating Hypothesis

Most quantitative studies are designed to test hypothesis. A hypothesis is a tentative statement of expected relationship between two or more than two variables. A research hypothesis is used when you wish to test the relationship between two or more than two variables. Hypothesis helps to draw conclusion for the study.

The Design and Planning Phase

This is the major stage in quantitative study. In this stage, research select and decide appropriate methodology and methods to carry out study. These methodological decisions are crucial implications for the integrity of the resulting evidence. Selection of rigorous research methodology may improve the research credibility. This phase includes following sub steps:

Selecting a Research Design

The research design is the heart of a research study. It is a formal plan to carry out a study. Research design is the architectural backbone of a research study. Various designs are available for quantitative research like experimental and nonexperimental research design. Non-experimental design further includes descriptive, correlational and exploratory design.

Developing Intervention Protocol

In case of experimental design, researcher has to develop a rigorous intervention protocol for delivering intervention with minimum biases. An intervention protocol must specify all the elements of intervention in details like who will deliver, when, frequency, timing, intensity, duration, etc. A well designed intervention protocol helps to get high quality evidence. For example, effect of yoga therapy on geriatric patient. Here, researcher has to specify certain points in protocol like; what is yoga therapy, who will deliver yoga therapy, how long yoga therapy will be delivered, how frequently yoga therapy will be given, and timing, etc.

Selecting the Population

Population is group of subjects who will participate in the study. Researcher should select a homogenous population group in order to generalize the findings. For example, caregivers of stroke survivors might be all caregivers providing care to stroke patient since one month of stroke episode.

Selecting the Sample

Studying whole population is not feasible and convenient for a researcher. Sample is a subset or a fraction of population which represent almost all characteristics of population. In a quantitative study, adequate size of representative sample should be selected for generalization of the result over target population. For example, caregivers who are more or equal to 18 years of age and providing care to stroke survivors for at least one month after discharge from hospital will be sample for the study.

Selecting the Specific Research Instruments

Based on variables of the research study, researcher will select the research instrument to measure or collect information about a variable under investigation. Questionnaire, rating scale and interview methods are the primary methods of data collection in quantitative studies.

Ethical Consideration

Nursing research conducted on human subject need to adhere to ethical principles. A researcher will present research proposal before ethical committee to obtain ethical permission. Informed consent, confidentiality and anonymity are the some common ethical principle to be followed in the research study. A formal written permission also collected from competent and concerned authority before gaining entry into setting.

The Empirical Phase

This phase includes collection of data and preparation of data for analysis.

Collecting the Data

Researcher collects data according to research plan. The researcher may use many methods to collect data like questionnaire, rating scale, checklist and interview method, etc. A formal designed research plan may guide the data collection process.

Preparing the Data for Analysis

Once the data collection is over, researcher has to code and prepare a coding sheet for analysis of data. For example, researcher may give code '1' for male participants and code '2' for females in the study.

The Analytic Phase

This phase deals with analysis and interpretation of the research findings for making information meaningful.

Analyzing the Data

The analysis is based on objectives or hypotheses of the study. In modern technology world, quantitative analysis maybe carried-out with the help of statistical software like SPSS and SYSTAT. The use of statistical tests is easy and may provide result on a very short notice.

Interpreting of Data

Once the data will be analyzed, it is important to know the meaning of the study findings. In interpretation, researcher attempt to explain the findings in light of the previous or existing findings. Interpretation provides direction for use of research evidence in concerned area of practice and education.

The Dissemination Phase

Research results are of little value unless they can be communicated to others. Once a researcher has completed a study, plans should be made to communicate or disseminate the results. This phase deals with the communication and utilization of research finding in concerned field or area of practice.

Communicating the Findings

A researcher may communicate the research findings by publishing in a scientific journal or presentation at professional scientific conferences.

Utilizing the Findings

Research findings may be utilized to improve the quality of nursing education and practice. Ideally, the main goal of conducting research study is to collect high quality evidence to overcome the barriers and other problems in practice settings. Nurses and other health care professionals may use research findings in concerned practice settings either to improve the knowledge or overcomes the burning problems. Research utilization (RU) and evidenced based practice (EBP) are the ways to utilize research findings at individual, organizational and clinical settings.

STEPS IN QUALITATIVE STUDY

Quantitative study follows a systematic and liner series of step. Qualitative studies in contrast to quantitative study follow a cyclic process than to a liner chain. Researcher plans in advance the steps to be taken to maximize study integrity and then follow those steps as truly as possible. Qualitative research is a flexible approach to examine an issue or life event to give

them meaning. Therefore, the process of qualitative studies is slightly differ than quantitative studies. However, a qualitative study has following steps (Fig. 3.2):
- Conceptual phase
- Design and planning phase
- Empirical and analytic phase
- Dissemination phase.

The Conceptual Phase

Qualitative researcher need to plan a study for a variety of circumstances, i.e. time, sample, equipments and human resources etc. Advance planning is especially useful with regards to followings:
- Selection of a broad framework or tradition to guide decision making
- Determine the amount of time available for the study, cost and other resources
- Plan a broad data collection strategy
- Collect relevant site material, i.e. maps, organization chart and phone directories, etc.
- Work of type of equipments that could help in data collection and recording i.e. audio-video recording device, camera, etc.
- Identifying personal biases, views and presumption and take measures to control them to explore the study.

Apart from above discussed points, a qualitative researcher may follow following steps to develop a concept for a qualitative study.
- *Identifying the research problem:* Qualitative research selects a broad research area that is poorly understood and about which little is known. Researcher uses his self-reflection and can have discussion with the experts to make the topic specific. For example, a study on life experience of Bhopal Gas tragedy survivors at Bhopal, Madhya Pradesh.

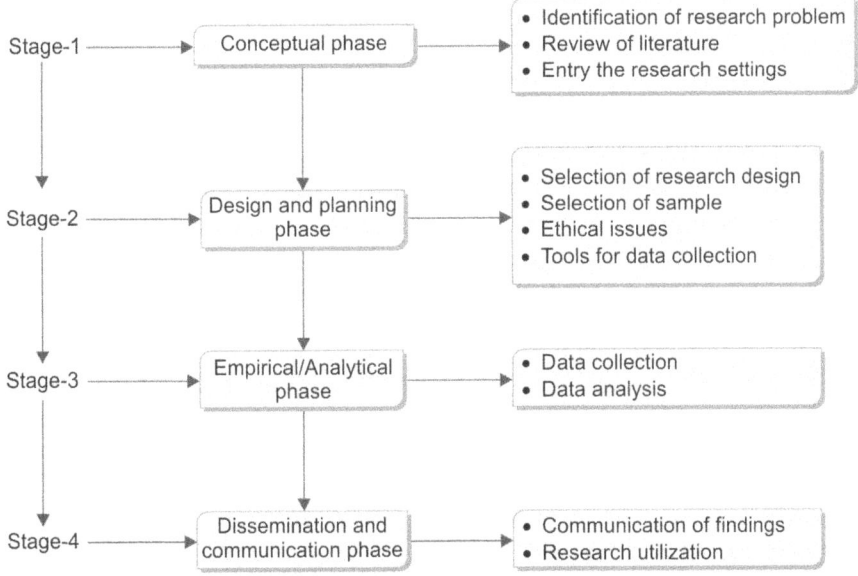

Fig. 3.2: Steps of qualitative research process.

- *Searching relevant literature search*: Qualitative researchers do not all agree about the timing of upfront literature review. Some researchers believe that researcher should not review literature in beginning or before conducting the study. It is been thought that reviewing literature before conducting study may change the mental image about the phenomena and may contaminate the result. Researchers sharing this opinion do the literature review at the end of the study. Other eminent researchers believe that a full literature review should be conducted before opening the study.
- *Entry in the research setting*: In qualitative studies, researcher must identify an appropriate site for conducting study. Once the site is defined, a researcher needs to gain permission to enter in the research setting. Gaining entry typically involves negotiation with **gatekeepers** who have the authority to permit entry into their world.

Design and Planning Phase

Although, qualitative researchers do not know in advance how and where the study will be carried-out. A qualitative researcher need to plan type of data, timing available for study, equipments needed for study, need of human resources and need of appropriate support staff, etc.

- *Developing research design*: Research design emerges during the course of data collection (emergent design).
- *Selecting sample*: Qualitative studies need a small sample to inquired an issue. Generally, the size of the sample in qualitative study are small than quantitative study. However, there are no defined rules for calculating sample size in qualitative study. For example, case study need single case and phenomenology confined to 10 samples to explore a phenomenon.
- *Addressing ethical issues*: A qualitative study need to adhere to ethical issues. Qualitative researcher need to develop a plan for addressing ethical issues to protect the participants. Qualitative studies need more rigorous ethical concern than quantitative studies because of the more intimate nature of relationship that typically develop between researcher and the study participants.
- *Selecting tools for data collection*: In qualitative research information collected through use of semi-structured or unstructured interview or focused group interview. The answer will be in descriptive or narrative format. Information may also be collected by using video-tape, recording device, cameras, photographs and diary, etc.

Empirical and Analytic Phase

In qualitative study, data collection is most time consuming and crucial step. Qualitative data collection begin by enrolling a very few participants initially and progress to enroll more number of participants until *'data saturation'* is not achieved. Data saturation occur when themes or phenomena under study become repetitive and redundant and no new information can be gathered by enrolling further participants. Data can be collected either through face to face interview or focused group interview. Researcher can use many recording devices to record or captures the phenomena.

Data analysis is an ongoing process in qualitative research. Since the beginning of data collection, researcher start thinking about the type of information he is getting and what all are possible measures can be taken for data analysis. In qualitative research, data analysis based on kind of information and type of participants selected for study. In data analysis, researcher read or listen the conversation and make relevant theme, template or category to prepare the data for further analysis. Therefore, data analysis is a challenging task in qualitative study.

Dissemination Phase

Qualitative researcher also want to share their study findings and expect to use them by others. These findings may be communicated either by writing in a scientific journal or by presenting findings in national or international conference or platform. Qualitative study findings sensitize other researcher's about understanding of the problem, their potential solution and their possible use in patient care.

REVIEW QUESTIONS AND ANSWER

Long and Short Answer Questions

1. Explain in detail steps in quantitative research. (RGUHS, MSc N-2003)
2. What are the various steps in qualitative research? (PGI, MSc N-2009)
3. Describe the elements in research. (KUHAS, MSc N-20013)
4. Explain each phases of quantitative and qualitative research. (AIIMS, MSc N-2000)
5. Define the terms. Abstract, variables, sampling, peer-review, operational definitions and pilot study. (TNMGRMU, MSc N-2017)

Multiple Choice Questions

1. It is an important phase of research process in quantitative study in which a researcher select and decide appropriate methodology and methods to carry out research study.
   - a. Conceptual phase
   - b. Design and planning phase
   - c. Empirical phase
   - d. Analysis phase

2. In this phase of quantitative research, a researcher attempt to explain the findings in light of the previous or existing findings?
   - a. Conceptual phase
   - b. Design and planning phase
   - c. Empirical phase
   - d. Analysis phase

3. It is a phase of qualitative research process in which data are collected from the participants?
   - a. Conceptual phase
   - b. Design and planning phase
   - c. Empirical and analytic phase
   - d. Dissemination phase

4. In quantitative research process overview, a researcher selects a homogenous population group in order to generalize the findings in the following stage?
   - a. Conceptual phase
   - b. Design and planning phase
   - c. Empirical phase
   - d. Analysis phase

5. In quantitative research process the selection of research problem and question take place in following stage?
   - a. Conceptual phase
   - b. Design and planning phase
   - c. Empirical phase
   - d. Analysis phase

6. Which of the following is initial and most significant step of the research process?
   a. Selection of research approach and design
   b. Finalize data collection plan
   c. Selection of statistical tests
   d. Selection of research problem

7. In quantitative research process, the literature review is done:
   a. At the beginning of research process
   b. Just before analyzing the data
   c. While disseminating the findings
   d. At the end of research process

8. Assumption and delimitation are identified in which stage of research process in quantitative research?
   a. Planning
   b. Implementing
   c. Writing report
   d. Critiquing

Answer Key

1.	2.	3.	4.	5.	6.	7.	8.
b.	d.	c.	b.	a.	d.	a.	a.

SUGGESTED READING

1. Boswall C, Canon S. Introduction to nursing research: incorporating evidence based practice. Sunbury, MA: Jones and Bartlett; 2007.
2. Burn N, Grove SK. Understanding nursing research: building an evidence based practice, 4th edition. St Louis: Saunders Elsevier; 2005.
3. Chinn PL, Kramer MK. Theory and nursing: integrated knowledge development, 5th edition. St. Louis: Mosby; 1999.
4. Gerrish K, Lacey A. The research process in nursing, 6th edition. United Kingdom: John Wiley and Sons; 2013.
5. Hockey L. The nature and purpose of research. In: Cormack DFs (Ed). The research process in nursing, 1st edition. London: Blackwell sciences; 1984. pp. 1-10.
6. James FA. Reading, understanding and applying nursing research (Google e-book): EA Davis; 2013.
7. Kedar P. Nursing research: principles, process and issues. New York: Palgrave Macmillan; 1997.
8. Polit DF, Beck CT. Nursing research: principle and methods, 7th edition. Philadelphia: Lippincott Williams Wilkins; 2004.
9. Treece EW, Treece JW. Elements of research in nursing, 4th edition. St. Louis: Mosby;1986.

Chapter 4

Ethical Issues in Research

INTRODUCTION

All research conducted on human being will bring some risk for subject; he might get injured in a road accident while traveling to participate in the research project; he might develop anxiety while filling up a questionnaire which makes him conscious about being at risk for heart disease, etc. The ethical justification for theses risk is that expected benefits from the research is far greater than risk. Being social sciences researcher does not give us any special power or entitlement to do anything with subjects.

Ethics are standard of professional behavior. In any discipline that involves research with human being or animals, researcher must address ethical issues. So, ethical concern is especially prominent in nursing research as well.

Ethical Violations in Research

Unethical research studies involve violation of rights of research subjects or involve scientific misconduct during study. The post of research filled with much research misconduct. However, some recent studies do included evidence of scientific misconduct with the violation of study subjects' rights and publication of fabricated and misleading informations.

The *Nazi Medical Experiment* of the 1930s and 1940s are the most famous example of research misconduct. In this research many subjects (prisoners) were used to test the limit of human endurance and human reaction to disease and tested drugs. The studies were unethical not only because prisoners were exposed to physical harm and death but selection was racial based, unfair and forced to take treatment.

Another recent example of unethical research involved the injection of liver cancer cells into elderly patients at *Jewish Chronic Disease Hospital, Brooklyn (1960)* without collecting consent of subjects and they were informed that some vaccine is been given.

CODE OF ETHICS

A Code of Ethics set out principles of behavior that professional should follow while carrying research. The misconduct in several research studies brought international attention towards formulation of Code of Ethics. After Nazi experiments, Nuremberg Code developed to evaluate consent process, protection of subjects from harm and maintain risk-benefits ratio (Nuremberg Code, 1986). This state's about informed consent, voluntary participation, right to withdraw from research and risk and benefits. The World Medical Association has developed the Declaration of Helsinki (1964, revised 2008) for medical research to protect the human subjects. The Belmont Report (1978) was also developed in response to Tuskegee Syphilis Study (1932) emphasized autonomy and beneficence (Katz and Garner, 2012) for human subjects in research study.

Box 4.1: Code of Ethics for Nurses (INC, 2006).
The nurses respect the uniqueness of an individual in provision of care
• Provides care for individual without consideration of caste, creed, religion, culture, ethnicity, gender, socioeconomic status and political status, personal attributes or any other ground • Individualizes the care considering the belief, values and cultural sensitiveness • Appreciates the place of individual in the family and community, and facilities participation of significant others in the care • Develop a trustful relationship with individual(s) • Recognize uniqueness of response of individuals to intervention and adapt accordingly
The nurse respect the right of individuals as partners in care and helps in making informed choices
• Appropriate individual rights to make decisions about their care and therefore gives adequate and accurate information for enabling them to make informed choices • Respect the decision made by individual(s) regarding their care • Protect public from misinformation and misinterpretations • Advocates special provisions to protect vulnerable individuals and groups
The nurse respect individual's right to privacy, maintains confidentiality and shares information judiciously
• Respect the individual's right to privacy of their personal information • Maintain confidentiality of privileged information except in life threatening situations and uses discretion in sharing information • Take informed consent and maintain anonymity when information is required for quality assurance/academic/legal reasons • Limit the access to all record written and computerized to authorized person only
The nurse maintain competence in order to render quality nursing care
• Nursing care must be provided only by a registered nurse • Nurses strives to maintain quality nursing care and upholds the standards of care • Nurse values continuing education, initiates and utilizes all opportunities for self-development • Nurse values research as means of development of nursing profession and participates in nursing research adhering to ethical framework
The nurse is obliged to practice within the framework of ethical, professional and legal boundaries
• Adheres to code of ethics and professional conduct for nurses in India developed by Indian Nursing Council (INC) • Familiarizes with relevant laws and practices in accordance with the law of the state
Nurse obliged to work harmoniously with members of the health team
• Appreciate the team work in rendering care • Cooperate, coordinates and collaborates with members of the health team to meet the needs of people
The nurse commit to reciprocate the trust invested in nursing profession by the society
• Demonstrate personal etiquettes in all dealings • Demonstrate professional attributes in all settings

Most disciplined developed their own Ethical Codes. The American Nurses Association (1968) Research and Studies Commission developed *'human right guidelines for nurses in clinical and other research'* and *'Ethical Guidelines in the conduct, dissemination and implementation of nursing research (1995)'.* The International Council for Nurses also developed Code of Ethics (ICN, 2006) for nurses for developing professionalism and accountability.

In India, The Indian Council of Medical Research (ICMR, 1980) formulated policy to safeguard the ethics of human subjects in research.

The central features of policy are given below:
- The right and welfare of human subject should be adequately prepared
- The risk to an individual participant is out weight by the potential benefits to him
- Informed consent should be obtained before conducting a research on human subjects
- The investigator should be competent and experienced enough to carried out research.

Indian Nursing Council (INC, 2006) also proposed the Code of Ethics for Nurses in India.

IMPORTANCE OF ETHICS IN RESEARCH

Health care researches are for the benefits of human and human society. Protecting the right of human being is a fundamental feature of a high-quality research. Followings are some of the important use of ethics in nursing research:
- Protect the research participants from exploitation (physical, psychological, social, financial and sexual, etc.)
- Use of ethics will helps to determine the feasibility of the research study in term of risk-benefit ratio and vulnerability of population
- It will help to protect the exposure of participants, its information and related things to others
- Use of ethical principles gives a sense of respect and dignity to the participants to cooperate in research.

ETHICAL PRINCIPLES FOR PROTECTING HUMAN RIGHTS

Human rights are claims or demands that have been justified in the eyes of an individual or by the consensus of a group of people (Fig. 4.1).

The Belmont Report (1978) given by National Commission for the Protection of Human Subjects of Biomedical and Behavioral Research, summarizes following three fundamental ethical principles for conducting a research:
1. Principle of beneficence
2. Principle of respect for human dignity
3. Principle of justice

Principle of Beneficence

Beneficence is the most fundamental ethical principle of 'doing good' for others. Beneficence means 'maximize benefits' to the participants with minimum or routine harm. A nurse researcher make the decision that research should do direct or indirect benefit to others. Similarly, a nurse researcher should act in the best interest of the participants and always function as advocate to protect the rights of the participants. Beneficence underpins both nonmaleficence and freedom from self-exploitation.

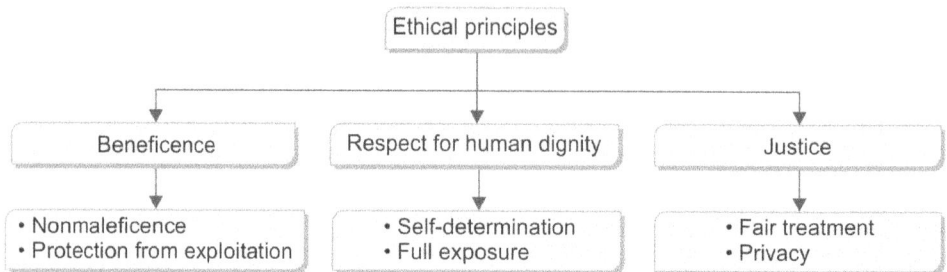

Fig. 4.1: Ethical principles.

- *Nonmaleficence*: Researcher have an obligation to follow all possible precautions to protect, avoid or minimize harm to study subjects. In research, harm can be of different types; physical (e.g. injury), emotional (e.g. crying and weeping), psychological (e.g. exaggeration of stress, depression and other existing problems), financial (e.g. loss of wages) and social (e.g. loss of social contact). The research process should be reviewed clearly to minimize all types of harm and discomfort to study subject and other who is going to affect with study.
- *The right to protection from exploitation*: Research study should not exploit the participants on any possible background. Exploitation can be in covert (e.g. emotional exploitation) and overt (e.g. Sexual or financial exploitation). Researcher should make ensure to participants that the information obtained in research will be used for research purpose only. For example, sharing information related to psychological disturbances should not make participant to feel inferior before other people. A competent researcher should also follow ethical and professional boundaries of interpersonal relationship during research study.

Principle of Respect for Human Dignity

Respect for human dignity has two components; the right to self-determination and right to full disclosure.
- *The right to self-determination:* A researcher should not impose any types of force on participants for their participation in research. The principle of self determination indicates that participants are voluntary and autonomous in nature to decide whether to participate in research or not. It also means that subjects have right to ask query, making their own decision and refuse to participate in the research.
- *The right to full disclosure:* Right to full disclosure means providing complete information of the study, purposes, duration, potential risk and potential benefits and responsibilities of a researcher. Informed consent encompass right of full disclosure and right to self-determination. A nurse researcher should provide complete information to participants to make decision to their participation.

However, as per ANA guidelines, concealment (collection of information without participant's knowledge and consent) and deception (providing false information or withholding true information about study) can be used in human research if the study contribute significant benefits to society or cause only minimal or routine harm to the subjects under study.

Principle of Justice

Belmont report proposed Justice as a third ethical principle, which underpins right to fair treatment and right to privacy to participants.

- *The right to fair treatment:* The right to self determination concern with the uniform distribution or potential risk and benefits to all participants. A nurse researcher should select the participants in the research as per needs irrespective of caste, creed, color, or socioeconomic status. Participants selection should be from a wide array of population and should not be forced. He should also cautious while selecting people from vulnerable or compromised community. Furthermore, participants not interested to participate in the study should also be treated in non-prejudicial manner.
- *The right to privacy:* A nurse researcher should use appropriate measures to protect the privacy of research subjects, such as use of coding sheet, and avoid collecting personal information, etc. Privacy encompasses veracity (truth telling) and confidentiality which refers to basic right of privacy of an individual. A researcher should avoid the invasion of privacy where the private information of the subject shared without his knowledge or wish. The Privacy Act, (1974) and The Health Insurance and Portability and Accountability Act, (HIPAA,1996) came into action to safeguard the invasion of privacy of research subjects.

MEASURES TO PROTECT THE RIGHTS OF STUDY PARTICIPANTS

The following measures can be taken to protect the violation of the rights of study participants in a study.

Informed Consent

It is primary measure to protect the rights of the study participants. Informed consent implies that participant should have adequate and complete information and ability to comprehend that information on right and wrong scale. Giving complete information about research study is worthless if a participant is not able to understand information completely. Participant understanding regarding purpose of study, duration, type of treatment, involvement, frequency and potential risk and benefits helps him/her to decide their participation in the study.

An experienced researcher should concern about the information given to the participants, especially about the risk component. However, it is equally essential to inform the participants about anticipated benefits and risk of the study.

Polit and Beck (2012) state that following major elements of informed consent should be inquired before proceeding to collect consent:

- *Participant status:* Level of understanding of the participants should be assessed before obtained consent. It is always good to explain the procedure or method in the participant's language for better understanding. This will allow the subjects to make a fair decision in their choice.
- *Study purposes:* The researcher should explain the study purposes in details.
- *Type of data:* A researcher should explain the types of information he is going to collect from the subjects. He should explain how and what types of information (i.e. numerical or narrative) will be collected from the subjects.
- *Procedure or intervention details:* Researcher should explained the intervention in detail. He should emphasize steps, duration, involvement, frequency and intensity of intervention to the participants. Researcher should also answer the queries or any doubts of the subjects.

- *Participant's selection:* A fair procedure for selection of study participants should be outlined and discussed with the subjects for their point of view. However, a researcher can decide the method of participants' selection considering the need and types of the research study.
- *Potential risk and benefits:* Researcher should explain risk and benefits of the study. However, a researcher should emphasize more on risk of the study rather than benefits. This will helps a subject to decide their participation in the study. Risk should be emphasized more clearly to study participants.
- *Privacy and confidentiality:* A researcher should take and explain to subjects the measures to protect privacy and confidentiality of information in the research.
- *It should be voluntary in nature:* The study participants should not be forced or coerced to participate in a research study. They should be given sufficient time to decide their participation in the study. The participants in research should be voluntary in nature.
- *Right to withdrawn from study:* The subjects should be informed for the right to withdrawn from study anytime without assigning any reason. However, a researcher may ask the reason for withdrawing from study to study participants.
- *Contact information:* Researcher should have detail contact information of subjects to contact in future for research purpose.

Types of Consent

In present era of consumer awareness, collecting consent became necessity for health care workers and nurses too to get rid out of any future unethical claims. A health care workers should have sound knowledge about the types of consent can be collected in health care setting. A details of types of consent is presented in this section:

- *Informed written consent:* This consent obtained after giving complete and detailed information to participant at his/her understanding level. This is more traditional and understood form of consent. However, the process of collecting written consent is more time demanding and laborious sometimes. Still, it is most commonly used types of consent in terms of proper recorded information, sole evidence and exchanged of information between authority and participant.
- *Process consent:* In qualitative research, consent is often viewed as ongoing and transactional process. Here, researcher comes in contact with participant many times and collect consent. In qualitative study, a researcher has to make multiple contact with participants and it became obsolete unnecessary to collect consent at each meeting point. So, this is an understanding between researcher and subject for their willingness to participate in the said procedure or project in future or until the research comes to conclusion.
- *Implied consent:* It is affirmative response of participants to participate in a procedure or research. Here, information is given to participants about the procedure or they get familiar with the procedure in due course. Implied consent is a indirect way to saying 'no' to participant in a study. For example, on a survey a response of 80 participants in response to distribution of 100 questionnaires indicate that only 80 participants are ready to participate or participated in the study and rest 20 refused for same. Venipuncture, a common procedure performed in clinical area is an another good example of implied consent.
- *Assent:* Assent refers to agreement to something after thoughtful consideration. The issue of assent describe special consideration. Children may not be able to assent to a procedure

because of lack of complete knowledge about the procedure. However, if a child is mature enough to understand and comprehend the intervention, it is advisable to obtain a written assent from the child to protect his right of self determination. Furthermore, a child above 12 years of age can only give consent only for medical examination but not for procedures.

Institutional Ethical Committee (IEC) or Institutional Review Board (IRB)

Every institution has an institutional ethical committee to review the research proposal to undertake various ethical issues. Institutional ethical committee must have at least five members from different professional background including one member from local community (Rothestein and Phuona, 2007). The researcher is asked to submit a copy of research proposal and curriculum vitae before institutional ethics committee. The IEC/IRB members will review the proposal for all possible risk and benefits before reaching on consensus for approval. However, Ethical committee or review board may call the researcher for a brief presentation before experts and ask him to clarify the doubts (if any) before giving approval for the study. The IRB members meet on regular interval at least once in a month to review and make informed decision about projected research proposal.

The IRB/IEC also discuss about the types of subjects in the study like vulnerable population; children, mentally challenged children, prisoner, laborer, mother, and geriatric population, etc.

IRB review focus on whether researcher has taken appropriate measures to protect the rights of research subjects. Review also decide the risk-benefit ratio of research in terms of time and potential benefits, and potential risk to participants.

Risk-Benefits Assessment

The researcher should evaluate the risk-benefits ratio before proceeding to research study. The benefits always ought to be higher than risk. However, all research involves some sort of risk to human subject, but risk is sometimes minimal. Minimal risk is defined as risk no greater than those ordinarily encountered in daily life, or during routine tests and procedure, i.e. pain during IM injection (Polit and Beck, 2012).

Protecting Basic Human Rights of Vulnerable Groups

A researcher should take additional measures to protect the rights of vulnerable group. US Federal Guidelines refers vulnerable group who may not able to give consent (e.g. mentally retarded children), or may be at higher risk of unwanted side effects because of their circumstances (e.g. pregnant women) or find themselves not comfortable in given environment (e.g. prisoners). Therefore, a researcher should pay special attention to protect the rights of vulnerable groups.

According to Federal Regulation regarding human research; the principal investigator holds the ultimate responsibility for protecting the safety; right and welfare of vulnerable groups. Vulnerable population maybe incapable of giving fully informed consent (e.g. mentally retarded people, pregnant women, terminally ill patients, institutionalized people, old age population, pregnant women and children) or maybe at risk of intended side effects because of their circumstances (e.g. pregnant women). A researcher while collecting informed consent should take special measures to protect the rights of vulnerable population such as protection of exploitation, and avoid situation which may compromise their safety or dignity or can place them in powerlessness while collecting consent.

ETHICAL ISSUES IN ANIMAL RESEARCH

Virtually, every major medical advances for both humans and animals has been achieved through biomedical research using animal models to study and find a cure for a disease and through animal testing to prove the safety and efficacy of new treatment.

Ethical considerations are clearly different for using animal and human being as participant in research. Concept of informed consent is not relevant to animal studies but at National level, certain guidelines given by the Indian Council of Medical Research (ICMR, 2001) under Institutional Animal Ethics Committee (IAEC), and Indian National Science Academy (INSA, 1999, revised in 2000) directs researcher for proper care and use of experimental animals. The salient features of IAEC guidelines are as follows:

- Review and approve research projects
- Prevent unnecessary suffering to animals during experimentation
- Proper accommodation/veterinary care
- Human disposal after termination of study
- Midterm termination if unnecessary suffering occur
- Adequate skilled personnel to do the experiments on animals.

At international level, International Committee for Laboratory Animal Science (ICLAS) with a membership of 100 countries is established to set-up international guidelines for animal husbandry, experimental procedures, teaching and training of researcher and professionals in the field.

REVIEW QUESTIONS AND ANSWER

Long and Short Answer Questions

1. Explain the importance of ethics in nursing research. (RGUHS, MSc N-2009)
2. What are the ethical issues in medical research? (AIIMS, MSc N-2003)
3. What are the ethical principles for human rights? (KUHAS, MSc N-2015)
4. Ethical considerations in nursing research. (PGI, MSc N-2012)
5. What are the measures to be taken by a nurse to protect the right of study participants? (TNMGRMU, MSc N-2008)

Multiple Choice Questions

1. It is a set of principles and guidelines that help a researcher to differentiate between right and wrong while conducting a research.
   a. Ethics
   b. Moral
   c. Belief
   d. Character

2. It is a written document, a research participant has to sign and handover to a researcher for his willing to participate in research before the study actually take place:
   a. Guidelines
   b. A commitment
   c. Informed consent
   d. Private information

Ethical Issues in Research

3. It is part of ethical issue in which a researcher not revealed any information of subject to anyone else researcher and staff:
   a. Confidentiality
   b. Anonymity
   c. Ethics
   d. Discretion

4. A process in which the participant's identity, although known to the researcher, is not revealed to anyone outside of the researcher and his or her staff.
   a. Anonymity
   b. Confidentiality
   c. Informed consent
   d. Discretion

5. What is the primary approach that is used by the IRB to assess the ethical acceptability of a research study?
   a. Utilitarianism
   b. Deontology
   c. Ethical skepticism
   d. Comparativism

6. Which of the following is the most fundamental ethical principle used in research?
   a. Beneficence
   b. Nonmaleficence
   c. Informed consent
   d. Privacy

7. This is the ethical principle indicates that participants are voluntary and autonomous in nature to decide whether to participate in research or not?
   a. Beneficence
   b. Nonmaleficence
   c. Self-determination
   d. Privacy

8. Which of the following types of consent is most appropriate to qualitative study?
   a. Informed consent
   b. Implied consent
   c. Assent
   d. Process consent

9. Code of ethic for nurses in India is given by which of the following body?
   a. Indian Nursing Council
   b. Trained Nurses Association of India
   c. Psychiatric Society of India
   d. Nursing Research Society of India

10. Which of the following detail is not a part of informed consent?
    a. Name of researcher
    b. Contact number of researcher
    c. Address of the researcher
    d. Income of the researcher

Answer Key

1.	2.	3.	4.	5.	6.	7.	8.	9.	10.
a.	c.	a.	a.	a.	a.	c.	d.	a.	d.

SUGGESTED READING

1. Burn N, Grove SK. The practice of nursing research: Appraisal, synthesis and generation of evidence, 6th edition. St Louis: Elsevier; 2009
2. Fouka G, Mantzorou M. What are the major ethical issues in conducting research? Is there a conflict research ethics and the nature of Nursing? Health Science Journal. 2011; 5(1).
3. Gerrish K, Lacey A (Eds). The research process in nursing, 6th edition. United Kingdom: Wiley Blackwell; 2010.

4. Indian Council of Medical Research (ICMR). Use of animals in scientific research. ICMR, Ministry of Health and Family Welfare, New Delhi; 2000.
5. Katz K, Garner Z. Respecting human subject: Responsibilities of the clinical investigator. In: Bercovitch L, Perlis C (Eds). Dermatuetics—contemporary ethics and professionalism in dermatology, 1st edition. London: Springer; 2012.
6. Nieswiadomy RM. Foundation of nursing research, 5th edition. New Delhi: Pearson Education; 2010.
7. Polit DF, Beck CT. Nursing research: Generating and assessing evidence for nursing practice, 8th edition. Philadelphia: Lippincott Williams and Wilkins; 2010.
8. Rothestein WG, Phuong LH. Ethical attitude of nurses, physician and unaffiliated members of institutional review board. Journal of Nursing Scholarship. 2007;39(1):79-85.
9. The code of ethics and professional conduct. Indian Nursing Council; 2006.

Chapter 5

Review of Literature

INTRODUCTION

Review of the literature are the foundation for theses, dissertation or any research papers. Era of computer technology produced a large number of scientific publications that became part of literature today. Literature review serve many purposes from selection of research topic to designing a research project, dissemination of findings to development of evidence-based proctorial. However, literature review process is not easy and reported a daunting task by many nurse researchers and students nurses. The most frequently asked questions of nursing student has been " How to search relevant literature for my topic?", "How much literature is too much?", "How to use appropriate keywords for searching literature?" What literature should I review for my research topic?" and so on.

Researcher should know the art of reviewing literature. A researcher should have sound knowledge of reviewing process to get in to relevant literature for the topic. He should also know about relevant sources, keywords, search strategies and skilled to synthesize the final literature to make it meaningful to audience.

This chapter present the purpose of literature in a research project, its importance as a independent section, suggestions to improve review strategy, synthesizing and organizing a draft of written review.

Definitions

A literature review consists of all written sources relevant to the selected topic. It helps a researcher to know about findings of previous studies, their authors, used theories, models and applied statistics, etc. A researcher can get ideas from similar existing work of others.

'A literature review is an objective thorough summary and critical analysis of the relevant available research and nonresearch literature on the topic being studies.' *(Hart, 1998)*

'An organized written presentation of what has been published on a topic by the scholars.' *(Burns and Grove, 2005)*

'It is a written summary of journal articles, book and other documents that describes that past and current state of information, organize the literature into topics and documents a need for proposed study.' *(Creswell, 2005)*

'An account of what has been published by accredited scholars and researcher.' *(Taylor, 2011)*

In nutshell, review of literature refers to identification of all published and unpublished material related to the problem area, studying the unfamiliar part, organizing and synthesizing it in a unique way to provide a strong basis for the present research.

CHARACTERISTICS OF A QUALITY REVIEW

A quality of review helps to direct the research process at each step. Literature must be clear and comprehensive in nature to other readers. An up-to-date literature helps to reflect current findings about the investigation. A good quality review should have following characteristics enlisted here:
- Review must be comprehensive and thorough incorporating up-to-date references
- It should be systematic
- It should be reproducible
- It should be free from bias and well written
- It should be in the form of 'sum of its parts'
- It should contain complete information on a particular topic and accessed from different sources
- It should be based on clear search and selection strategy
- Review should be structured well to enhance the readability flow
- Accurate use of terminology and no scope of jargon make the review effective for others
- References should be accurate throughout the review.

FACTORS AFFECTING LITERATURE REVIEW

Review of literature is not an easy job for a researcher. Literature review is bit similar to a full-fledged study. Literature search is an art and science examine expertise and skills of a researcher. A high quality of review is the result of rich experience, resources availability and support of others. There are many factors that may affect depth and breadth of literature, including following:
- *Researcher's background:* It is a well known facts that reviewing literature is an easy job for an experienced researcher than a novice. To conduct a high quality literature search, knowledge of review process, keywords and reference management is needed. A novice investigator may not be able to collect in-depth review of literature due to lack of knowledge and experience of review process.
- *Complexity of research project:* Literature search is an easy job for a simple and well defined research topic/variable as compare to ill defined and complex one. A research may have one or more than one variables under investigations and reviewing literature for a research contains more than one variable is tedious and challenging for a researcher, e.g. literature search will be easy for a topic *'physical exploitation'* in elderly in comparison to *'exploitation in elderly,'* as exploitation is very complex variable encompass verbal, physical, financial, sexual and many other different types of exploitations in it. Therefore, a researcher should define the variable operationally before starting to review it.
- *Availability of resources:* This is the primary factor that may hinder or facilitate search of relevant literature. A high quality literature review is a collective result of knowledge and experience of researcher and availability of resources like computer, internet facility, reference management software and subscription of online and offline journals, etc.

- *Study time frame:* Literature search is a time consuming process and lack of time may affect quality literature search. Studies which are time bound (e.g. undergraduate and postgraduate project) allow limited time for a researcher to in depth review and explore the topic.
- *Availability of support system:* Relevant literature is the end product of contribution of many experts. A motivational research environment is necessary for reviewing relevant literature. Indeed, researcher may get information from other about certain things like sources, library and accession of journals, which may enable to complete the review on time.

PURPOSES OF LITERATURE REVIEW

A comprehensive literature review can serves the following purposes:
- It helps to discover newer knowledge about the research problem
- The review aim to know the work already done by others in the area and provides vision to distinguish between what has been done and what need to be done
- The review add to vast storehouse of knowledge and acquaints us with latest and other existing related and unrelated theories, principles and laws
- It helps to understand different ways of conducting a research study
- It attempt to enable us to locate the comparative data and therefore, helpful in interpretation and discussion of study results
- It is oriented to provide us with the insight of study and acquaints us with the strength and limitations of previous study
- It enables critical thinking and develops expertise; determine the relevance of study and establish credibility.

IMPORTANCE OF LITERATURE REVIEW

A literature review in a research report reflect the background of current knowledge of a researcher and helps to understand the significance of the new study. Literatures search play a key role in a research from identification of problem to till dissemination of findings. A few important uses of literature review are enlisted here:
- The review enables us to build the foundation of knowledge and develop a sound background to understand the problem under investigation
- It determines gaps, consistencies and inconsistencies in existing body of knowledge
- It helps to discovered unanswered question about the phenomena under investigation
- It helps to generate and refine relevant research question
- It helps in identification of variables and define them appropriately for easy research
- It helps to formulate theoretical or conceptual framework for the study
- It helps to choose resource of funding agencies for present study
- A quality review also help to formulate hypotheses and their testing to develop and refine theory and practice
- It provides assistance to design, develop and refine intervention protocol for a research problem
- It provide guidelines for selection of research instruments for the study
- It suggests the appropriate procedure, sources of data and statistical techniques for the research

- It helps in data analysis, interpretation and comparison of study findings with the earlier work on similar topic or area
- A standard and quality review assist in selection of appropriate research design and methodology to study a problem
- It imparts divergent thinking and save time, money and energy in research study
- It shows the ways for dissemination and communication of research findings to target audience.

TYPES OF LITERATURE REVIEW

Broadly, the literature review can be classified (Table 5.1) under following headings:
1. Integrated literature review
2. Systematic review
3. Meta-analysis
4. Meta-synthesis

Integrated Literature Review

Integrated review is the most basic form of literature review. It is popular in nursing and other allied health professions. In integrated review, authors review the existing work to come on conclusion on many different studies. This review aims to synthesize the existing relevant literature on a topic to draw a logical and meaningful conclusions.

The primary purpose of integrated review is to give comprehensive overview of the problem to develop insight in to problem and impose the significance of new research in area.

Systematic Review

In contrast to integrated review, systematic review use more well defined and rigorous approach to review a problem under investigation. Evidence based medicine publications more frequently used the term 'systematic review'. Systematic review are meant specifically for clinicians to provide strong base for practice of evidence-based medicine. Systematic review focused on development of treatment, protocol, cause identification, diagnosis and prognosis. Parahoo (2006) suggests that in order to improve reliability and validity of review, the reviewer need to select the precise criteria.

Table 5.1: Overview of literature reviews.

Integrated review	• Selective review that broadly cover a specific topic
	• Does not follow strict systematic methods to locate and synthesize articles
Systematic review	• Utilizing extracting search strategies to make certain that the maximum extent of relevant research has been considered
	• Original articles are methodologically appraised and synthesized
Meta-analysis	• Quantitative methods to sum up the results of similar studies
	• Capable of performing a statistical analysis of the pooled result of relevant studies
Meta-synthesis	• Nonstatistical technique to integrate, evaluate and interpret the findings of multiple qualitative research studies

Table 5.2: Integrated and systematic review: A comparison.

Feature	Integrated review	Systematic review
Topic	Usually, focus on a broad area or topic	Focused research question
Authorship	A single expert or reviewer, sometimes a team	A team of experts with methodological expertise
Article selection criteria	Typically not specified	Use stringent exclusion and inclusion criteria for article selection
Appraisal of included article	Indefinite; may be variable	Critical appraisal is meticulous
Synthesis	A qualitative summary is usually provided	Quantitative summary is provided
Inferences	Sometime evidence base	Usually evidence based

For example, impact of varied amount of normal saline instillation on physiological parameters during tracheal intubation in unconscious patients. Here, a reviewer should choose following criteria to make an ideal systematic review:
- Select a specific research question for the problem
- Set time frame (duration) for the review
- Formulate stringent inclusion and exclusion criteria
- Select source of literature review
- Select the types of statistical methods will be used to analyze results.
  Comparison of integrated and systematic review is discussed in Table 5.2.

Meta-analysis

Meta-analysis is distinct from other types of reviews. In meta-analysis, reviewer use a precise quantitative methods to sum up the results of similar studies. The reviewer should choose specific research question, and purpose of review before careful selection of papers and evaluation to announce the results. A reviewer use statistical technique to analyse the findings of similar existing studies. Meta-analysis applicable to analysis of quantitative information only (Polit and Beck, 2006).

Meta-synthesis

In recent era, there is a growing demand for methods of synthesing the findings of qualitative studies. This is especially relevant to nursing and midwifery. Meta-synthesis is a non-statistical techniques used to evaluate, integrate and interpret the findings of similar types of qualitative studies. Meta-synthesis focus to identify a common themes on many different but similar types of qualitative studies. Meta-ethnography, meta-study and meta-summary are examples of meta-synthesis of qualitative studies.

SOURCES OF LITERATURE REVIEW

Libraries are obvious resource for a student performing a literature search, but other sources may be explored to search relevant review. Regardless of the sources you see, *keep a bibliographic trail*, track title, authors, publication information, page numbers, library call number (LCN), International Standard Book Numbers (ISBN) and International Standard Serial Numbers (ISSN), so that search can be duplicated if necessary (Fig. 5.1).

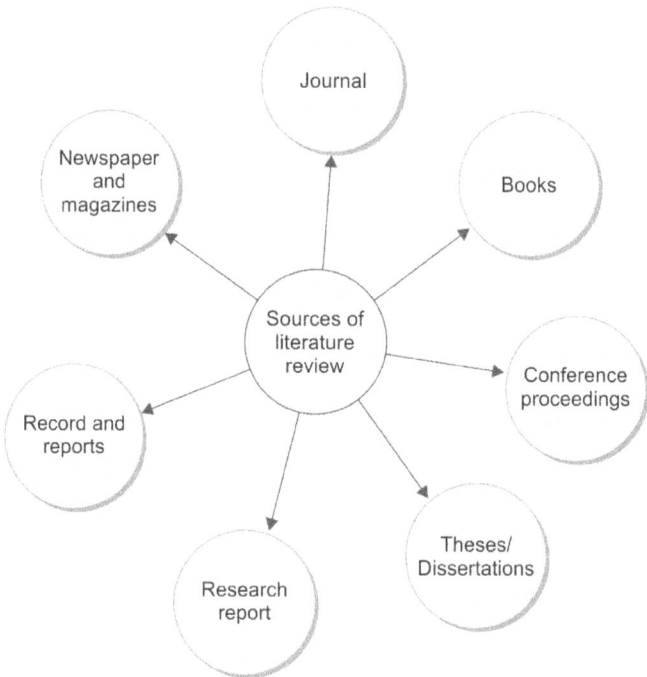

Fig. 5.1: Sources of literature review.

Types of Sources

Deciding an authentic source determine the credibility of your review. Selection of appropriate source is an important step of literature search. Broadly, there are two main sources:
1. Primary sources
2. Secondary sources

Primary Sources

These are first hand information generated by the person who is sole responsible for originating and conducting of the work. It is research publication written by the person or people who conducted the research or developed the theories. In review, primary sources preferred over secondary sources to avoid problem of bias, and any other distortion beyond the control of a researcher.

Advantages of Primary Sources

- These are first hand information considered real and reduce the chance of bias and other distortion.
- First hand information will help to supplement the minute details of the work.
- Interpretation of the first hand information is easy.

Box 5.1: Example of Primary Sources.

Research article, unpublished thesis/dissertation, workshop or conference abstract, conference proceedings, personal diary, artifacts, hand written record and reports, etc.

Review of Literature

Box 5.2: Sources of Literature Review.

Source	Definition
Primary source	A report prepared by the original researcher
Secondary source	Summary of the work done by someone other than original researcher.

Secondary Sources

A secondary source is one which summarise the information of primary sources belongs to other authors. Secondary sources summarise the information provided by the primary sources. Thus, a researcher should understand, and interpret the work of other researchers, paraphrase the information and cite the work of other in their own work. Citing a research work of other author in the review of literature division is an example of secondary source. Secondary sources should not be considered substitution to the primary sources because of higher chances of bias, distortion and subjectivity of the information.

Disadvantages of Secondary Sources

Secondary sources may not be a good choice for a research work because of following reasons:
- The second hand information may be influenced by researcher's own bias and perception
- Interpretation of second hand information is challenging and may leads to errors
- Possibility of errors in presentation of findings
- Sometimes, secondary sources fail to give a detail description of work.

Box 5.3: Example of Secondary Sources

Newspaper, book chapters, television/radio, magazines, wikipedia, and journal articles, etc.

Online Sources

The following sources also helpful to search a relevant and quality literature for a research study.
- *Electronic sources:* Use of computer brings the revolution in history of literature search and made the task easiest for a researcher. Most of electronic databases can be accessed either online or by help of CD-ROM. Use of computer made the literature search easy, convenient and comfortable at one hand. However, it has many disadvantages in terms of more time consuming, need of special knowledge and skills to operate computer and searching literature, appropriate use of keywords search and search strategy, etc. Search engine like Google (www.google.co.in), Yahoo (www.yahoo.in), CINAHL (www.cinahl.com), PubMed (www.pubmed.gov), and Science Direct (www.sciencedirect.com) can be used to search relevant literature review (Fig. 5.2).
- *Electronic databases:* A nurse researcher can explore many databases for searching good literature. A details of commonly used online databases is provided here for your ready reference:
    - *CINAHL (Cumulative Index to Nursing and Allied Health Literature):* It is most important database for nurse researchers. It provides reference of more than 1200 journals covered from 1982 to the present. It can be accessed online or by using CD-ROM. It is also known as *'Red Book'*.
    - *MEDLINE (Medical Literature Analysis and Retrieved System Online):* It is developed by US National Library of Medicine (NLM). Medline cover more than 4300 journals and contains more than 100 million records. The Medline databases can be accessed

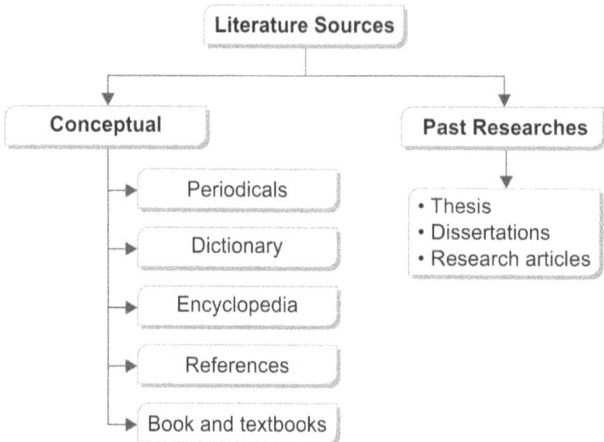

Fig. 5.2: Literature sources.

online or by using CD-ROM through commercial vendor (e.g. Ovid Search). A list of other important electronic databases is given here.

- *Social work abstracts:* Social work and related journals on topic such as homelessness, AIDS, child and family welfare and aging, etc.
- *Sociological abstracts:* Sociological and related discipline, both theoretical and applied areas.
- *ERIC:* Abstracts of journals, articles, books, research hypotheses, conference paper and technical report of education (including research and practice) and other education related materials.
- *Nursing studies index (NSI):* Yale university prepared the nursing studies index under direction of Virginia Henderson. It consists English literature on historical and biographical material concerning nursing. NSI has a records of around 1959 by 1963.
- *Index medicus (IM):* Index medicus is a well known index of medical literature. It cover literature on biomedicine including nursing and allied health field. IM has last publication in December 2004.

Box 5.4: List of Electronic Databases.

- PubMEd (www.pubmed.com)
- CanerLit (Cancer literature)
- CHILD (Combined Health Information Databases)
- EMBASE (Exerpta Medica Database)
- Radix (Nursing and Managed Care Database)
- ETOH (Alcohol and Alcohol problems Science databases)
- Health STAR (Health Services, Technology, Administration and Research)
- Ovid
- Science Direct
- British Nursing Index (BNI)
- Midwives Information & Resource Service (MIDIRS)
- Nursing Studies Index (NSI)
- Index Medicus (IM)

Table 5.3: List of nursing journals

National Nursing Journals	International Nursing Journals
• The Nursing Journal of India	• Clinical Nursing Research
• Journal of Nursing Science and Practice	• Nursing Science Quarterly
• Indian Journal of Continuing Nursing Education	• Applied Nursing Research
• Nursing and Midwifery Research Journal	• Journal of Emergency Nursing
• International Journal of Nursing Care	• Accident and Emergency Nursing
• International Journal of Nursing Education	• Archives of Psychiatric Nursing
• Asian Journal of Nursing Science and Practice	• Nursing Research
• Nightingale Nursing Time	• American Journal of Nursing
	• International Journal of Nursing Studies
	• Research in Nursing and Health
	• Journals of Obstetrics, Gynecology and Neonatology in Nursing
	• Western Journal of Nursing Research
	• Journal of Nursing Scholarship
	• American Journal of Maternity and Child Nursing
	• Advances in Nursing Sciences

- *BIOSIS:* Research databases in life sciences information including biodiversity, biotechnology, drug discovery, gene therapy and other topics.
- *Cochrane library:* A researcher can directly access Cochrane database directly from The Cochrane Library at www.cochrane.org. The Chochrane prepare, maintain and disseminate high quality independent evidence of the interest of health care. It has 4000 records.

- *Journals (online and offline):* A large number of national and international journals also available to review the literature. Usually, a reviewer can access abstract or full article free of cost, but sometimes accession of some journals need membership or fees. A detail list of national and international nursing journals can be accessed by clicking the given link https://en.wikipedia.org/wiki/List_of_nursing_journals (Table 5.3).
- *Obtaining information from literature sources*
  - Unpublished Bachelor, Master and Doctoral dissertation and theses
  - Magazines and newspaper
  - Hospital record and reports
  - Minutes of meetings
  - Year books
  - Periodicals
  - Biography
  - Research Information Center (RIC)
  - Dictionary
  - Abstracts: Nursing research abstracts, psychological abstracts, and masters abstracts international, etc.
  - Theses: Unpublished or published graduate, master and PhD theses.

STEPS OF LITERATURE REVIEW

Reviewing literature is not simple as it looks. A review process begins with a specific research question, clinical or any education related. Based on the types of question, a reviewer select the literature sources and search the literature by using appropriate keywords and search strategy. Once the review process over, relevant literature will be organized and presented. Usually, a systematic process of literature review consists following steps:

- *Selection of topic for review:* Selecting a topic for review can be daunting task for the students and novice reviewer (Timmins and McCabe, 2005). Usually, students select a very vague topic for review. As a thumb rule, it is better to start with narrow and focused topic and if necessary broadens the scope of review as you progress. It helps you to focus on topic of interest and refine your search strategy. Usually, it is challenging for a reviewer to cut short the topic progressively over a short span of time. Hence, selecting a specific topic will help a reviewer to choose appropriate source in the beginning and review the topic in depth. For example, myocardial infarction (MI) is not a good topic to review and therefore, a researcher may select a specific section related to myocardial infraction such as pain, etiology, manifestations or treatment for a comprehensive review and save time.

- *Searching the literature:* Topic selection proceed the literature search. The researcher should select an appropriate search engine, keywords and define search strategy to review a topic from each angle. Furthermore, it is also important for a reviewer to check comprehensiveness and relevancy of the review sources before proceeding literature search. Nowadays, use of computer and electronic databases made the literature search convenient. Computer databases offer access to vast qualities of information, which can be accessed quickly and easily than using manual search (Younger, 2004). Therefore, it is very important to identify relevant databases to search review. A sound knowledge of relevant sources will speed up the review process.

  Research should familiar with different types of search strategy such as keyword search, bibliographic search, ancestory search, decendancy approach and grey literature sources for a comprehensive literature search. Appropriate keywords use can also helps the process easy and time efficient. It is always good to keep a store of alternative keywords for a topic under review such as use of pressure ulcer, decubitus ulcer or pressure sore keywords for searching literature on bed sore among unconscious patients (for example, for pressure ulcer, decubitus ulcer and pressure sores also can be used as keywords). In conducting literature review search, it is important to keep a record of the keywords and methods used in searching the literature.

Box 5.5: Steps of Review of Literature.

1. Selection of specific review topic/question
2. Search the literature
3. Assemble, read and interpret the literature
4. Write down the literature
5. References the sources

- *Analyzing and synthesizing the literature:* At this stage, it is advisable to collect all review articles to get a sense of what they are about. It is necessary to classify and group the similar and related articles together. Use of PQRS approach may be helpful to interpret and summarize the literature. This methods helps in easy identification of relevant literature from a bunch of retrieved published articles.

Box 5.6: PQRS Approach for Literature Review.	
P-Preview	This is screening step helps a reviewer to keep the relevant review and exclude the heaps of irrelevant published articles.
Q-Question R- Read	Steps Q and R go side-by-side. Reviewer read the literature and question to each publication about types of sources, relevancy, inclusion criteria used, use of methodology in article, etc. This strategy help you to decide good and poor quality of articles at this stage.
S-Summary	Write summary in your own words, reporting your own key thoughts, i.e. weakness and strengths of review

- *Writing the review:* Once the appraisal of review is over, a researcher may structured and start writing the literature. The reviewer may have to write one or more draft of review to make it comprehensive before proceeding to final draft. The basis of good writing is to avoid long and confusing words and keep jargons to minimum. Use of short sentence in a literature will make it impressive to audiences. Similarly, a reviewer should mind grammatical errors and spelling mistake before writing final draft. The organization of material should be objective and comprehensive in nature.

Primarily, the written report includes an introduction, main body and conclusion (Burns and Grove, 2007). The length of literature may vary but it should follow a defined word limit. Review can be presented in the form of abstract (Fig. 5.3).

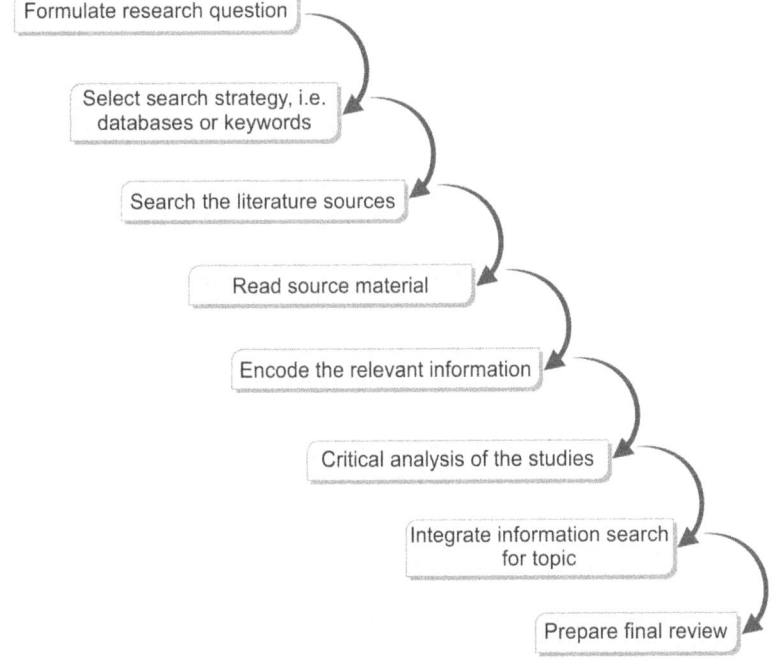

Fig. 5.3: Review process.

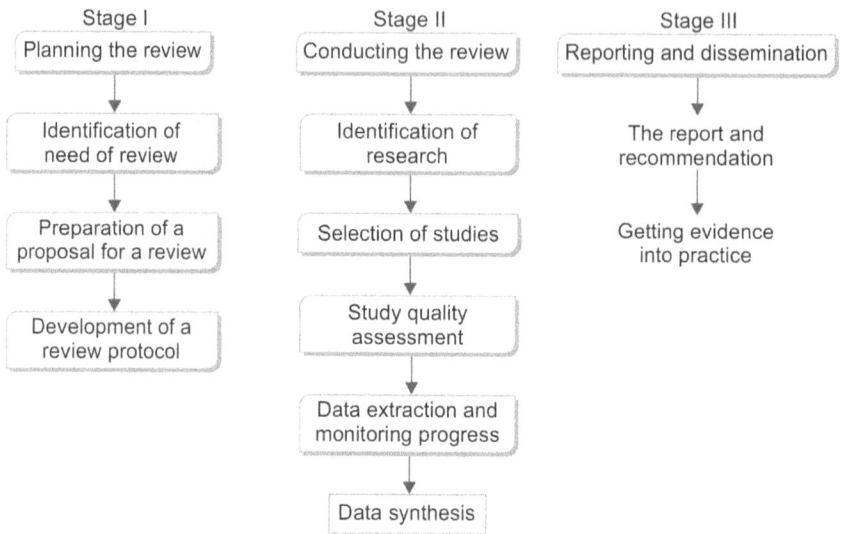

Fig. 5.4: Stage of systematic review.

ORGANIZATION OF LITERATURE REVIEW

A review of literature may be undertaken as an art of research project. The steps in review process involves selection a specific review question, searching literature, appraising strengths and weakness and writing the review with its used resources. A well framed literature may be presented in following format (Fig. 5.4):
- *Introduction:* Introduction part present purpose and central theme of the literature review. This gives reader an insight in to the breadth and depth of literature sources. This part should explain what is the purpose and why literature review has been taken over.
- *Main body:* This is the central and longest part of the review. It includes important concepts and arguments of the literature. Main body focus on critical review of methodology and discussion of the study findings. It is recommended to use tentative language to depict the findings in a literature. Furthermore, use of own language to write review is good to attract the target audience.
- *Conclusion:* It is the last section describe the summary of your major findings. It also focus on overall pitfalls of the review. Conclusion should follow the aims and objectives of your review and should say whether they are achieved or not.
- *References:* A literature should contain list of all resources used in writing review. A details of references, bibliographic database, journal articles, and other media cited in your work should be there in the list. Failing to acknowledge the earlier work lead to plagiarism, a serious misconduct.

TIPS FOR WRITING LITERATURE REVIEW

A review is a summary of findings and critical appraisal of number of research studies on a specified topic. A comprehensive review should be succinct, logical and objective in nature. A researcher may use following tips to make the review comprehensive and objective.

- *Based on primary source:* An objective and valid review should be based on primary sources. Primary sources provide more valid and bias free review than secondary and tertiary sources. Although, a reviewer may take helps of secondary sources for reviewing literature but, primary sources should be preferred for their objectivity.
- *Comprehensive:* A review must be comprehensive in nature. Comprehensive review of literature aims to provide a pluralistic approach to conduct a research. A comprehensive review of literature use an array of sources (published quantitative, qualitative and mixed methodology research as well as grey literature). It provides a detail of empirical and non-empirical literature for a selected review topic/question.
- *Avoid technical jargon:* A well written and concise review should avoid technical jargon and abbreviation. Use of technical jargon and abbreviations makes the review ambiguous and less useful.
- *Easy and simple:* A review must be written in simple language with short sentences use of short sentence make the review more meaningful. Using very long sentences and paragraphs make the review unable to use.
- *Record of review sources:* A reviewer should keep a record of review sources, i.e. citation and references for readymade availability for self and others to verify the things.
- *Focus in current review:* A comprehensive review must be based on current evidences. Adding the old evidences might not be useful or contradictory for current practices.
- *Maintain order of year:* A reviewer should maintain a logical order of year while writing literature. For example, writing review of current year first and then subsequent year of literature.
- *Systematic and organized:* A review must be systematic and organized. It should be written in a systematic manner like introduction, methodology, results, discussion and conclusion. Systematic review enables a researcher or audience to make it more meaningful.
- *Reference citation:* A list of references cited as a sources must be included in bibliography or reference section. It helps readers to locate the exact source of review.

CRITICAL APPRAISAL OF REVIEW

A critique is the process of critical appraisal the review on objectivity, strengths and weaknesses for its scientific merit and application to practice. Critical appraisal need an in-depth knowledge of the subject matter and skills of how to critically read and appraise a review. The following questions may be answered to appraise a review article. To assist the appraisal of review articles in general, the following question can be answered.

Box 5.7: Critical Appraisal of Review.
- Was a clear study question asked?
- Was the study question was specific enough?
- Was an appropriate search strategy planned?
- Does the review rely on appropriate materials (i.e. primary sources)?
- Were the inclusion and exclusion criteria were followed?
- Was an adequate literature search conducted?
- Was the validity of the studies included in the review assessed?
- Do the reviews follow a systematic and logical order and flow?
- Were the directions for future research offered?

REVIEW QUESTIONS AND ANSWER

Long and Short Answer Questions
1. Explain the purpose, scope, source and steps in Review of Literature. (KUHAS, MSc N-2002)
2. Enlist the sources of literature review, importance and steps in reviewing literature and utilization of nursing theories in research. (AIIMS, MSc N-2017)
3. Explain the methods of review of literature. (PGI, MSc N-2007)
4. Describe the importance of review of literature in nursing research. (RGUHS, MSc N-2014)
5. Enlist the various factors affecting the review of literature. (PGI, MSc N-2008)

Multiple Choice Questions
1. Which of the following is an example of secondary source for review of literature?
   a. Unpublished thesis/dissertation
   b. Workshop or conference abstract
   c. Personal diary and artifacts
   d. Book chapters

2. Which of the following is the example of primary sources in literature search?
   a. Newspaper
   b. Book chapters
   c. Television/radio
   d. Personal diary

3. The primary sources are more preferred over secondary sources because of following reason:
   a. Objectivity
   b. Subjectivity
   c. Ease availability
   d. Possibility of more errors

4. Which of the following is most important database for nursing literature?
   a. MEDLINE
   b. CINAHL
   c. Psych Info
   d. EMBASE

5. Which of the following is the database to review literature?
   a. Scopus
   b. Google Scholar
   c. MEDLINE
   d. PubMed

6. Which of the following is a search engine used for literature review?
   a. Scopus
   b. Google Scholar
   c. PubMed
   d. All of the above

7. It is a types of literature review in which a reviewer uses a precise quantitative method to sum up the results of quantitative studies:
   a. Meta-analysis
   b. Meta-synthesis
   c. Narrative review
   d. Cochrane review

8. It is a types of literature review use non-statistical techniques to evaluate, integrate and interpret the findings of qualitative studies:
   a. Meta-analysis
   b. Meta-synthesis
   c. Narrative review
   d. Cochrane review

9. Which of the following database is also known as 'red book' for nursing literature?
   a. CINAHL
   b. EMBASE
   c. MEDLINE
   d. PubMed

10. Which of the following is considered bibliographic database for biomedical literature?
    a. Medline
    b. Google
    c. MSN search
    d. Yahoo

Answer Key

1.	2.	3.	4.	5.	6.	7.	8.	9.	10.
d.	d.	a.	b.	c.	d.	a.	b.	a.	a.

SUGGESTED READING

1. Beyea S, Nicoll LH. Writing an integrative review. AORN J. 1998;67(4):877-80.
2. Burn N, Grove SK. Understanding nursing research: Building an evidence-based practice, 5th edition. St Louis: Saunders Elsevier; 2010.
3. Burn N, Grove SK. Understanding nursing research: building an evidence-based practice, 4th edition. St Louis: Saunders Elsevier; 2007.
4. Cooling J. Demystifying the clinical nursing research process: the literature review. Urol Nurs. 2003;23(4):297-9.
5. Coughlan M, Cronin P, Ryan F. Step-by-step guide to critiquing research, Part-I: Quantitative Research. Br J Nurs. 2007;16(11):658-63.
6. Creswell JW. Educational research: Planning, conducting and evaluating quantitative and qualitative research, 2nd edition. Upper Saddle River, NJ: Pearson; 2005.
7. Cronin P, Ryan F, Coughlan M. Undertaking a literature review: A step-by-step approach. Br J Nurs. 2008;17(1):38-43.
8. Hart C. Doing a literature review. London: Sage publication, 1998.
9. Parahoo K. Nursing research: Principles, process and issues, 2nd edition. Palgrave, Houndmills; 2006.
10. Polit DF, Beck CT. Essential of nursing research: Methods, appraisal and utilization, 6th edition. Philadelphia: Lippincott Williams Wilkins; 2006.
11. Polit DF, Beck CT. Nursing research: Principle and methods, 7th edition. Philadelphia: Lippincott Williams Wilkins; 2004.
12. Taylor RB. Medical writing: A guide for clinicians, educators and researchers, 2nd edition. Springer Sciences and Business media; 2011.
13. Timmins F, McCabe C. How to conduct an effective literature search. Nurs Stand. 2005;20(11): 41-7.
14. Younger P. Using the Internet to conduct a literature search. Nurs Stand. 2004;19(6):45-51.

Chapter 6

Theories and Conceptual Models in Research

INTRODUCTION

When asked about nursing theories and conceptual model application in research, many nurses and nursing students, and often even nursing faculty will respond with a furrowed brow, a pained expression, and a responding 'ugh'. When questioned about their negative response, most will admit the idea of studying theory is confusing, seems no practical value and too much complexity. Use of application of nursing theories in research becomes a major item in the last century and it continues today to stimulate phenomenal professional growth and expansion of nursing literature, education and research.

Nurses of early eras delivered excellent care to patients; however, much of what was known about nursing was focused on skills and functional tasks. Therefore, a major goal put forward by nursing leaders in the 20th century was development of evidence-based knowledge through research and application of knowledge in practical areas by using appropriate theory application.

THEORY

Theory refers to set of logically interrelated concepts, statements, proposition, and definitions which have been derived from philosophical belief of scientific data from which question, hypotheses can be deducted and tested.

'A theory is an organized, coherent and systematic articulation of a set of statements related to significant questions in a discipline and communicated as a meaningful whole.'

'A systematic explanation of an event in which constructs and concepts are identified and relationship are proposed and prediction made.' *(Streubert and Carpenter, 1999)*

Nursing Theory

Definition of nursing theory has been most problematic, as demonstrated by many exchanges in the nursing literature. Many concepts have been used interchangeably with the term theory such as conceptual framework, conceptual model, paradigm, metapardigm, theorem and perspective.

'Nursing theory defined as conceptualization of some aspects of nursing reality (invented or discovered) communicated for the purpose of describing phenomena, explaining relationship between phenomena, predicting consequences, or predicting nursing care.' *(Meleis, 2012)*

TERMINOLOGY OF THEORY

Concept

A concept is a general idea that is created through the process of abstracting which involves removing all the characteristics that are uncommon and retaining those aspects that are common.

Chin and Kramer (1999) define a concept as a 'complex mental formulation of experience'. A concept is the statement or components of phenomena necessary to understand the phenomena.

They are abstract and derived from impressions of the human mind receives about phenomena through sensing the environment. Concept may be theoretical, empirical and abstract in origin. The person, health, environment and the nurse are common concepts used in nursing.

For example, notice the difference between describing the phenomena of what happens to individual who travel from one time zone to another through detailing their sleep disturbances, and change in their moods, eating habits, bowel movements, routines and summarizing all those details through the concepts of *'Jet-leg'*. The latter is a more concise and more efficient way of communicating the ideas contained in, and related to, *Jet-leg*, that is a concept. In *Jet-leg*, a group of symptoms experienced by a person is a *phenomenon*.

Construct

Construct are most complex type of concept. They comprised of more than one concept and typically built or constructed by the theorists or philosopher to fit a purpose.

For example, *'hand-washing'* is a concept but hand washing before each procedure, with using 2–3 mL liquid soap for 3–4 mints under running tap water by following 7 steps of hand-washing is a construct. Here, many concepts merge together to make a complex construct.

IMPORTANCE OF THEORY IN NURSING

Nursing theory helps a nurse to prepare and plan nursing care and evaluate the extent to which the nursing process is successful to achieve the goals. Theory serve following purposes in nursing:
- To determine the need of the patient
- To demonstrate effective use of interpersonal and communication techniques
- Help in assessment of patient's condition
- Theory help in preparation of nursing care plan based on identified needs of the patient
- Nurse use appropriate nursing theory to meet the need of the patient
- Theory help in evaluation of nursing process and provide feedback for re-planning.

MODEL

Model are representation of relationship among and between the concepts showing pattern. Model bring different individual concept together and knit to each other to make successful application to nursing practice. They are prepare background of thinking behind theory and helps in application of theory in to nursing practice. Schematic model represent concepts and their linkage between each other through use of arrows, boxes and other symbols, i.e.

Myra Estrin Levine: The Conservation Model; which stated that nursing is a human interaction, her model deals with interaction of nurse and client as shown in Figure 6.1.

Models provide a means for ordering, clarifying and analyzing concepts and relationship; they provide analogs to reality and stimulate the scientific process by identifying new possibilities. A model primarily express structure, whereas theory provides substance. Model used in nursing must represent the ordered reality of focus on human being, their environment, their health and nursing itself.

CONCEPTUAL FRAMEWORK

While reading research article, you may come across a sentence stating 'a conceptual framework used to underpin' this study. The Oxford dictionary defines 'framework 'as 'frame, structure, upon or into which casing or contents be put in,' and 'underpin' as 'support from below with masonry strengthen'.

'A conceptual framework is a written or visual presentation that explains either graphically or in a narrative form, the main things to be studied such as the key factors, concepts, or variables and the presumed relationship among them.' *(Miles and Huberman, 1994)*

'A conceptual framework is a basic structure developed to organize a number of concepts that are focused on a particular set of questions.' *(O' Toole, 2003)*

Conceptual framework refers to a set of interrelated concepts that symbolically represent or convey a mental image of a phenomenon. Conceptual model of nursing identify concepts and describes their relationship to the phenomena of central concern to the discipline.

A conceptual framework is an organized grouping of ideas or concepts that assists in providing overall structure to the research project and the nursing process. A conceptual framework is defined as, by analogy as unifying central theme that provides the mechanism for articulating and relating all parts of the curriculum.

A conceptual framework is a clearly organized and presented literature review that explicitly identifies the concepts and hypothesized relationship among these concepts. These concepts are then defined both conceptually and concretely so that reader can fully understand the effect of one variables on other. Unfortunately, in many studies, the framework remain vague and unclear and only implicitly developed at best.

This reference to building and construction can equally apply to research. One can say that the function of a conceptual framework is to provide a structure that strengthens the study. Novice researcher may think of themselves as unqualified to develop conceptual scheme of their own. Many times a researcher study lacks a theoretical framework.

The nursing process is an example of conceptual framework; it has four components (concepts)—assessment, planning, implementation and evaluation. These components represent the structure to which nurses attach the contents (such as information gathered in the process of assessing a patient). Thus, the nursing process can be used as a conceptual framework in a study of nursing care. The direction of the study may be presented in the form of Figure 6.2.

A conceptual framework for a research study can be derived from conceptual definition, models or theories. For example, in a study, 'student nurse's view of health', the researcher can use concept of *health* given by World Health Organization (WHO, 1946) of physical, mental, spiritual and social well-being.

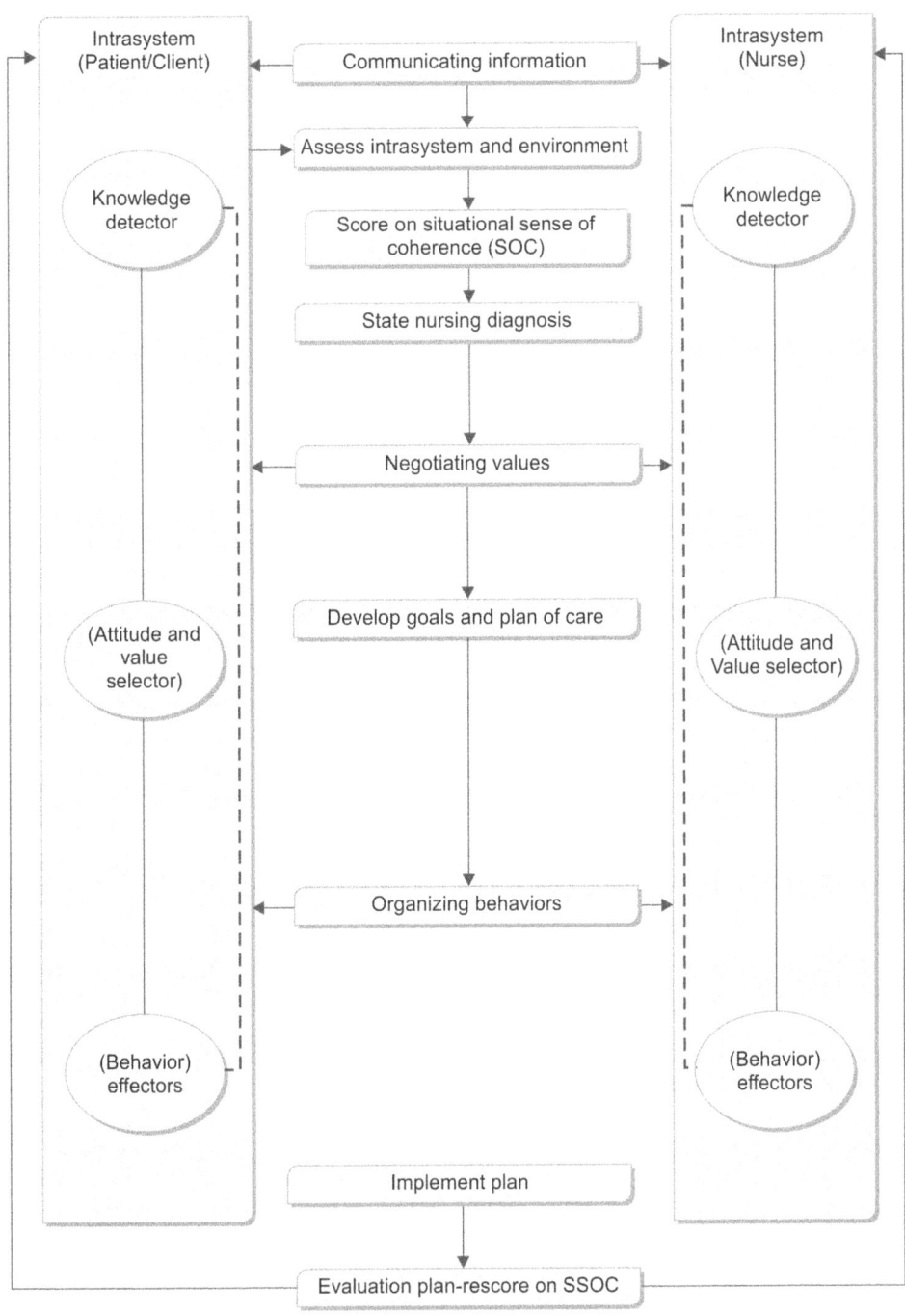

Fig. 6.1: Myra Estrin Levine: The conservation model.

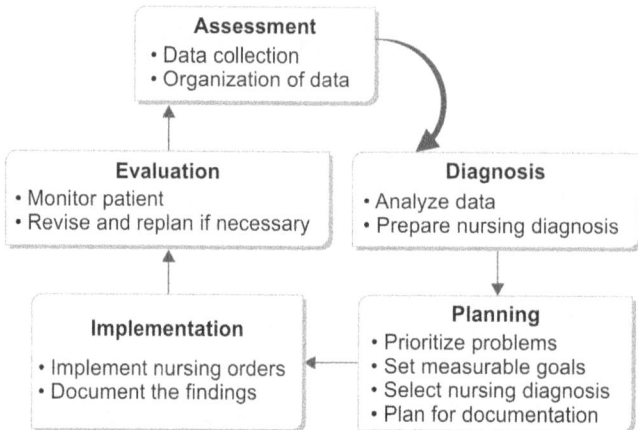

Fig. 6.2: The nursing process.

These four components of health will help a researcher to base his questionnaire of health in his study. Although, he may also choose 'progressive model of health contains four components of health for devising questionnaire for same study. Alternatively, she could combine both the definitions and provide his own conceptual framework.

The nursing literature reveals a number of ways in which researcher make a link between existing knowledge and their own studies. For example, Kumar R (2012) studied 'attitude of urban and rural community population towards patients with mental disorders'. An attitude scale consists of 35 items was used to determine stigmatization, stereotyping, benevolence, separatism, restrictiveness and pessimistic prediction. Here, each concept of the scale based on some theory or exploratory model. Therefore, a researcher use nursing theories in multiple ways in conducting research.

Purposes of Conceptual Framework

Bordage (2009), Nieswiadomy (2008), Smyth (2004) and Trafford and Leshem (2007), enlisted the following purposes of conceptual framework:
- Helps the researcher to explain why we are doing a project in a particular way. For example, the sequence of the steps in the data collection
- Helps to see and differentiate the variables clearly, for example in the *study of stress and coping among nursing students*, the researcher is clear about the concept *stress* and *coping strategies*
- Provides the researcher a general framework for data analysis. For example, in a study to assess the effect of structured training program on self-assertiveness skills in staff nurses, researcher should compare the level of assertiveness skill score before and after structured training program
- Gives direction to research methodology, therefore promotes clarity of the research topic
- Shows the relationship of the different constructs or concepts a researcher interested to investigate. For example, in a study to assess the effect of *structured training program* on *self-assertiveness skills* in staff nurses, *structured training program* is an independent variable and *assertiveness skills* is a dependent variable.

Basic Elements of Conceptual Framework

Miles and Huberman (1994) suggested followings as a basic elements of a conceptual framework.
- Concept/variables
- Relationship
- Statement hierarchy

Concepts/Variables
Based on the degree of abstractness of a term, they maybe termed as construct, concept, or variable. A construct is something which has a general meaning.

Relationship
This declares some kind of connection between and among two or more than two concepts. It is center part of a conceptual framework. The statement of relationship in a conceptual framework maybe made of objectives, hypothesis, research question, study design, statistical analysis and the findings.

Statement Hierarchy
Statement hierarchy deals with abstractness of conceptual ideas. The levels of abstractness are as follows:
- *General proposition:* Highest level of abstractness (conceptual models)
- *Specific proposition:* Moderate level of abstractness (theories)
- *Hypothesis:* It is very specific and lowest level of abstractness.

THEORETICAL FRAMEWORK

A framework is the overall representation of a study. Every study may not have a theory or a conceptual model but every study has a framework. The research study based on a theory framework called theoretical framework. The research study can also base on conceptual model often called conceptual framework. In literature, the word conceptual framework and theoretical framework are used interchangeably.

Table 6.1 briefly explains the differences in conceptual framework, theoretical framework, theories and conceptual model.

Table 6.1: Conceptual framework, theoretical framework and conceptual model: A comparison.

Feature	Conceptual framework	Theoretical framework	Conceptual model	Theory
Meaning	It is the researcher's idea on how the research problem will have to be explored	It is a theory that serves as a basis for conducting research	It is a set of highly abstract related constructs, that broadly explain a phenomena	Consists of an interrelated coherent set of concepts and model that propose testable outcomes
Scope	Specific for a study	Provide a relation between concept for a given phenomena	Explain the phenomena broadly	It is useful for nursing education, practice and administration

Contd...

Contd...

Feature	Conceptual framework	Theoretical framework	Conceptual model	Theory
Purpose	Describes the relationship between specific variables identified in a study	It guide the research process	It provide conceptual perspective regarding interrelated phenomena	Describes broader relationship between concepts
Outcome	It is a theory in the making and to be tested and confirmed	It is based on established theory that has been tested for it fit in the current study	Helps to express abstract ideas in a more understandable form	Explain, describe, predict and prescribe phenomena
Example	Conceptual framework of the image of nursing among plus two science students	The system model (Ludwig von Bertalanffy)	Roy's adaption model	Theory of cultural care diversity and universality

TYPES OF THEORIES

Theories and conceptual models are the primary mechanism by which a researcher can organizes findings into broader conceptual context. Theories and conceptual model have much in common, i.e. origin, purpose, and role in research, etc. A theory is a set of integrated concepts and proposed relationship statements between concepts.

Over the last 40 years, a number of methods for classifying theory in nursing have been described. These includes based on range/scope or abstractness (grand theory and middle range theory) and purpose of the theory (descriptive, predictive or situation producing theory).

Theory Classification by Level or Scope

Abstractness refers to the complexity of the nursing theory and concreteness and specificity of the concepts and propositions used in the theory. For example, grand theory are most complexed used to explain the discipline of nursing and includes very broadly defined concepts. Similarly, the concept of health, for example, is a broad, with potentially broad interpretations. Therefore, it is difficult to test theories because of complex and broad concepts (Fig. 6.3).

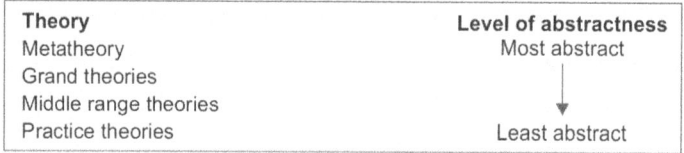

Fig. 6.3: Scope of nursing theories.

- *Metatheory:* Metatheory refers to the theory of theory. In nursing, metatheory focuses on broad issues such as development of knowledge and development of theory, etc. Metatheory helps to develop and analyzes methods for creating nursing theories.
- *Grand theory:* Grand theory are most complex and broadest in scope. Grand theories developed through thoughtful and insightful appraisal of existing theories. The majority

of nursing theories are grand theories, i.e. Orem's self-care theory, Roy's adaptation theory and Roger's theory, etc.
- *Middle range theory:* Middle range theory lies between nursing models and practice theories. These are specific and consists a very limited number of concepts. These theories relatively consists concrete concepts that are operationally defined and empirically tested, i.e. theory of peaceful end of life, public health nursing practice model, Benner's model of skill acquisition in nursing, Leininger's cultural care diversity and universality theory and Pander health promotion model, etc.
- *Practice theory:* Practice theory also known as situation specific theory, circumscribed theory or microtheories. These theories are least complex and most specific than middle range theory, i.e. symptoms focused diabetes care, theory of health promotion for preterm infants, theory of breastfeeding, migration transition model and model of maternal HELLP syndrome, etc.

Theory Classification by Purpose (Table 6.2)

Theory serve many purpose in research and hence classified as descriptive, explanatory or predictive. The research designs that generate and test these theories are descriptive, explanatory and experimental, respectively (Fawcett, 1999).

Table 6.2: Types of theories and corresponding research.

Type of theory	Type of research	Research example
Descriptive	Descriptive/Exploratory	Description of stress and coping strategies among nursing students (Kumar R, 2011)
Explanatory	Correlational	Relationship between internet addiction and psychosomatic symptoms among engineering students (Kumar R, 2014)
Predictive	Experimental	The effect of reminiscence therapy on cognition, depression, and activities of daily living for patients with Alzheimer disease (Dura AG, et al. 2016)
Prescriptive	Randomized control trails (RCT)	Trails under controlled environment

IMPORTANCE OF THEORY, MODELS AND FRAMEWORK IN RESEARCH

Theory is the integral part of research. Use of theory help to assimilate and structure the nursing knowledge to explain, understand and predict nursing practice. Use of theory also promotes rational and systematic practice by collecting research evidence. It is important to use theory as a framework to provide perspective and guidance to a research study. Indeed, theoretical framework provides direction regarding selection of research design, identify approaches, method of data analysis and specify criteria for acceptability of findings as valid.

Fitzpatrick (1998) summarize the use of theory to improve research process and develop more empirical evidence for nursing practice. He point out following ways a theory can guide research:
- Identify meaningful and relevant areas for research study
- Develop or reformulate middle range theory linked to research

- Define the concepts and propose relationship among concepts
- Helps in interpretation of research findings
- Develop clinical practice manual
- Develop evidence-based nursing diagnosis.

USE OF THEORY IN RESEARCH

In the past few decades several models and theories have been formulated in nursing. Beginning in the 1970s, nurse scholars encouraged researchers to provide a theoretical or conceptual framework for research studies. At the same time, a growing number of nurse theorists were seeking researchers to explore way to test their models in research and clinical applications. As a result, there was a push to combine research and nursing models. This emphasizes using nursing models as the framework for research to provide research into unique perspective of nursing.

Theory brings organization to the variables of interest and the concepts reflected in a study. It provides a guide for developing a study and allows the findings to be placed in or linked to, large body of knowledge. Theories tend to show up in the research process in one of three ways:

1. Theory generating research
2. Theory testing research and
3. Use of theory as research framework

Theory Generating Research

Research that generates theory is designed to develop and describe relationship between and among phenomena. Theory generation is an inductive approach that includes grounded theory, field observation and phenomenology.

Norwood (2000) explained the following steps used in theory generation:

1. Identification of observation shared a common characteristics and themes
2. Translation of identified observation into more abstract concepts
3. Translation of observational relationship into propositional statements and weaves the concepts and propositions together into a framework or theory.

Theory Testing Research

Some studies conducted to test a theory. In theory testing research, theoretical statements translated into research question and hypotheses. Theory testing is a deductive approach and consists following steps:

- Selection of a theory or a part of (concept) theory
- Development of research question and hypotheses to measures the variables
- Conduction of study and interpreting the findings
- Development of implications for further use of the theory in research.

Theory as Conceptual Framework in Research

This is the most common way of incorporating a theory in research. In this case, problem being investigated is fitted into an existing theoretical framework, which guide the study and enriches the value of its findings.

Norwood (2000) mentioned following steps of use of a theory as a conceptual framework in a nursing study.
- Selection of a research problem consistent with the framework
- Writing conceptual definitions derived from the framework
- Selection of research instruments congruent with the framework
- Interpretation of findings in light of explanation provided by the framework
- Implications for advanced practice nursing are based on the explanatory power of the framework
- Relationship for future research address the concepts and relationship designed by the framework.

Application of a theory as a conceptual framework in research is possible in two ways.
1. *Theory fitting:* If the concepts or variables of the research are fitting in the existing framework completely.
2. *Forced fitting:* The concepts or relationship from original theory maybe incorrectly applied, the work may appear 'forced' or the study may fail to reach on a meaningful conclusion.

Use of Theoretical Framework in Research

A conceptual framework was used in a research study entitled, *'a descriptive study to assess stress and coping strategies among nursing students.'* (Kumar R, et al. 2012). This conceptual framework was based on Betty Neuman System Model as depicted in Figure 6.4. The model explain how the research concepts and variables knit to each other in the model.
- *Client system:* According to Betty Neuman, each individual or group is unique. Each system is a composite of common known innate characteristics with in a given range of responses contained within a basic structure. In the present study, the basic structure is a student-nurse with all its innate and acquired characteristics.
- *Stressors:* Neuman defined stressors as 'tension-producing stimuli with the potential for causing system instability'. Stressors can be interpersonal, intrapersonal and extrapersonal.
- *Intrapersonal stressors:* Forces occurring within the individual. In the present study, intrapersonal factors are adolescence age of the nursing students and the related physical, physiological and psychological changes.
- *Interpersonal stressors:* Forces occurring between one or more individuals. In the present study, interpersonal factors are peer-group acceptability and social support system.
- *Extrapersonal stressors:* Forces that occur outside the system. In the present study, extra-personal factors are academic and clinical stressors encountered by the nursing students.
- *Flexible line of defense (FLD):* Neuman defined FLD as a rapidly changing situational variable which buffers the stressors. The strength of FLD is determined by the interaction of person's variables inherent within it (psychological, physiological, developmental, sociocultural and spiritual). If the stressors are numerous and powerful, they create pressure on FLD and can make it more close to the NLD that can make stress response (NLD invasion) more likely. In this study flexible line of defense were stressors.
- *Normal line of defense (NLD):* According to Neuman, each individual client/client system, overtime, has evolved a normal range of responses to environment that is referred to as normal line of defense, or usual wellness/stability state. In the present study, the nursing students are subjected to intrapersonal, interpersonal and extrapersonal stressors which

Nursing Research and Statistics

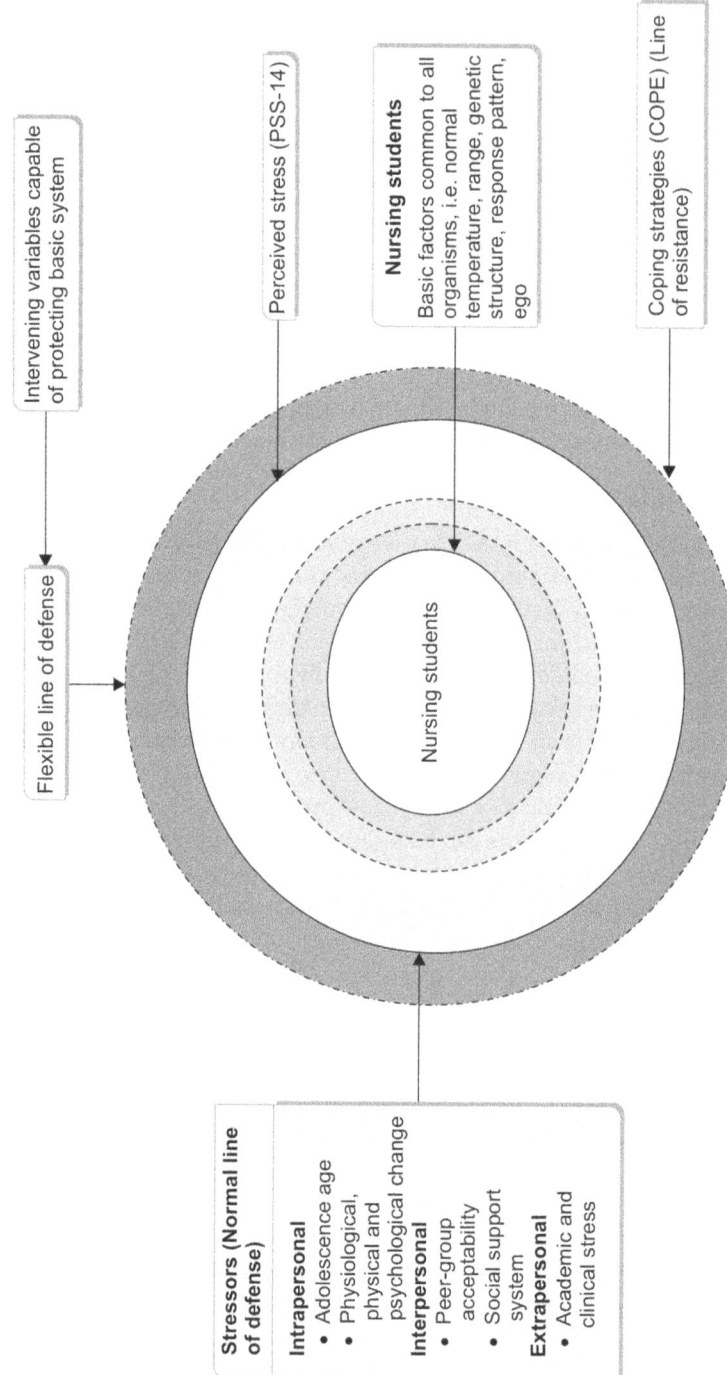

Fig. 6.4: Conceptual framework based on Betty Neuman System Model.

can invade normal line of defense (NLD) in the presence of weak flexible line of defense (FLD) and is measured as a perceived by perceived stress scale-14 (PSS-14).
- *Line of resistance (LOR):* LOR are the internal factors defending against the stressors. In the present study, the protective qualities of a student nurse developed overtime and are called as coping strategies such as, ventilating feelings, seeking diversions, relaxing, self-reliance, developing social support, solving family problems, avoiding, seeking spiritual support, investing in closed friends, seeking professional support, engaging in demanding abilities and being humorous. The coping strategies are measured by using Adolescent Coping Orientation for Problem Experiences (ACOPE).

In this study, the basic structure is a student nurse with all its innate and acquired characteristics. In college life, nursing students come across various stressors like intrapersonal, interpersonal and extrapersonal. Nursing students use FLD, NLD and LOR as buffer to maintain a balance between self and environment.

RELATIONSHIP BETWEEN THEORY, RESEARCH AND PRACTICE

Majority of nursing professionals lack a true understanding of the interrelationship of theory, research and practice. Indeed, at that time nursing professionals urged that nursing research be combined with theory development to provide a rational basis for practice (Fig. 6.5).

Theory, research and practice have reciprocal cyclic relationship to each others. Research validates and modifies theory. In nursing, theories stimulate nurse scientists to explore significant problems in the field of nursing. In this process, development of nursing knowledge increases. Result of research helps to refine or replace outdated clinical practice.

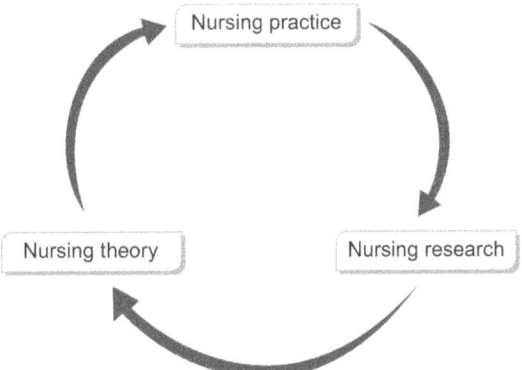

Fig. 6.5: Nursing theory, research and practice.

PROCESS OF CONCEPTUAL FRAMEWORK DEVELOPMENT

The process of development of conceptual framework has been described by many nursing scholars. Development of conceptual framework requires researcher's knowledge, theory and model experience, practical application and involvement in conduction of research study(s). In addition, the brain storming, intuition and creativity are other skills required for identification and establishing the relationship between two or more than two variables. However, use the following steps may help a researcher to come up with a conceptual framework.

- *Identification or development of concept:* This is the step of conceptual framework development involves identification of concepts in research statement. This provides foundation for conceptual framework development and includes specifying, defining and clarifying the concepts used to describe phenomena. For example, *'A study to assess stress and coping strategies among nursing students at a selected private college, Amritsar, Punjab'*. In the statement the concept 'stress' and 'coping strategies' to be defined operationally and clearly to fit into possible application in existing model.
- *Develop relationship between concepts:* Relational statements are the skeleton of framework. This is the means by which the concepts come together and framework skeleton will be developed. The process of formulation and validation of statement involves developing the empirical statement.
- *Development of logical construct or hierarchical statement:* This step includes formulating systemic linkage between and among concepts, which result in a formal, coherent theoretical structure. In above given example of research study, construct is combination of characteristics of subjects, stress and coping strategies used by nursing students.
- *Validating and conforming relationship (showing the direction of the study):* Validating involves empirically refining concepts and theoretical relationship. After validation, revision may be made before development of a framework. It is also important to establish the congruity between conceptual model, its components, the research problem, hypotheses, concepts, design and subjects. In most of research, force fitting method use to apply theory in research in which researcher deliberately fit research concept in the conceptual framework.

REVIEW QUESTIONS AND ANSWER

Long and Short Answer Questions

1. Explain what is theory along with its nature and its types (KUHAS, MSc N-2002)
2. Explain the role of theory in research in detail. (PGI, MSc N-2011)
3. Define conceptual framework and its importance in nursing research. (PGI, MSc N-2001)
4. What is the process in conceptual framework development? (RGUHS, MSc N-2014)
5. Explain the relationship between theory, research and practice. (AIIMS, MSc N-2013)
6. What are the steps in developing, using and testing conceptual framework?
   (TNMGRMU, MSc N-2016)

Multiple Choice Questions

1. These theory refers to the theory of theory and focus on broad issues such as development of knowledge and development of theory are called:
   a. Metatheory
   b. Grand theory
   c. Middle range theory
   d. Practice theory

2. The central concepts of conceptual models in nursing includes:
   a. Human, heart and hand
   b. Man, environment, nursing, health
   c. Agent, host reservoir, environment
   d. Human, disease, health, environment

3. Orem's self-care theory is an example of which types of theory in Nursing?
   a. Metatheory
   b. Grand theory
   c. Middle range theory
   d. Practice theory

4. It is a types of theory which help to establish relationship between two or more than two variables in a research is called:
   a. Descriptive theory
   b. Explanatory theory
   c. Prescriptive theory
   d. Predictive theory

5. It is a systematic explanation of an event in which constructs and concepts are identified and relationship are proposed and prediction made is called:
   a. Concept
   b. Construct
   c. Phenomenon
   d. Theory

6. In which of the following ways theory may help in research process?
   a. Theory generate research
   b. Theory test research
   c. Research use theory as conceptual framework
   d. All of the above

7. Which of the following is the first step in development phase of a conceptual framework?
   a. Develop relationship between concept
   b. Arrangement of concept in hierarchy
   c. Identification of concepts
   d. Validating concepts and relationship

8. All of the following are building block of theory, *except:*
   a. Theoretical proposition
   b. Concept
   c. Construct
   d. Conceptual definition

Answer Key

1.	2.	3.	4.	5.	6.	7.	8.
a.	b.	a.	b.	d.	d.	c.	d.

SUGGESTED READING

1. Bordage G. Conceptual framework to illuminate and magnify. Med Educ. 2009;43(4):312-9.
2. Burn N, Grove SK. The practice of nursing research: Appraisal, synthesis and generation of evidence, 6th edition. St Louis: Elsevier; 2009.
3. Chin PL, Kramer MK. Theory and nursing: Integrated knowledge development, 7th edition. St. Louis: Mosby; 2008.
4. Constitution of the World Health Organization. In: World Health Organization: Basic documents. 45th edition. Geneva: World Health Organization; 2005.
5. Dorothy D Theodore. Conceptual framework: A road map for nursing research. Indian journal of continuing nursing education. 2013;14(2):15-22.
6. Duru Aşiret G, Kapucu S. The effect of reminiscence therapy on cognition, depression, and activities of daily living for patients with Alzheimer disease. Journal of Geriatric Psychiatry and Neurology. 2016;29(1): 31-7.

7. Fawcett J. Conceptual models and nursing practice: The reciprocal relationship. Journal of Advanced Nursing. 1992;17:224-8.
8. Fawcett J. The relationship of theory and research, 3rd edition. Philadelphia: FA Davis; 1999.
9. Fawcett J. Thoughts on concepts analysis: Multiple approaches, one result. Nursing Science Quarterly. 2012;25:285.
10. Fitzpatrick JJ. Encyclopedia of nursing research. New York: Springer; 1998.
11. Kerlinger FN, Lee HB. Foundation of behavioral research. New York: Harcourt; 2000.
12. Levine ME. Introduction to clinical nursing, 2nd edition. Philadelphia: FA Davis; 1973.
13. McEwen M, Wills EM. Theoretical basis for nursing, 2nd edition. Philadelphia: Lippincott Williams and Wilkins; 2007.
14. Meleis A. Theoretical Nursing: Developmental progress, 3rd edition, Philadelphia: JB Lippincott company; 2007.
15. Miles MB, Huberman AM. Qualitative Data Analysis: An Expanded Sourcebook, 2nd edition. Beverley Hills: Sage; 1994.
16. Nieswiadomy RM. Foundation of nursing research, 5th edition. California: Pearson Prentice Hall; 2008.
17. Norwood SL. Research Strategies for Advanced Practice Nurses. Upper Saddle River, NJ: Prentice Hall Health; 2000.
18. O' Toole MT (Ed). Miller-Keane Encyclopedia and Dictionary of Medicine, Nursing and Allied Health, 7th edition. Philadelphia: Saunders; 2003: pp. 1421, 705.
19. Polit DF, Beck CT. Nursing research: Generating and assessing evidence for nursing practice, 8th edition. Philadelphia: Lippincott Williams and Wilkins; 2008.
20. Rajesh K, Nancy. Stress and coping among nursing students. Nursing and Midwifery Research journal. 2011;7(4):141-51.
21. Rajesh K, Santosh M, Raminder K. A study to identify the learning needs of staff nurses working in psychiatric nursing unit regarding legal and ethical responsibilities in the field of psychiatric nursing. An unpublished Master in Nursing (MN) thesis, Delhi University, New Delhi; 2010: pp. 13-5.
22. Rajesh K. Attitude to people with mental illness—A survey from Punjab state. International Journal of health science and research. 2012;3(12):135-45.
23. Rajesh K. Relationship between internet addiction and psychosomatic symptoms among engineering students. Delhi Psychiatry Journal. 2014;17(2):202-9.
24. Smith JA. The idea of health: A philosophical Inquiry. Advance in Nursing Science. 1981;33:43-50.
25. Smyth R. Exploring the usefulness of a conceptual framework as a research tool: A researcher's reflection, issues in educational research. 2004;14(2):167-80.
26. Streubert-Speziale HJ, Carpenter DR. Qualitative research in nursing: Advancing the humanistic imperative, 3rd edition. Philadelphia: Lippincott Williams and Wilkins; 2003.
27. Trafford V, Lesham S. Overlooking the conceptual framework. Innovation in education and teaching International. 2007;44(1):93-105.
28. Walker LO, Avant KC. Strategies for theory construction in Nursing. New Theory: Person Prentice Hall; 2005.

Chapter 7

Research Designs

INTRODUCTION

Common sense and research both involve an attempt to understand various aspects of the world. However, research but arguably not common sense, involves an explicit, systematic approach to finding things out, often through a process of testing out preconceptions. This process begins with deciding on a research question. It is then necessary to conduct a literature review and to decide on a research design which addresses the research question. Decisions made at this point include considering what kind of data will be collected, how they will be collected, who will be invited to participate and how the data will be analyzed.

Research Approach

When starting a research study, it is best to identify clearly what you wish to attain and then think at the best way of achieving it. Selection a research approach for study is an initial step and all further steps are based on it. All research approaches are possible to manage once you learned how to do that. Research approach is a broad plan to explore a phenomenon under study. A researcher may use qualitative, quantitative and mixed method approach to answer a research question. Selection of research approach enable the researcher to decide certain methodological aspects for study like design, sample size, data collection strategy and type of statistical application.

Research Design

A research design is the framework or guide used for the planning, implementation, and analysis of a study. It is the plan for answering the research question or hypothesis. It is important to have a broad preparation and understanding of the different types of research designs available to answer different types of questions and hypotheses. However, it is becoming more popular to use a mixed method design in nursing studies nowadays. Research designs are most often classified as either experimental or non-experimental.

Definitions

A researcher's overall plan for obtaining answers to the research questions or for testing the research hypotheses is referred to as the research design.
'It is a blueprint for conducting a study with maximum control over factors that may interfere with validity of the findings.' *(Burns and Grove, 2003:195)*

'It is a plan that describe how, when and where data are to be collected and analyzed.'
(Parahoo, 1997:142)

'It is decision regarding WHAT?, WHERE?, WHEN? HOW MUCH?, by WHAT? Means concerning an inquiry or a research study constitute research design.' *(Kothari, 1988)*

'Research design is researcher's overall for answering the research question or testing the research hypothesis.' *(Polit, et al. 2001:167)*

Characteristics of a Good Research Design

A good research design is characterized by the followings:
- The design chosen should be appropriate to the nature and objective of the problem to be studied
- It must be economical, considering the available time, money and researcher's skill for research work
- The design supposed to be flexible enough to permit consideration of varied aspects of the phenomena
- The measuring tool/instrument should be yield objective, reliable and valid data
- The design must minimize the bias and maximize the reliability of the data collected
- The information should obtain from requisite size of the sample
- The design should ensure appropriate statistical analysis of the collected data
- The selected design must ensure generalization of the findings of the research study.

Factors Affecting Selection of Study Design

The following are some factors that may affect selection of study design. These are as follows:
- *Availability of resources:* To conduct a research, researcher need different types of resources like manpower, material, money, time and other technical resources. Needs of resources are vary from one design to other. For instance, to conduct a longitudinal study, a researcher needs to have enough time. Therefore, selection of research design affect with the availability of resources.
- *Aim and purpose of study:* The selection of research design influenced with the aim and purpose of the study. For instance, to test a drug sensitivity, a true experimental design is needed than non-experimental design.
- *Availability of scientific information:* Selection of research design depends on the availability of scientific information. To get more empirical information on an attribute, choice of experimental design is much better than non-experimental one.
- *Knowledge and experience of investigator:* Knowledge and experience of researcher may also influence selection of research design, for instance a well experienced researcher may be more confident in choosing a familiar research design. Therefore, selection of research design influenced with the knowledge and experience of researcher.
- *Interest and motivation or researcher:* Interest and motivation are key attribute that helps in selection of research design. A researcher's interest helps to choose and complete the study on or before time.
- *Ethical issues:* This is another important factor that may influence selection of a research design. The studies which are stand to ethical issues are more commonly accepted and selected rather than unethical studies.

- *Subjects related issues:* Usually, in nursing and allied sciences, research studies are conducted on human being. A researcher should see the availability of subjects, their participation or cooperation before selection of research design.
- *Implications of the study:* The basic purpose of research in nursing is to improve quality education and client care in practice. Therefore, designs which are more concerned to meet the nursing problems are easily accepted and appreciated than other designs.
- *Users of the study:* Sometime, research study is conducted to serve the purpose of a specific group of professionals. Therefore, while selecting a research design, a researcher should know about the users of the study findings.

QUANTITATIVE AND QUALITATIVE RESEARCH

Nurse investigators conduct both quantitative and qualitative studies. Quantitative research is concerned with objectivity, rigid controls over the research situation and the ability to generalize results. Qualitative research is concerned with the personal meaning of an experience to an individual.

In the past, nurse researchers have mostly conducted quantitative research. Quantitative research has been the traditional methodological approach used by many of the other disciplines. A few investigators do not consider qualitative research to be scientific. Others view quantitative research as hard science and qualitative research as soft science.

For example, consider subjects who are experiencing chronic pain, quantitative research would be concerned with the level of pain that these people were experiencing, and qualitative research would be concerned with what it means to be living with chronic pain. For more details refers chapter 1 for comparison between qualitative and quantitative research.

QUANTITATIVE RESEARCH

Quantitative research designs adopt objective, rigorous, and systematic strategies for generating and refining knowledge.

Quantitative research is most often about quantifying relationships between or among variables—the independent or predictor variable(s) and the dependent or outcome variable(s). Broadly, quantitative research designs are classified as either non-experimental or experimental.

Definition

'Quantitative research is a formal, objective, systematic process in which numerical data are used to obtain information about the world.'

Validity of Quantitative Research

In experimental studies, as well as in other types of research, the researcher is interested in controlling extraneous variables that may influence study results. The extraneous variables, or competing explanations for the results, in experimental studies are labeled threat to internal and external validity (Campbell and Stanley, 1963). The internal validity of an experimental design concerns the degree to which changes in the dependent variable (effect) can be attributed to the independent variable (cause). In general, it is show the strength of relationships between independent and dependent variable in a quantitative study. External validity refers

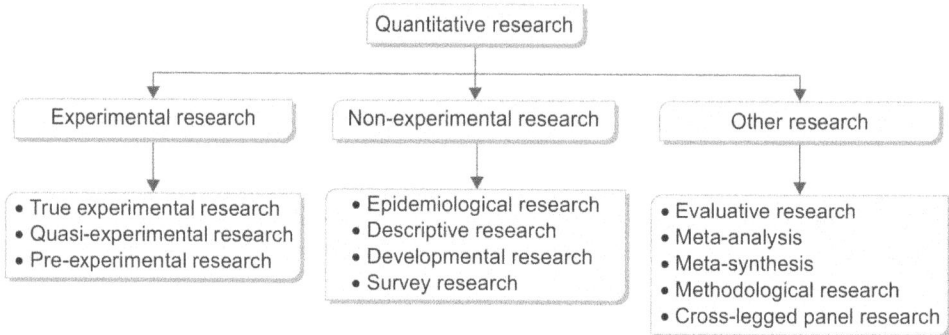

Fig. 7.1: Quantitative research.

to the degree of generalization of results to other population in different context. Internal and external validity are related in that as the researcher attempts to control for internal validity, external validity is usually increased.

Factors Affecting Internal Validity (Threats to Rigor)

Campbell and Stanley (1963) have identified threats to internal validity. A researcher should mind following threats before designing the study in order to improve generalization of the findings.

- *Selection bias effect:* Selection bias is most common threat than other threats in quantitative study. It refers to the extent to which the selection of sample influence the final result of the study. A researcher may impart the selection bias at the screening process (use of inclusion and exclusion criteria) or at the time of random allocation of subjects to experimental or control groups.
- *History effects:* The threat history occurs when some event beside the experimental treatment occurs during the course of the study, and influence the dependent variable. Suppose a researcher might be interested to see the effectiveness of 2 weeks structured teaching program on hazardous effects of alcoholism in a community. During the time of the study is being conducted, an article is published in the newspaper concerning the harmful effects of alcoholism. This 'history' event could result in an increase in knowledge related to hazardous effects of alcoholism.
- *Maturation effects:* It refers to changes in participants status over a period of time. Maturation effects refers to the developmental, biological or psychological processes that operate with in an individual as a function of time, and are external to the concept of investigations (LoBiondo-Wood, 2006). For example, a school health nurse trying to looking the impact of hot breakfast on weight gain among under 10 years children. Simultaneously, she should also understand that weight gain is a natural phenomena over the age.
- *Testing effects:* Testing effects refers to the degree of extent to which repeated administration of the same instrument bring changes in responses of the participants. It is also known as *sensitization* effects.

    For example, if subjects were weighed and told their weight before an experimental weight reduction program, these subject may reduce their weight because they are been informed that they are overweight.

- *Instrumentation effects:* This is refers to degree to which changes in instrument bring change in response of participants. This issue should also deal with data collection by means of biophysiological methods. Therefore, calibration of equipments is necessary before after data collection. Similarly, all data collectors or team member should be trained in same manner to ensure uniformity in data collection.
- *Mortality or attrition effects:* It is also known as *attrition or drop out effects*. It refers to the extent of drop out or attrition of sample from one data collection point to another point in a study. It also refers to difference in mortality between experimental and control group. Mortality effect should be seen if the attrition rate goes more than 20% in a study (Polit and Beck, 2008). Therefore, a researcher should take anticipatory measures to prevent the drop out effect on study findings.
- *Statistical regression effects:* It is also called as regression to mean. It refers to the extent to which low or high scores of an instrument move towards the sample mean at the second time administration of the instrument. Statistical regression happens because of very high or low score occurs by chance and the chances of this happening is lower than for score (that) reflect the average or mean. Statistical regression occurs because of administration of an instrument more than once.
- *Interaction of threats effects:* Cambell and Stanley (1963) pointed out interaction of threat effects, for example, interaction of selection bias effects with any of the other effects leads to interaction of threats effects.

Factors Affecting External Validity

Campbell and Stanley (1963) identified four threats to external validity. These threats are considered alternative explanation to the explanation that study findings are true and unbiased.
- *Hawthorne effects:* Hawthorne effect occur when research participants behaved in different way because they are aware of presence of researcher or by being observed by someone. Mayo (1953) coined this term at the Western Electric Hawthorne Works located in Cicero, Illinois. It might be possible to control this threat by single blind or double blind study approach, where neither the researcher nor the participants are aware of presence of researcher or observation of their behavior.
- *Experimenter effects:* This refers to the impact of behavior or characteristics of researcher on the response of behavior of a participant, e.g. dressing sense, language, gesture and posture may have impact on response pattern of a participant. The term experimenter effect only implemented to experimental studies, a term similar meaning is used in the non-experimental studies called as Rosenthal effect.
- *Reactive measurement effects/testing:* Taking a test multiple times could change the response of the subjects. The effect of taking a pretest on the post-test is called testing effects. The pretest may sensitize the subjects. Generally, subjects score higher score in post-test because of sensitization to pretest. A researcher should paper-pencil technique of data collection to control testing effects.
- *Novelty effects:* Use of new treatment strategy may change the behavior of participants. Subjects might be curious to know about new intervention strategy and may do the things differently. Once the participants get familiar with treatment, result might be different.

EXPERIMENTAL RESEARCH

Experimental method is an empirical research method used to examine a hypothesized causal relationship between independent and dependent variables. It is a scientific investigation in which observations are made and data are collected according to a set of well defined criteria. In an experiment, a researcher works as an active agent not passive observer.

Experimental designs typically use random assignment, manipulation of an independent variable(s), and strict controls over extraneous condition to see the desired effect of independent variable on dependent variable. These characteristics provide increased confidence of cause and effect relationships. The most common experimental designs are: true experimental, quasi-experimental and pre-experimental design.

Characteristics of Experimental Research

An experimental design have following important characteristics:
- They involves testing of clinical treatment
- There is random assignment of subjects to experimental and control conditions
- Collection of information on treatment outcomes from all groups
- They generally use large and heterogeneous sample of subjects, frequently selected from multiple, geographically dispersed sites to ensure generalization of result
- The required sample size is usually calculated from equation that include a measure of the power of the study, i.e. the ability of the study to detect existing relationship among variables.

Types of Experimental Research

The investigator planning an experiment has many experimental design options to choose. Experimental designs fall into three major categories:
1. True or classical experimental design.
2. Quasi-experimental design.
3. Pre-experimental design.

TRUE EXPERIMENTAL RESEARCH

True experimental designs examine the cause and effect relationships between independent and dependent variables under strict controlled conditions. To review, 'true' experimental design provides the strongest evidence in support of hypothesized casual relationship between variables, because they include the following basic features:
- Researcher manipulates one or more independent variables that are hypothesize to generate a change in the dependent variable
- Use of at least one control or comparison group (or occasion)
- Random assignment of study participants into experimental and control group
- Control over the relevant environmental features that could otherwise provides competing explanation for the seemingly effective intervention.

To be classified as true experimental, there must be randomization, a control group, and manipulation of a variable in an experiment. When any of above mention requirements is not met, the design is no longer a true experiment and is classified as quasi-experimental or a pre-experimental.

Characteristics of True Experimental Research

A true experimental research should have following three key features: (1) Random assignment of subjects (randomization), (2) Manipulation of independent variable and (3) Use of control group.

Random Assignment (Randomization)

Randomization refers to assignment of study participants to either experimental or control group to investigate the treatment condition at random. Randomization provides an equal and independent chance to participants of being assigned to any groups, therefore, it helps to eliminate systematic bias.

Although randomization is a preferred scientific method for equalizing the groups, still, there is no guarantee that the groups will be comparable. Therefore, a researcher should also used other method simultaneously for generating comparable groups. Such as use of control group or manipulation of independent variable. Following methods are commonly employed for random assignment of subjects.

Methods of Randomization

A researcher may use following methods for random assignment of participant into experimental and control group:

- *Flipping coin:* It is common method to assign the participants in control and experimental group. A researcher may flip the coin for assignment of participants to control and experimental group.
- *Matching:* Sometimes, researcher may create groups of participants with comparable characteristics. For example, if a researcher develop group on the basis of gender, then, men and women would be randomly assigned to condition separately.
- *Draw of lots (pulling name from hat):* It is also known as *lottery method*. A researcher may write the name or code number of participants on slips and ask someone else (individual not a part of research project) to pull the name of participants for experimental and control group.
- *Table of random numbers:* A table of random number will be developed to decide control and experimental group. To draw the participants from random table, researcher blindly put the finger/pencil on anyone number then move the finger/pencil up/down or right and left to device experimental and control group.
- *Cluster randomization:* It involves random assigning clusters of participants to experimental and control group. In case of large sample size, cluster randomization may enhance the feasibility of conducting an experiment.
- *Computer generated random numbers:* Computer generated table of random numbers may also be used to categories the participants in control and experimental condition. In this method, a random number of table is created with the help of computer software to draw a desired number of participants for experimental and control group. It is similar but advanced method of creating a table of random number with the help of computer software to minimize bias in random selection of participants.
- *Randomization.com:* A researcher may go online to create experimental and control group for study.

Manipulation of Independent Variable

It is the process of doing something to study subjects (independent variable) to see the desired effect on outcome variable. In experimental designs, the causative variable must be amenable to manipulation by the researcher that is 'does something', to subjects in the experimental condition. However, while manipulation, a researcher should see the followings:

- *Manipulation strength:* It is an assessment of the 'likelihood that the treatment could have its intended outcome', independent of the actual effect of the treatment on the dependent variable.
- *Manipulation checks:* This is checking to see whether the manipulation had its intended effect on dependent variable or perhaps resulted in an unintended effect(s) that could compromise the validity of an experiment.

For example, a researcher might be interested to see the effect of yoga therapy on blood pressure change among hypertensive patients. Here, the independent variable is yoga therapy which could be manipulated by giving to some patients and withholding it from others. Therefore, it is possible to compare the blood pressure (dependent variable) in the two groups to see the desired effect of independent variable on dependent variable.

Use of Control Group

Control refers to use of one or more strategies to controls over the experimental situation to see the desired effect of independent variable on dependent variable. Control in experimental research may be achieved by using a control group, manipulation, developing rigorous experimental protocol and using randomization to divides participants in experimental and control group. Using control in experimental research will help to reach on an objective conclusion. Control group used as a basis of comparison in a study is referred to as the *counterfactual*.

For example, a researcher is interested to see the effect of a specially designed nutrient therapy on weight gain among low birth weight neonates at the end of 2 weeks. In case of lack of control group, the weight gain at the end of 2 weeks would tell us nothing about the treatment effectiveness as gaining weight in a newborn is a normal growth process. If we really want to know about the effect of a nutrient therapy on weight gain, then, we have to have a control group along with experimental group to compare the findings. In case of lack of control group, findings seem furious and cannot be justified.

Control in Experimental Research

Control is one of the key features of true experimental research. A researcher may use certain methods to control on external environment to have a desired effect of independent variable on outcome variable. Some of the following methods used for control in experimental study are discussed here:

- *Blocking:* In blocking, potential confounding variable is incorporated into the study design as an independent variable. The level of this variable are considered blocks on the basis of their value on the blocking variable. Next, in each block, subjects are randomly assigned. For example, randomized block study.

- *Matching:* Matching may be fixed or propensity in nature. Fixed matching is weaker but common method to control on extraneous variables. In fixed matching, the researcher identifies one or more extraneous variable (usually up to three) to be controlled. As soon as the subject is recruited for one of the treatment group, the researcher then tries to find out subject for the other groups identical to the subject on the specified matching variables.

   In propensity matching, all known or presumed confounding variables are used to calculate propensity score for each subject. Subjects are then matched on this propensity score.
- *Homogeneity testing:* Another method of controlling confounding variables is through statistical analysis. The concept of statistical analysis based on procedure called analysis of covariance (ANCOVA).
- *Counterbalancing:* Counterbalancing occur when the researcher is concerned that the order in which treatment are administered may influences the result. When counterbalancing is used, all subjects receive all treatments; however, the order of administration of treatment is varied.

Intervention Protocol in Experimental Research

In designing an experimental research, researcher makes many decisions about the intervention to get fair test. The goal of most interventional research is to have an identical intervention for all participants in experimental group. The intervention protocol should be fairly developed with all necessary information. A full fledged intervention must be delineated explicitly in intervention protocol with all possible necessary informations. A researcher should keep a crystal clear answer for following question to get a fairer result of an experiment.
- What is the intervention and How does it differ from routine intervention?
- What procedure to be used to deliver intervention?
- What time the intervention will be delivered?
- Who will deliver intervention?
- Amount or intensity of intervention.
- When, Where and How long a intervention will be delivered?
- How frequently the intervention will be delivered?
- Under What circumstances, intervention will be stopped or withdrawn?
- What will be the alternative intervention for control group like placebo, standard method of intervention, different dose of intensity intervention or delayed intervention, etc.?

Steps in Experimental Research (Fig. 7.2)

- Delineate the population or universe to be studied (i.e. the set of subjects or objects that share a common observable characteristics)
- Select a sample from the population by random sampling
- By random assignment, subdivide the sample into two subsamples
- Specify one subsample, the experimental group and other the control group
- Before introducing the independent variable, observe and record all important characteristics of the two groups (baseline parameters)

- Introduce the independent variable into the experimental group and withholds it from the control group
- After introducing the independent variable, observe the dependent variable in both experimental and control group
- Compare the changes that occur in the experimental group with those that may have occurred in the control group
- Record the difference
- Compare these values with statistically computed values that judge the significance of the difference, and indicate whether or not the observed differences could have occurred by chance.

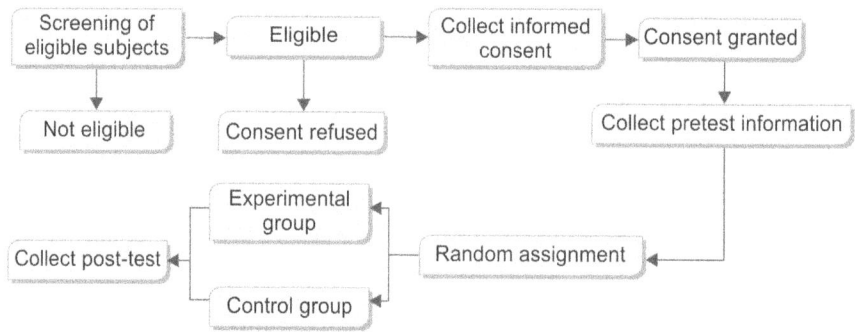

Fig. 7.2: Steps of true experimental design.

Types of True Experimental Designs

Most common used true or classical experimental designs are discussed here. These are:
1. Pretest-Post-test control group designs
2. Post-test only control group designs
3. Solomon four group design
4. Factorial design
5. Cross-over/repeated measure design
6. Randomized block design.

Pretest-Post-test Control Group Designs

It is also known as *classical experimental design*. The experimental and control groups are both randomly assigned from the sample that was randomly selected. The treatment is under control of the researcher, and the dependent variable is measured twice before and after manipulation of the independent variables. The researcher observes the two groups to determine effect of manipulation (post-test).

Box 7.1: Example of Pretest-Post-test Design (Symbolic).

$$R \quad \frac{E \quad O_1 \quad X \quad O_2}{C \quad O_1 \quad \ldots \quad O_2}$$

> **Box 7.2:** Symbols in Experimental Designs.
>
> X = Independent variable or intervention (sometimes written as T for treatment, but this can lead to some confusion where 'T' or 't' is also used to denote time)
>
> R = Randomization or random assignment
> NR = Nonrandom assignment
> M = Group matching
>
> O = Observation or measurement
> O_1 = Baseline or pretest observation
> O_2 = Outcome or post-test observation

Post-test only Control Group Designs

This design also called *after only control group design*. In this design treatment administered on experimental group and only post-test performed to see the desired effect of treatment on an experimental group by comparing it to control group. In this design pretest cannot be established. Usually, in certain situation pretest is not feasible to record, including followings:
- The administration of pretest often can overly sensitize the people to find that something very unusual is going to happen to them, making generalization to unsensitized people hazardous
- It is more expensive to take measurement both before and after an experiment
- The analysis of the data is necessarily more complicated because of the additional variables
- Sometime, certain clinical condition impose barrier to collect pretest information, for example, effect of moist heat therapy on pain reduction, swelling, and would healing after episiotomy. In said example, pretest is not possible to conduct. So, to explore such kind of issues, post-test only experimental design is used.

> **Box 7.3:** Example of Post-test Only Design.
>
> Effect of hydrocolloid application in preventing occurrence of angular stomatitis on orally intubated patients.
> - Forty patients randomized to experimental and control groups
> - E–Hydrocolloid application at the angle without changing the position
> - C–Control group (routine treatment).
>
> | R | | | | |
> |---|---|---|---|---|
> | | E | | X | O_2 |
> | | C | | XO | O_2 |

Solomon Four Group Design

It is a combination of pretest post-test control design and post-test only experimental design. Solomon four group design is especially helpful to see the effect of pre-test sensitization on subjects. Solomon four group as name implies includes two experimental and two control groups. Initially, the participants are randomly assigns to the four groups. Out of four groups, only experimental group 1 and control group 1 receives the pretest, followed by the treatment to the experiment group 1 and experimental group 2. Finally, all the four groups receive post-test, where the effects of the dependent variables of the study are observed and comparison is made between four groups to assess the effect of independent variable on the dependent variable. In this design, one group work as control group to each other.

> **Box. 7.4:** Example of Solomon Four Group Design.
>
> | | | | | | |
> |---|---|---|---|---|---|
> | R | Group 1 | E_1 | O_1 | X | O_2 |
> | | Group 2 | E_1 | XO | X | O_2 |
> | | Group 3 | C_2 | O_1 | ... | O_2 |
> | | Group 4 | C_2 | XO | ... | O_2 |

Factorial Design

This design enables the researcher to investigate the effects of two or more variables simultaneously. Factorial design enables the researcher to test the multiple hypotheses in a single experiment. In factorial design, subjects are randomly assigned to specific combination of conditions. The investigator would randomly assign individuals to each of the experimental conditions. Each experimental condition in this design represents a different treatment protocol.

Box 7.5: Example of Factorial Design.

'A study on effectiveness of music and relaxation therapy on pain relief among cancer patients.'
One factor (type of treatment) at two levels (frequency of treatment) can be studied with another factors music therapy and relaxation therapy. A total of 180 cases are available for the study.

	Type of treatment	
Daily dosage	Music therapy (B_1)	Relaxation therapy (B_2)
One daily (A_1)	$A_1 B_1$ (30)	$A_1 B_2$ (30)
Twice daily (A_2)	$A_2 B_1$ (30)	$A_2 B_2$ (30)
Thrice daily (A_3)	$A_3 B_1$ (30)	$A_3 B_2$ (30)

This design indicates that 60 cases are available to compare music therapy and relaxation therapy once daily and another 60 cases are available for the same comparison at twice daily followed by 60 cases are available for thrice daily exposure to treatments. If the difference in effectiveness between the music therapy and relaxation therapy at once daily is the same as at the twice daily, there is no interaction between the two factors, viz. type of treatment and frequency.

This analysis brings out the existence of effects due to two factors, i.e. type of treatment as well as dosage (*main effects*) and also *interaction effects* between the two factors.

Factorial design may be of following types:

1. *Simple factorial designs:* Here the effects of varying two factors on the dependent variable are considered. It is also called two—factor factorial design. It may be a 2 × 2 simple factorial design or 3 × 4 or 5 × 3 type of simple factorial design.
2. *Complex factorial design:* When experiment is done with more than two factors, it is called as complex factorial design. Experiments more than two factors at a time involve the use of complex factorial designs. A design which considers three or more independent variables is called as complex factorial design.

Cross-over/Repeated Measure Design

It involves the exposure of the same subjects to more than one experimental treatment. The subjects are randomly assigned to one of two groups. This type of within subjects design has the advantage of ensuring the highest equivalence among subjects exposed to different experimental treatment. In crossover design subjects serve as their own control. One group receives the experimental treatment first and the other group receives the second experimental treatment at same time. After a period of time the treatments are crossed over or shuffle for the groups. A researcher may use the *counterbalancing* to overcome the effect of ordering. For example, if there are three conditions (X, Y, Z), participants would be randomly assigned to one of six counterbalanced orders:

X	Y	Z
Y	Z	X
Z	X	Y

X	Z	Y
Y	X	Z
Z	Y	X

While administering the experimental treatment second time, a researcher should keep in mind the *washout time* period between two interventions administration. Washout period enable the researcher to control *the carry-over effect* (influence on the second intervention by their experience in the first intervention) on shuffled groups.

For example, effectiveness of two alternative backrest positions (supine vs 30° head elevation) on intracranial and cerebral perfusion pressures in brain injured adults.

Box 7.6: Example of Cross-over/Repeated Measure Design.

'A study to see the effects of soy protein rich diet on renal function in young adults with insulin dependent diabetes mellitus'. *(Stephenson TJ, et al. 2005)*
- Twelve type I DM patients
- Four weeks assessment of baseline data
- Assigned to soy or control diet for 8 weeks
- Crossed over to alternative diet for 8 weeks
- Outcome measures: GFR, LDL cholesterol, urinary excretion of soy is of isoflavones at the end of each 8 weeks period

---

Randomized Block Design (Levels-by-Treatment Design)

It is similar to factorial design in which one of two factors is not experimentally manipulated. Randomized block design enable the researcher to reduce the variability among the treatment groups by selecting a more homogeneous combination of the subjects. Investigator divides subjects into subgroups called *blocks* to reduce the variability within blocks. Then, subjects within each block are randomly assigned to treatment conditions. The categorical variable, (i.e. gender, blood group) which cannot be manipulated by the investigator, is known as *blocking variable*.

Box 7.7: Example of Randomized Block Design.

'A study to see the effect of three different types of tea ingestion on blood sugar level in adolescents at a nursing college'.

Gender	Treatment		
	Green tea	Lemon tea	Milk tea
Men	150	150	150
Women	150	150	150

In above said example the subjects were assigned to blocks, based on gender. Then, within each block, subjects are randomly assigned to treatments (either green tea, lemon tea and milk tea). Here, we can see that out of two factors (gender and type of tea), only type of tea can be manipulated and gender cannot be manipulated and called as *blocking variable*.

Strengths of Experimental Research
- It is a powerful method for testing hypotheses of cause and effect relationships
- It provide highest quality evidence regarding effects of specific interventions
- 'If....then' relationship important because of implications for prediction and control
- Experimental strength lies in the confidence with which causal relationship is inferred
- Through the controls imposed by manipulation, comparison, and randomization, alternative explanations to a causal interpretation can often be ruled out or discredited
- It improve precision and minimize bias
- It helps in generalization of results.

Limitations of Experimental Research
- It looks artificial in nature as researcher control over many things in experimental method that may constraints human experience, therefore, transferring the findings from the artificiality constructed experiments into realities of practice may be impractical
- It is based on randomization and then equal treatment within groups to be created. Recruitment of enough people to form control and experimental groups of sufficient size to achieve meaningful result can be problematic
- Experimental method does not answer 'Why' the intervention resulted in the observed outcome (if without a guiding theoretical framework)
- A researcher feel difficult to maintain the integrity of the intervention and control conditions if study extends overtime
- In experimental study, it is rarely possible that experimenter have full control over the clinical environment. So, chances of bias may be there
- Ethically, it may be inappropriate to withhold intervention or knowledge about which group people belong to (this is particularly important in drug trails when placebo medication is given)
- Awareness of researcher may launch 'Hawthorne effect' in the study and therefore, chances of biased findings will be more (to avoid Hawthorne effect a researcher may use masking- single blind or double blind study).

QUASI-EXPERIMENTAL RESEARCH

True experiment with random assignment thought to provide the most powerful test of research hypotheses concerned with cause and effect relationship, because of the extent to which extraneous influences may be controlled.

There are many instances, however, when a true experimental research is not feasible; because of unethical random assignment of subjects or sometimes a researcher has to withhold subjects from a special treatment. However, a quasi-experimental research has manipulation and some amount of control on environmental condition but does not have random assignment of subjects to treatment condition. However, the boundaries of experimental and quasi-experimental studies have blurred. Often investigator like to define their study as experimental when in fact it is quasi-experimental. The limitations of quasi-experimental research lies in the increased threat to internal validity.

Still, quasi-experimental designs are useful in testing the hypotheses and are considered closer to natural settings. However, exposure to a greater number of threats may decrease confidence and generalization of study's findings.

Quasi-experimental Designs

Quasi-experimental designs further classified under following headings:
1. Non-equivalent control group pretest post-test design
2. Non-equivalent control group post-test design
3. Time series design
4. Counterbalanced design.

Non-equivalent Control Group Pretest-Post-test Design

The most common quasi-experimental design is the nonrandomized control group design. It is also known as *non-equivalent control group pretest post-test design*. It is structured like a pretest post-test control group design, but it lacks the random assignment, a true feature of the true experimental design. This type of quasi-experimental design is useful when it is not possible to randomly assign subjects into different interventions. Despite the absence of randomization, nonequivalent control group design can be considered relatively a strong design.

> **Box 7.8:** Example of Non-randomized Pretest Post-test Design.
>
> 'A study to see the effects of physiotherapeutic instructions on anxiety of CABG patients'.
>
> (Garbossa A, et al. 2009)
>
> $$NR \quad \frac{E \quad O_1 \quad X \quad O_2}{C \quad O_1 \quad XO \quad O_2}$$

Non-equivalent Control Group Post-test Design

This research design suitable when the researcher not able to collect baseline parameters before the intervention. However, this design have comparison group to see the definitive impact of intervention on study variables. Here, non-equivalent group means that subjects are not assigned to either the experimental and control group in a random manner. There is no basis for determining the baseline equivalence of the groups, therefore, an alternate explanation for the post-test differences could be used to justify the study findings.

> **Box 7.9:** Example of Non-equivalent Post-test Only Design.
>
> 'A study to determine the effect of the electronic health record system on the morale of nurses.'
>
> $$NR \quad \frac{E \quad X \quad O_1}{C \quad XO \quad O_1}$$

Here, it is impossible to divide the nurses in a hospital into two groups (there is constant contamination), so it is decided to use an adjacent hospital for control. It is, however, difficult to ascribe any differences between pretest and post-test to the effect of manipulation.

Time Series Design

It is also known as *interrupted time series design*. In times series design, the investigator collects the information over an extended period of time before and after exposure to a treatment.

A group of subjects is pretested at a different period of interval to establish any change in the baseline performance. Then, the intervention is introduced and further post-tests are administered at different time interval to determine any change in baseline performance of underlying phenomena. Although, randomization and control are lacking in this design, but the longer period of time reinforces the indication of change that has been brought out.

Types of Time Series Design

- *Single group interrupted time series designnw*

  E   O1   O2   O3   O4   X   O5   O6   O7   O8

> **Box 7.10:** Example of Prospective Time Series Design.
>
> A prospective time series study to test the adverse reactions of alcohol based antiseptic among neonatal care nurses. Result reported that nurses with adverse reactions had been employed in the study unit and work for shorter duration in nursing profession than those with no reactions and were significantly more likely to report history of itchy and sore skin.   *(Cimiotti JP, et al. 2003)*

- *Control group interrupted time series design:* When several assessments are made on experimental and control group, it is also called *multiple group time series design*. In this study, experimental group receives intervention at defined period of interval but control group is not.

	E	O1	O2	O3	O4	X	O5	O6	O7	O8	O9
Non-equivalent	C	O1	O2	O3	O4	X	O5	O6	O7	O8	O9

- *Time series with multiple institution of treatment*

  O1   O2   X   O3   O4   X   O5   O6   X   O7   O8

- *Time series with intensified treatment*

  O1   O2   X   O3   O4   X+1   O5   O6   X+2   O7   O8

- *Time series with withdrawn and reinstituted treatment*

  O1   O2   X   O3   O4   (–X)   O5   O6   X   O7   O8

Strengths of Time Series Research
- It is easy to conduct on small sample size
- It helps to give a serial record of underlying phenomena after administering intervention
- It is convenient and simple to plan a time series study
- Even small numbers of measurement points can provide better information than cross sectional studies.

Limitations of Time Series Research
- Long time of study may create problem in maintaining consistency in record keeping and therefore, can be a problem at the end of study
- Study may face problem of attrition
- Seasonal variations or other cyclical influences can be interpreted as treatment effects
- Maturation threat can also influence the study findings
- It takes long time as compared to other interventional research.

Counterbalanced Designs

Counterbalanced design is the deprived version of crossover design without the random assignment of subjects to different groups.

Latin square design is most common in counterbalanced design where four different treatments are applied to four naturally non-randomized groups or individuals. Each group receives post-test after intervention. However, a researcher should try to keep the number of intervention and groups equal for empirical findings. A researcher should try to keep the number of intervention and groups equal for empirical findings. However, all groups receive all form of treatment in the research. Strength of counterbalanced design lies in that some degree of control can be achieved because the same subjects serve as their own equivalent control group. *Testing effect* makes the design weak.

Box 7.11: Example of Counterbalanced Design.

'A clinical trails of the effectiveness of water as a conductive medium in electrocardiography'.

(Birks M, et al. 1993)

	Group								
	Group 1	X1	O	X2	O	X3	O	X4	O
NR	Group 2	X2	O	X4	O	X1	O	X3	O
	Group 3	X3	O	X1	O	X4	O	X2	O
	Group 4	X4	O	X3	O	X2	O	X1	O

Strength of Quasi-experimental Research

- It is more practical approach than true experimental
- It is difficult to conduct true experiments in nursing research in real life setting, therefore quasi-experimental design are most suited to profession
- Quasi-experimental research introduce some research control when full experimental rigor is not possible
- It justify several rival hypotheses competing with intervention for the results
- Researcher take the weaknesses into account in interpreting results.

Limitations of Quasi-experimental Research

- Conclusion depend in part on human judgment rather than more objective criteria, cause and effect inferences may be less convincing
- Lack of key features of experimental design makes the result of the study less reliable and generalizable.

PRE-EXPERIMENTAL RESEARCH

Campbell and Stanley (1963) first time use pre-experimental design considered very weak with little or not control over the research. Their use is strongly discouraged because they do not permit even remote inference about the direction and dynamic of change and causality. The validity of pre-experimental designs is threatened by inadequate control during implementation of intervention. Therefore, researchers should be especially cautious when interpreting and generalizing the results of pre-experimental research.

Types of Pre-experimental Designs

The following types of pre-experimental design are possible:
1. One Group Pretest Post-test Design
2. Single Group Post-test only Design
3. Static Groups Comparison.

One Group Pretest Post-test Design

In this design, only one group will be observed before and after the intervention is introduced. This is weakest type of experimental design. The one-group pretest post-test design is employed when the nurse investigator does not have access to an equivalent group and cannot use random assignment. The design lacking two important characteristics of experimentation—randomization and control over the extraneous variables. Although, lack of the control group decreases the usefulness of the study but it is a good choice where it is not possible or feasible to create control group.

Box 7.12: Example of One Group Pretest Post-test Design.

'A pre-experimental study to see the effect of yoga exercise on blood pressure reduction in the elderly'.
(Windartik E, et al. 2018)

In this study, researcher selects a group of elderly with hypertension and administers yoga therapy as defined in the protocol. Once the treatment is over, post-test is collected and compared to pretest findings to conclude the study findings.

NR   E O_1 X O_2

In above said example, researcher select a group of elderly with hypertension and administers yoga therapy as defined in the protocol. Once the treatment is over, post-test is collected and compared with pretest to find the difference in the findings.

Single Group Post-test Only Design

It is also known as *one shot case study design*. It is useful in studying naturally occurring events that could not be manipulated by the nurse investigator. In this study, a group of respondents are identified based on one or more preexisting criteria and are administered questionnaire that is then measured. In this design, a treatment is given and measurement is made. This is considered weakest design among all because of no control on selection of participants in the study. Most of surveys can be characterized as one shot case studies.

Box 7.13: Example of Single Group Post-test only Design.

'A study to determine the impacts of use of simulation based hand hygiene practices on infection load at high dependency unit at a tertiary care hospital, North India'.

E   X O_1

Static Groups Comparison

It is also called *two group post-test only design without random assignment*. In static group comparison, a group which is already exposed to an intervention is compared to another group which is not. This will help to determine the effect of intervention by comparing the difference between two groups. There is nor pretest in this design. The design use two naturally occurring groups. The merits of static group comparison lies to compare different practices and to make conclusion for best one. However, this design is discouraged due to lack of evidence about group equivalence information.

> **Box 7.14:** Example of Static Groups Comparison.
>
> 'A study examined the effect of intravasation in women undergoing hysteroscopic procedure. An intervention group with intrauterine pressure during hysteroscopy was compared to a control group. Results reveals significant reduction in complication in intervention group.' (Bennet, et al. 1996)
>
> NR $\dfrac{E \quad\quad \ldots\ldots \quad\quad X \quad\quad O_1}{C \quad\quad \ldots\ldots \quad\quad XO \quad\quad O_1}$

Strengths of Pre-experimental Research
- These studies are convenient to conduct in natural setting where true experiment not feasible
- It is safe, simple and less expensive research design
- A large group of people can be easily studied and hence, less time consuming.

Limitations of Pre-experimental Research
- It is considered weak design to establish cause and effect relationship between independent and dependent variables
- It has higher threat to internal validity
- It has very little control over the research variables
- Higher risk of erroneous interpretation of results.

NON-EXPERIMENTAL DESIGNS

Non-experimental study do not have manipulation of independent variables, control group and random assignment of subjects to control and experimental groups. These research study the variables in naturally occurring setting to describe or explore the variables under study. A researcher may go for non-experimental studies because multiple reasons. First, it is not possible to manipulate few variables in controlled conditions. Second, a number of variable not amenable to experimental manipulation. Third, ethical issues do not allow to manipulate many variables, etc. Non-experimental design is somewhat similar to Post-test design where the independent variable or outcome is already present and you have to measure it. Non-experimental designs are focused to describe, explore and compare the underlying construct in the study.

Non-experimental research is quite popular in nursing. In trying to determine client's perceptions of pain, the only way to obtain this information would be to ask the client about their pain rather than going for an experimental study would not be an appropriate idea.

Types of Non-experimental Research

Many scholars classified the non-experimental research in their own ways. Still, there is lack of consensus for classification of non-experimental research. A more simplified classification non-experimental research is given in Table 7.1.

Table 7.1: Classification of non-experimental research.

Broad categories	Types of research designs
Descriptive research	• Univariate descriptive designs • Comparative studies • Exploratory studies
Epidemiological research	• Case control studies (retrospective studies) • Correlational studies • Cohort studies (prospective studies) • Cross-sectional studies
Developmental research/time related studies	• Longitudinal studies • Cross-sectional studies
Survey research	• Different types of surveys, i.e. descriptive, comparative, evaluative, correlational, and exploratory, etc.
Other research designs	• Evaluative studies • Meta-analysis • Ex-post facto design • Secondary analysis • Methodological studies • Cross legged panel design

DESCRIPTIVE RESEARCH

It is a broad class of non-experimental research. The basic purpose of descriptive studies to observe, describes, and documents aspects of a situation without undue manipulation in natural setting. Three basic research designs are undertaken in descriptive studies: Univariate descriptive studies, exploratory studies and comparative studies.

Univariate Descriptive Designs

The aim of descriptive research is to describe the frequency of occurrence of behavior or condition rather than to study relationship. Two types of descriptive studies come from the field of epidemiology: *Prevalence studies* and *incidence studies*.

1. *Prevalence studies:* The primary purpose of prevalence study on estimation of prevalence rate of a disease (e.g. stroke, epilepsy, etc.) or condition (e.g. smoking, substance abuse, etc.). Usually, prevalence studies are cross-sectional in nature and obtained data from population at risk.

Box 7.15: Prevalence Rate.

$$PR = \frac{\text{Number of cases with the condition or disease at a given point in time}}{\text{Number in the population at risk of being a case}} \times K$$

K is the number of people for whom we want to have the prevalence rate (e.g. 100, 1000 or lakhs, etc.)

---

2. *Incidence studies:* Incidence studies estimate the occurrence of number of new cases of condition at a time.

> **Box 7.16:** Incidence Rate.
>
> $$IR = \frac{\text{Number of new cases with the condition or disease over a given period of time}}{\text{Number in the population at risk of being a case}} \times K$$
>
> K is the number of people for whom we want to have the incidence rate (e.g. 100, 1000 or lakhs, etc.)

Comparative Designs

Comparative studies also known as *ex-post facto* or *casual-comparative studies*. The primary purpose of comparative studies is to describe and compare the difference in variables between two unit, cases or groups in naturally occurring setting. Comparative study state the hypothesis to test the difference between two or more than two units or groups. Comparative studies do not have control group.

Comparative studies can be qualitative and quantitative. Comparative studies are usually field studies in which the independent variable already exits and the sample is selected on the basis of the independent variable.

In the comparative descriptive design, control over the data is accomplished through the subject's selection methods, the situations under which variables are observed and measured.

> **Box 7.17:** Examples of Comparative Study.
>
> Aggarwal A, et al. (2012) used a comparative study design to compare the knowledge, attitudes and behavior of dental and nursing students towards HIV/AIDS. This questionnaire based survey included a total of 300 nursing and dental students. Results concluded that dental students have significantly greater knowledge than nursing students. However, both nursing and dental students had very good attitude regarding the known patient of HIV/AIDS. A few misconceptions were reported common in nursing and dental students.

Exploratory Designs

Exploratory research provides an in-depth explanation of a single event, case or variable. Such as job satisfaction or role conflict. For example, you might be trying to examine the caregiving needs of the family members of stroke patient. You will conduct a literature search to know a bit more about the phenomena to fame research questionnaire or checklist. It is likely that you would find a brief information on the topic. An exploratory research would be best solution to explore the phenomena in depth.

Use of flexible approach is much more useful than structured approach to collect data (mixed approach). Sometimes, qualitative information also collected in exploratory study. Usually, hypotheses are not prepared in exploratory study.

> **Box 7.18:** Example of Exploratory Research.
>
> Kumar R, et al. (2016) used an exploratory research design to identify the family needs of the caregivers of stroke survivors in a selected community setting, Punjab. Hundred participants were enrolled purposively. Modified family needs questionnaire (FNQ) was used to identify the needs of the caregivers. Results concluded that 'Health information', 'Professional support' and 'Involvement of care' sub scales were the most important needs areas of the caregivers. Study recommended that assessment of family needs amongst the caregivers of individuals with stroke is important for all health care professionals in understanding problems from the caregivers' perspective.

EPIDEMIOLOGICAL RESEARCH

The purpose of epidemiological approach is to study the distribution and determinants of health problems in groups or populations. A nurse also use epidemiological research to collect information on different hospital and community indicators. The community health nurses must therefore become familiar with both epidemiological literature and clinical nursing research in order to integrate both into practice. This section provides an overview of different types of epidemiological designs used in nursing.

Descriptive Studies

Descriptive studies focus on description of distribution of disease, health outcomes, morbidity and mortality in a defined population in a period. These studies report the phenomena in terms of Who, What and Where. Descriptive study describes a phenomenon with the help of frequency, percentage, incidence rate, mortality and prevalence rate, etc. Descriptive studies also help to show trends of a specific health problem or outcome in a defined population over a period of time.

> **Box 7.19:** Example of Descriptive Study.
>
> Patten SB, et al. (2006) used descriptive epidemiological approach to estimate the life time prevalence of depression in population aged 15 years or over living in private occupied dwelling. Every alternate house was selected through random approach. The survey concluded that overall prevalence of major depressive episode (MDE) was 4.8% (95% CI, 4.5–5.1%). The life time prevalence was 12.2% (95% CI, 11.7–12.7%).

Correlational Research

In correlational research, the focus is to examine the strength of relationships between two or more than two variables. Further, it examine that how changes in one variable is associated with change in another variable and in which direction (positive or negative). A correlation indicates degree to which one variable (A) is related to another variable (B). Further, relationship between two variable may be negative (–) or positive (+). This relationship range from +1.00 (perfect positive) to –1.00 (perfect negative). However, correlation research never answer causation of this relationship between variables.

Types of Correlational Research

- *Simple correlation studies:* It helps to examine the relationship between two or more variables in a single group of subjects. A relationship between two or more variables does not mean one causes the other, e.g. a study to assess the effectiveness of teaching methods and student performance.
- *Prediction studies:* It examines the predictive nature of the relationship between the variables. It is further classified into two studies which are as follows:

> **Box 7.20:** Example of Prediction Research.
>
> 1. Simple predictive studies: The performance of one variable is used to predict the performance on another variable.
>   A correlational study on psychological factors as predictors of suicidal ideation among adolescents in Malaysia.
>   **(Ibrahim N, et al. 2014)**

Contd...

Contd...

> 2. Multiple predictive studies: It examines the impact of multiple variables on a single variable.
>   – A correlation study on depression and quality of life in caregivers of individuals with mental illness.
>   *(Aarti, Ruchika, Kumar R, 2018)*
>   – A correlation study on personality traits, academic stress and adjustment styles among nursing students.
>   *(Kumar R, 2018)*

Strengths of Correlational Research

The strength of correlational design lies in the followings:
- Correlational study are relatively uncomplicated to plan and implement
- The researcher has flexibility in exploring relationships among two or more variables
- The outcome of correlational study have practical implications in nursing practice
- Correlation studies provides framework for examining relationship between variables that cannot be manipulated for practical or ethical reason
- An effective and efficient method of collecting a large amount of data about an issue of interest
- Explore direction and strength of relationship between variables.

Limitations of Correlational Research

- The researcher is unable to determine the causal relationship between the variables: why one variable cause change in another variable
- Correlational designs lack control and randomization between the variables, therefore, researcher unable to draw solid conclusion for their research.

ANALYTICAL STUDIES

Analytical studies are next version of epidemiological research focus on determinants of pattern—the how and why. These studies identify the factors, determinants, characteristics or behavior might responsible for particular pattern of health outcomes in a study population. An election polls or survey are example of cross-sectional study.

> **Box 7.21:** Analytical Studies.
>
> 1. Cross-sectional study (Prevalence study)
> 2. Case-control study (Retrospective, Case comparison)
> 3. Prospective cohort (Concurrent cohort, Longitudinal follow-up)
> 4. Retrospective cohort (Nonconcurrent cohort)

Case-control Designs (Retrospective Design)

In case-control study, a researcher select a case with and without exposure to a particular disease or event of interest and go backward in their history to find out that how these two cases were different in regards to possible exposure and occurrence of a disease.

Strengths of Case-control Designs

- Case-control approach do not expose a case to unnecessary risk
- Case-control approach is helpful to study a rare case phenomena.

Limitation of Case-control Designs
Case-control studies are more prone to susceptibility and observation bias.

Box 7.22: Example of Case-control Study.

Marcin JP, et al. (2005) used a case control approach to determine the association between unplanned extubation and years of experience and nurse to patient ratio in pediatric intensive care unit (PICU). Unplanned extubations were identified from January 1999 through December 2002. Three control patients for each of the patients experiencing an unplanned extubation were selected on three matching factors: age, intubation duration, and severity of illness as defined by the Pediatric Risk of Mortality (PRISM) III. Study concluded that pediatric patients are more likely to experience an unplanned extubation when being cared for by a nurse assigned to two patients compared with a nurse caring for one patient.

Cohort Designs (Prospective Design)

Cohort refers to a group of people share common characteristics. These characteristics might be their date of birth, place of loving or something collectively happen to the group. These studies are prospective and longitudinal in nature in which a researcher look forward and track a cohort for health and illness trends for a longer period. The cohort will also be traced for possible factors that might be responsible to the trends in health and illness (Fig. 7.3).

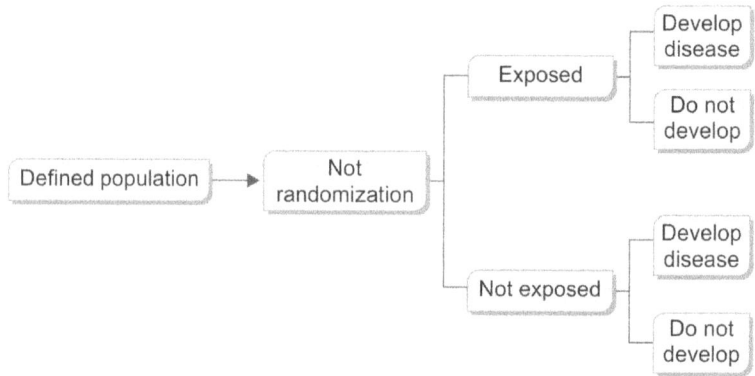

Fig. 7.3: Process of cohort studies.

Box 7.23: Example of Cohort Study.

Thai nurses—cohort study is a longitudinal prospective cohort study initiated in 2009 and expected to run until 2027. Cohort comprised Thai nurses holding registration in nursing and midwifery in Nursing and Midwifery Registration Council, Thailand. The study first round used self-administered questionnaire to elicit response on intention to leave their nursing carrier and associated factors. *(Sawaengdee K, et al. 2016)*

■ DEVELOPMENTAL RESEARCH

The purpose of developmental research is to assess changes over an extended period of time. It is a non-experimental research approach that not only examines the present status of the variables and progressive developmental changes in variable over a period of time. It is further classified here:

Longitudinal Design

A design in which nurse investigator study the same subjects or the same population over a period of time to study the emergence of disease or long-term effects of treatment. Subjects are followed over a period of time and data collection occurs at prescribed intervals over the period.

Box 7.24: Example of Longitudinal Study.

DiMattio MK, et al. (2003) used a single-group longitudinal design to describes changes in functional status and the influence of comorbidity, household composition, fatigue, and surgical pain on functional status in women during the first 6 weeks at home following coronary artery bypass surgery. Women were interviewed in person before hospital discharge and by telephone at 2, 4, and 6 weeks after discharge. Results revealed that women experienced significant gains in functional status over 6 weeks, particularly between 2 and 4 weeks. They engaged most frequently in personal care and low-level household activities during the study period, and most reported improvement in their overall functional status.

Longitudinal studies may be of following types:
- *Trend studies:* Trend studies are investigation in which samples from a defined population are studied over a period of time with respect to some phenomena. The long-term trends in the use of a particular intervention or nursing care technique could be researched using trend techniques. These studies enable a researcher to examine pattern of change, rate and to predict future prediction.
- *Panel studies:* Panel is a group of people providing information on a phenomena. Panel studies use the same respondents at each progressive time period for providing information about the underlying phenomena. It is longitudinal and prospective in nature. Panel studies naturally yield more information than trend studies. However, limitation of panel studies are lies in subjectivity and maturational bias.
- *Follow-up studies:* Follow-up studies are similar to panel studies and are used to determine subsequent change after administering a specific intervention. For example, follow-up of stroke patients at outpatient department for subsequent recovery or deterioration in health status.

Strengths of Longitudinal Study
- Longitudinal studies are good choice to study a developmental or historical trends
- These types of studies are cost-effective and cost-efficient
- These studies enables a researcher to establish cause-effect relationship
- Longitudinal studies are appropriate to study the dynamics of a phenomenon or concept.

Limitations of Longitudinal Study
- These studies are more prone for higher sample attrition rate
- It takes very long-time to complete
- Large sample size are expensive to access
- Long-time nature of study can create problem of maintaining records of information
- Longitudinal study are not easy to design and plan.

Cross-sectional Design

A cross-sectional design is one in which data are collected from different groups of people who are at different stage in their experience of the phenomena at same time. However, cross-sectional design allow researcher to access a cross section of the population. Cross-sectional design are appropriate for describing the status of phenomena or for describing relationship among phenomena at a fixed point in time. These deigns helpful to study a large population in very less time.

> **Box 7.25:** Example of Cross-sectional Design.
>
> Kumar R, et al. (2014) in a cross-sectional survey to identify the caregiving needs, burden, coping styles and health related quality of life in caregivers of stroke survivors. Using Purposive sampling techniques, 22 caregivers of survivors of stroke were interviewed. Results shows that Health Information (HI) related needs were most important followed by seeking need of Professional Support (PS), and need of having a Community Support Network (CSN). Caregivers reported higher level of burden in financial area followed by burden in terms of disturbed relationship. Acceptance was most frequently used coping strategies reported by caregivers followed by problem solving and distraction positive. Study reported good quality of social life in caregivers.

Strengths of Cross-sectional Studies
- Cross-sectional studies are quick, easy to do and inexpensive
- It is comparatively easy to design and plan
- It helps to study a large population in limited time
- Study cover a large population, hence, chance of generalization of findings will be more.

Limitations of Cross-sectional Studies
- Cross-sectional studies fail to establish cause and effect relationship
- These studies are more for selection bias
- Cross-sectional studies are not a good choice to study a rare disease, concept or phenomena.

SURVEY RESEARCH

Survey is old and ancient in use as long as mankind has been in existence. Survey studies are commonly undertaken in nursing and social sciences. In fact, everyone who is going through this content has been involved in some kind of survey.

Survey is the use of self-report methods to collect the information on variables of interest. A judicious use of sampling technique and large sample size enable a researcher to generalize the findings. Surveys conducted for fulfilling different purposes. However, use of survey in assessment of knowledge, attitude, opinion, and perception is common. A clinical nurse may also employ survey to identify nursing needs of the patients, satisfaction to nursing care, and perception of hospital services, etc.

Survey may be conducted by using telephone, mail, online (web-survey) or through personal contact. Questionnaires and interviews are the most preferred methods used in survey research. Cross-sectional and longitudinal approach are common in surveys to study the participants.

Types of Survey
According to the objective of survey, it can be classified as follows:
- *Descriptive survey:* It is used to describe a phenomena. It describe the question in terms of what, when, where, and what. However, it does not answer *'why'* of a question. It usually collect the information about the concept in natural setting.

- *Correlational survey:* It collect information on multiple variables at a time. Therefore, enables the nurse investigator to find relationship between variables.
- *Comparative survey:* This survey used to collect and compare information of two or more groups at one or more than one variables.
- *Cross-sectional survey:* It is used to collect information on a population at a single point of time. This design is useful to take a snap shot or cross-section of a population at a time.
- *Exploratory survey:* This survey approach is good to study a concept about which little is known. Exploratory survey helps to provide an in-depth detail about the concept of interest.
- *Explanatory survey:* It provides fundamental explanations of a phenomenon or circumstances. The nurse investigator should be familiar with the literature to identify the fundamental relationship specific to the projects as it involves hypothesis testing.
- *Evaluative survey:* Evaluative survey determine how well a program, policy or practice is going on. The major objective of this survey is to determine the progress of a program. This survey helps to provide information on why a particular program was failed or successful.
- *Longitudinal survey:* It is used to gather data over period of time. These surveys are particularly helpful for assessment of developmental or historical trends.

Strengths of Survey
- Survey is easy to design and plan
- Survey is a good source for developing hypothesis
- Survey help a researcher to study a large population in a limited time frame
- Survey helps to provide a large volume of information
- A higher degree of representativeness make the findings more generalizable on other population.

Box 7.26: Examples of Survey.

- A descriptive survey to assess stress and coping strategies among nursing students at a selected nursing institute, Punjab, India. (Descriptive Survey)   *(Kumar R, et al. 2011)*
- A cross-sectional survey to identify needs, burden and coping strategies among caregivers of stroke survivors at selected community settings, Amritsar Punjab. (Cross-sectional Survey)
  (Kumar R, et al. 2014)
- A longitudinal survey to observe changes in perception of nursing students towards care of a HIV patient at AIIMS Rishikesh, Uttarakhand (Longitudinal Survey)*
- An exploratory survey to determine family needs of caregivers of stroke survivors at selected community settings, Punjab India. (Exploratory Survey)   *(Kumar R, et al. 2016)*
- A correlational survey on academic climate, academic stress and self esteem among baccalaureate nursing students at AIIMS Rishikesh, Uttarakhand. (Correlational Survey)   *(Kumar R, et al. 2018)*
- A comparative survey to find out the level of satisfaction among patient attending psychiatric and medicine out patient services at AIIMS Rishikesh, Uttarakhand. (Comparative Survey)

Note: *Hypothetical statements

Limitations of Survey
- Survey only provide a superficial background information about the concept
- Survey do not have control over extraneous variables and bias may be possible
- Survey is not feasible for a small sample size study
- Survey not helpful to establish cause and effect relationship

- Survey only relies information accessed through closed ended questionnaires or checklist, hence response are often limited.

ADDITIONAL TYPES OF QUANTITATIVE RESEARCH

There are some other research designs used in social and allied health sciences. Although, some scholars categorized theses design under non-experimental studies but on the other hands they are kept separate from any classification. These designs are discussed in this sections.

Evaluative Studies

Evaluative studies have great importance in current era of evidence-based practice. Patient centered care and consumer awareness also influence the importance of evaluative studies over other types of research. Clinicians can reflect upon their practice and refine as per the research evidences. Evaluative studies tend to focus on a particular practice, policy or event. They are normally carried out when the researcher wants to find out if, how and what extent the objectives of particular interventions have been met or are being met. These interventions could be provision of a service, a teaching program or a series of therapeutic session.

Box 7.27: Example of Evaluative Study.

Gupta SN, et al. (2007) conducted an evaluative survey to assess—(1) treatment outcomes of Revised National Tuberculosis Program (RNTCP), (2) to identify gaps and underlying contributing factors and (3) to suggest appropriate measures to minimize the gaps. A system approach was used to record inputs, processes and outputs of the program and its outcomes.

Meta-analysis

Meta-analysis is a statistical technique which involves taking the findings from several studies on the same subjects or topic and analyzing them using standardized statistical procedures (Polit and Beck, 2006).

Box 7.28: Example of Meta-analysis.

Darvishi N, et al. (2015) in a meta-analysis investigated the effect of alcohol use disorder (AUD) on suicidal thought and behavior. The main bibliographic data bases, including PubMed, Scopus, and web of science, were searched until February 2015. Cross-sectional, cohort and case control studies were included in the meta-anaylsis,. Finally, 31 studies out of 8548 full text retrieved studies were included in the analysis. Results depicted that there was a significant association between AUD and suicidal ideation (OR = 1.86; 95% CI:1.38, 2.35), suicide attempt (OR = 3.13; 95% CI:2.45, 3.81) and completed suicide (OR = 2.59, 95% CI:1.95, 3.23 and RR =1.74; 95% CI:1.26, 2.21). Therefore, meta-analysis found that AUD can be considered an important predictor of suicide.

A meta-analysis involves an examination of studies conducted in a particular area to try to better understand the overall outcomes of available research. Criteria are usually developed regarding the research methods used. It is extremely useful in health care for judging the clinical and practical significance of any effects the intervention may have had. The challenge of meta-analysis is to find a sufficient number of studies that used similar populations and measures.

Meta-synthesis

Meta-synthesis is used to integrate the findings of qualitative studies. It is a non-statistical techniques used to integrate, evaluate and interpret the findings. Meta-synthesis helps to detect and depict a common them from a pool of studies. Meta-synthesis is preferred for phenomenology, grounded theory and ethnography.

> **Box 7.29:** Example of Meta-synthesis.
>
> LeSure P, et al. (2015) in a meta-synthesis explore the explore the experience of caregivers who were caring for cancer patients, including their perceptions and responses to the situation and describe the context and phenomenon relevent to the experince. Five databases were used: CINAHL, MEDLINE, Academic Search, Science Direct, and a Thai database known as the Thai Library Integrated System (ThaiLIS). Three sets of the context of the experience and the phenomena relevant to the experience were described. The contexts were (1) having a hard time dealing with emotional devastation; (2) knowing that the caregiving job was laborious; and (3) knowing that I was not alone. The phenomenon showed the progress of the caregivers' thoughts and actions. A general phenomenon of the experience—balancing my emotion—applied to most of the caregivers; whereas, more specific phenomenon—keeping life as normal as possible and lifting life above the illness—were experienced by a lesser number of the caregivers. This review added a more thorough explanation of the issues involved in caregiving for cancer patients.

Secondary Analysis

The secondary analysis of the existing data has become rapidly popular in health sciences. Secondary analysis is a useful research strategy which makes use of pre-existing findings to test new research question or hypotheses. Secondary analysis can be used for both quantitative or qualitative findings. However, a researcher has to prepare a fresh proposal with different research questions and hypotheses. Previous data are re-examined and re-analyzed by using desired statistical techniques. Secondary analysis helpful in number of ways. It helps to re-examine the existing research projects to serve new and important purposes. It may be helpful to examine the unanalyzed concepts, subsample or a particular unit of existing data. A researcher can choose 'researcher question driven' or 'data driven' approach for analysing the existing data. The analysis of data is cost-effective in terms of time and money. However, sometimes choice of variables were not available for the analysis. Social surveys, census, institutional administrative records and public records would be best used in secondary research.

Methodological Studies

In present era of evidence-based nursing (EBN), nurse investigators become increasingly interested in conducting methodological research. Methodological research use to develop and evaluate data collection tools, instruments, protocol or techniques. Methodological research are differ to other routine research because it does not follow all steps of research process. These research focus on development of a valid and reliable instrument to measure a construct under study. However, these studies are time consuming and laborious in nature.

> **Box 7.30:** Steps in Methodological Research.
>
> - Selection and definition of construct or behavior under study
> - Formulation of items for instrument development
> - Writing instruction for users and respondents
> - Testing the validity and reliability of the instrument

> **Box 7.31:** Example of Methodological Study.
>
> Bandana, et al. (2009) used a methodological research design to develop an audit tool to audit the family health records. The audit tool developed in six phases. This developed tool was used to audit 500 family folders to check their content and construct validity. This study has made a significant contribution to evaluate the family health records maintained by the nursing students of NINE, PGIMER, Chandigarh with minimum time.

QUALITATIVE RESEARCH DESIGN

Qualitative research design is a form of social inquiry that focuses on the way people interpret and make sense of their experiences and the world in which they live. It is used to gain insight into people's attitudes, behaviors, value systems, concerns, motivations, aspirations, culture or lifestyles and what lies at the core of their lives. Qualitative research methods have become increasingly important as a way of developing nursing knowledge for evidence-based nursing practice. Qualitative research answers a wide variety of questions related to nursing's concern with human responses to actual or potential health problems (Ploeg J, 1999).

The intent of qualitative research is to gather data that illuminate the meaning of an event or phenomenon. The main purpose is to develop an understanding of meaning from the informants point of views. Qualitative research has been called constructivist research because it is grounded in the assumption that individuals construct reality in the form of meaning and interpretation.

There is no universally accepted definition of qualitative research, because it is a field of enquiry rather than a single entity. Qualitative research is a broad term for a variety of research approaches, just as quantitative research that encompasses a variety of research designs, such as experimental, non-experimental designs and surveys.

According to Denzin and Lincoln (1994), qualitative research focuses on interpretation of phenomena in their natural settings to make sense in terms of the meanings people bring to these settings. Qualitative research involves collecting information about personal experiences, introspection, life story, interviews, observations, historical, interactions and visual text which are significant moments and meaningful in peoples' lives.

Qualitative research seeks to provide understanding of human experience, perceptions, motivations, intentions, and behaviors based on description, observation and utilizing a naturalistic interpretative approach to a subject and its contextual setting (Encyclopedia.com 2009).

Validity of Qualitative Research Study

Quality is as important to qualitative work as it to quantitative work. *Rigor* is the term used to describe both the process and end product of qualitative research. Morse (2003) said that rigors refers to appropriateness of methods and design adopted for qualitative research. Linconn and Guba (1989) state that trustworthiness involves the following elements: credibility, dependability, conformability and generalizability.

Credibility (Internal Validity)

Credibility refers how extensively research methods raise the confidence in the truth of data and in the researcher's interpretation in the findings.

Credibility may be sought by using following measures:
- Prolonged engagement in the field of setting
- Triangulation
  - *Investigator triangulation:* A type of triangulation in which more than one investigator used to collect, analysis or interpret a set of data.
  - *Theory triangulation:* A type of triangulation in which multiple perspective are obtained and used from other researcher or published literature.
  - *Method triangulation:* A use of multiple data collection method (e.g. interviews, observation and document review) results in method triangulation.
- Peer debriefing
- Persistent observation
- Negative case analysis (e.g. search and account disconfirming data)
- Member checking: A method of ensuring validity by having participants review and comment on the accuracy of transcripts, interpretation, or conclusions.

Dependability (Reliability)

Findings of the study need to be consistent and correct to be dependable, so that anyone reading the study will be able to evaluate the self-sufficiency of the analysis and results from the research process. For dependability, an auditor can inspect the inquiry process (audit trail) and the records relating to the inquiry in order to judge its authenticity. An audit trail is a through, conscientious reflection on and documentation of the decision that were made, the procedure that were designed, and the questions that were raised during analysis of data.

Transferability (Generalizability)

Transferability is equivalent to generalizability in quantitative research. Transferability refers to application of findings of one qualitative study to similar other population in different situation. Although, quantitative research use many measures such as use of purposeful sampling and sample size estimation to improve generalizability. However, use of these measures are not possible in qualitative research. In qualitative research, following measures are use to improve transferability:
- *Thick description* refers to provision of detailed database. It provide rich description of experiences shared by the people under study. Rich description is a vehicle to communicating to the reader a realistic and holistic picture
- The concept of applicability (applying result of a study to another population when the sample is very similar)
- *Fittingness:* When findings fit into contexts different from the research situation and other find the findings meaningful and applicable to their own experiences.

Confirmability (Objectivity)

Confirmability refers to measures used to attain objectivity in qualitative research. However, confirmability is never fully achieved in any types of research. The *reflexive journal* and *audit trail* are two important strategy to achieve the objectivity in qualitative research. These strategies helps to schedule the activities, maintain log of data collection and methods used and personal reflections.

Types of Qualitative Research

Qualitative research are commonly used to explore health or illness related issues about which very little is known. It also used to develop insight about previously explored issue or concept. The methods used in qualitative research are less structured and primarily includes participant observation, detail interview, narrative records, and handwritten diary and notes, etc. The following qualitative designs are commonly used in nursing and allied health profession.
- Phenomenology
- Ethnography
- Grounded theory
- Historical research
- Case study
- Action research

PHENOMENOLOGY

Edmund Husserl proposed the concept of descriptive phenomenology. Later on, Husserl and Heidegger developed an approach to study the life experiences of people. Typically, phenomenology deals with the human experiences as described by people involved. These experiences are called lived experiences. The phenomenologist investigates subjective phenomena in the belief that essential truths about reality are grounded in people lived experiences. The goal of phenomenological studies is to gives the meaning to experiences hold for each subject. Phenomenology in nursing is well suited to the investigation of experiences important to nursing practice.

Phenomenological studies are primarily relying on in-depth interview for data collection, but they may go beyond a traditional approach to gather and analyze data. Phenomenologies are limited to small sample size (usually 10 or fewer).

Definitions

'The study of people's conscious experience of their life-world, that is, their everyday life and social action'. *(Schram, 2003)*

'Phenomenology is defined as research methodology that is rigorous, critical, and systematic in its investigations of a human experience in context'. *(Fain, 2009)*

'Phenomenology is an investigation of the meaning of an experience among a group that has lived through it'.

Types of Phenomenology

Phenomenology has two main school of thoughts: (1) Descriptive phenomenology and (2) Interpretive phenomenology (hermeneutics).

Descriptive Phenomenology

Descriptive phenomenology was proposed by Husserl (1962). Descriptive phenomenology concerned to careful description of usual day-to-day life experiences. For example, hearing, seeing, feeling, remembering and acting, etc. Descriptive phenomenology studies often involves following four steps:
1. *Bracketing:* It is the process of identifying and holding in abeyance preconceived belief and opinions about the phenomena under study. Although, it is very difficult to achieve complete bracketing in descriptive phenomenology.

2. *Intuiting:* Intuiting occurs when researchers' remain open to the meaning attributed to the phenomena by those who experienced it.
3. *Analysis:* It is the process of analysis of phenomenological findings. It consists extracting information, making category, and giving the phenomena essential meaning.
4. *Describing:* Phenomenologist describe the experiences what he/she collected from a group of people involved.

Interpretive Phenomenology

Heidegger (1962) given the concept of interpretive phenomenology. He shifted his focus on interpretation and insight development of experience to unveil otherwise concealed meaning in the phenomena. His assumption is that lived experience is inherently an interactive process and everyone has different meaning for it. The interpretive phenomenology interprets the experience and infers the meaning of experience for an individual. Interpretive phenomenology is a valuable method for the study of phenomena related to nursing practice education and research.

Interpretative phenomenology studies rely primarily on in-depth interviews with the individual who have experienced the phenomena of interest.

Steps of Phenomenology Studies

- *Study of phenomena of interest:* The researcher needs to understand the philosophical perspectives behind the approach, especially the concept of studying how people experience a phenomenon. A detail knowledge of phenomena of interest will develop insight to explore the phenomena in-depth.
- *Writing research question:* The investigator writes research questions that can explore the meaning of life experiences for individuals and asks individuals to describe their everyday lived experience.
- *Data collection:* The investigator collects data from individuals who have experienced the phenomenon under investigation. Typically, this information is collected through detail and in-depth interviews.
- *The phenomenological data analysis:* The protocols are divided into statements or horizonalization, the units are transformed into clusters of meaning, tie the transformation together to make a general description of the experience, including textural description, what is experienced and structural description, i.e. how it is experienced.
- *Report writing:* The phenomenological report ends with the reader underlying better the essential, invariant structure of the experience.

Box 7.32: Example of Phenomenology Study.

Cassol H, et al. (2018) conducted a phenomenology to explore near death experience (NDE) in 34 cardiac arrest survivors. Participants are requested to complete sociodemographic information (gender and age at interview), their age when they experienced the NDE, the time elapsed since the NDE and if the NDE has occurred during a life-threatening event. The Greyson NDE scale was then used to identify the presence of a NDE. Apart from this, participants were asked to write a detailed narrative of their experience. Triangulation, theoretical validation and an iterative process was followed to test validity of data. The analysis conducted on the 34 narratives distinguishes 11 main themes, among which we identified 10 timebounded themes and 1 transversal theme. The division of narratives into themes provides detailed information about the vocabulary used by NDEs to describe their experience.

Strengths of Phenomenology
- It is valuable tool to understand the meaning of life experiences of people involved in research
- Phenomenological findings helps to contribute in development of nursing theories.
- It helps to collect a real life experiences of people.

Limitations of Phenomenology
- Data collection and analysis is a laborious task and need lot of time and money
- A researcher has to develop different skills to conduct interview and elicit accurate information on life experiences
- The analysis and interpretation of data required special skill and may be a challenging task for a researcher
- Data interpretation may influenced by personal bias and prejudice of a researcher.

Table 7.2: Qualitative research overview.

Type	Question	Focus
Phenomenology	What is the life experience of people undergoing chemotherapy?	Summary of experiences
Grounded theory	What are the process by which elderly with depression live happily?	Concept and theory building
Ethnography	What are the practice, value and belief of people living in Himalayan region?	Describe experience of a particular culture

ETHNOGRAPHY

Ethnography is one of the oldest qualitative research approach. This qualitative research approach focus on study of social interaction, behavior, and perception of a group, team, society or communities. The assumption underlying this approach is that every individual or group evolve a culture that guide the individual to structure their experience and view about others. Ethnography is a form of social research encompass explanation of a social concepts, unstructured data and interpretation of meaning of human action. It focus on describing a culture and to understand another way of life from the (other person's) point of view (Spradley, 1980).

It is a qualitative approach examine the cultural patterns and perspectives of participants in their natural settings. Ethnographers seek to learn from members of a cultural group to understand theirs's world view. Ethnographic researchers sometimes refer to *'emic'* and *'etic'* perspectives. An *emic* perspective refers to the way the members of the culture perceive their world (insiders view). The *emic* is the local language, concepts or means of expression used by the members of the group under study. The *etic* perspective, by contrast, is the outsider's interpretation of the experiences of the culture under study.

Definitions

'Ethnography is a descriptive account of social life and culture in a particular social system based on detailed observations of what people actually do. It is a research method that is used by sociologists often when studying groups, organizations, and communities that are a part of a larger complex society.' *(Crossman A, 2013)*

'A qualitative research approach that emphasizes observation in the natural environment and that focuses on detailed and accurate description of reality in term of the people being observed.' *(Rubin, 2009)*

Box 7.33: Salient Features of Ethnographic Study.

- With its origins in anthropology, ethnography is the study of social interactions, behaviours and perceptions that occur within groups, organisations and communities
- Ethnography has an underlying research methodology and an associated toolbox of methods (participant observations, interviews, documents) which shape both and generate detailed understanding of the social action
- Ethnographers employ a number of key techniques (e.g. thick description, reflexivity, triangulation) to enhance the quality of their work
- Ethnographic research has generated a number of insightful accounts into the development and delivery of medical education.

Box 7.34: Example of Ethnographic Study.

Seabrook's (2004) work was part of a longitudinal ethnographic study of a single UK medical school between 1995 and 2000. A grounded theory approach was used to develop themes. Seabrook observed curriculum committees, teaching, assessment and evaluation activities; conducted in-depth semi-structured interviews with doctors and students; and participated in informal discussions with staff and students. The major themes reported included teachers' concerns about the students, the infrastructure for teaching and their relationship with the medical school.

Ethnographic studies limited to a small sample size (20–25). An ethnographer need to record a variety of elements in their field notes. Use of participant observation, direct engagement and involvement with people under study are common methods to collect information. Ethnographer routinely use conversational or informal interview to discuss, probe or to ask question about unusual event in natural setting. Use of 'casual' interview approach helps to elicit highly sincere explanations from individuals. Ethnographers also gather formal in-depth interviews and documentary data such as minutes of meetings, diaries, artifacts, and photographs. Participants or situations are sampled on an opportunistic or purposive basis. Use of triangulation and reflexivity in ethnography are important key elements used to establish rigor/quality of data. A details of triangulation method in ethnography is given in box.

Box 7.35: Triangulation in Ethnography (Denzin, 1970).

- *Data triangulation* involves the use of different sources of data to examine phenomenon across settings and at different points in time
- *Method triangulation* entails the use of multiple research methods to compare and contrast different insights each method may provide
- *Investigator triangulation* involves different investigators gathering data to produce more complex empirical explanations by understanding possible differences
- *Theory triangulation* use different concepts and theoretical perspectives to see how each illuminates the data in different ways

Strengths of Ethnography
- It is only research approach facilitate the study of culture and behavior of a group or community
- It generate a rich understanding of social action and its subtleties in different contexts
- Ethnography findings sensitize about how a particular group react in health and sickness conditions
- This approach help to study human behavior in natural setting
- Ethnographic research can identify, explore and link the social phenomena, which, on the surface, have very little connection to each other
- This method also gives ethnographers the chance to gather empirical insights into social practices which are normally 'hidden' from the public awareness.

Limitations of Ethnographic Studies
- Ethnographic studies relatively consume long period of time
- Obtaining formal ethical approval in ethnography approach is a complicated job
- It is a challenging task to record the multifaceted nature of social action that occurs within a clinical or ward
- An ethnographer need to be flexible, patient and persistent to face unpredictable nature of social (or clinical) life.

GROUNDED THEORY

Barney Glaser and Anselm Strauss first proposed the concept of grounded theory. Grounded theory had its root in social research but it has gained popularity in various other disciplines such as business research, marketing, organization and leadership studies. The use of grounded theory procedures leads to a coherent, well-connected set of concepts that describes as well explains the phenomenon under study. Grounded theory is a commonly used qualitative method in health research. It primarily focus on development of theory.

Typically, grounded theory purposively select participants who they believe can offer valuable insight in to the topic under study. Ideally, theoretical sampling is a choice in grounded theory. This mean starting by interviewing a small number of people whose characteristics match to study participants and selecting further participants on the basis of information provided from the early interview.

Qualitative interview is the most commonly used method for data collection in ground theory. However, it can also collect data through observational visits, unstructured or semi-structured interview methods. Unstructured interview is preferred to inquire a very poorly understood topic of a phenomenon to get maximum inputs related to the concepts.

In grounded theory, data are collected and analyzed in tandem. A well-established coding procedure is followed to code and interpret the data. Following steps help to understand data analysis in grounded theory.
- Data are broken down in the part to represent individual segment of the data. Each segment will represent a unique concept or theme. This stage is called 'open coding'
- In the next step, researcher make a tentative proposition about the relationships between emerging categories and postulate how variation in context might shape participants' experiences. This is referred as 'axial coding'. During coding, the first author wrote reflexive and theoretical memos (written record of analysis)

- The final phase in grounded theory data analysis is 'selective coding'. Selective coding involves the identification of a core category that incorporates other categories or supersedes them in explanatory importance. Theses relationship between categories constitutes substantive theory. However, the refinement in coding is continue and relationships between categories after interviewing has ceased.

Definitions

'Grounded theory is a systematic set of techniques and procedures' that enable researchers to identify concepts and builds theory from qualitative data.'   *(Corbin and Strauss, 2008)*
'The discovery of theory from data systematically obtained and analysed in social research'
(Glaser and Strauss, 2009)
'Grounded theory focus on psychosocial process of behavior and seek to identify and explain how and why people behave in certain ways, in similar or different context.'
(Corbin and Strauss, 2008; Dey, 2008; Charmaz, 2006)
'The discovery of theory from data systematically obtained and analysed in social research.'
(Glaser and Strauss, 2009)

Strengths of Grounded Theory

- Grounded theory provide opportunity to use single or multiple sources of data and provide enormous flexibility to the researcher to understand phenomenon in detail
- It is an effective approach to build or refine existing theory or model in nursing
- It helps to understand influence of context on experience of an individual and therefore, is an appropriate approach to study patients' behavior in hospital.

Limitations of Grounded Theory

- Grounded theory is a difficult approach require utmost care, diligence, sensitivity and conceptualization ability
- Data are collected in natural setting, hence difficult to control influence of extraneous factors on findings
- Sometimes, a researcher feel challenging to segregate and study a large volume of data.
- It is time consuming and laborious research.

HISTORICAL RESEARCH

Historical research is the type of qualitative research that examines past events or combinations of events has happened in the past. Historical research can show the trends of events occurred in the past and changes in the events over a period of time. This trends develop insight about where we came from and where we are today. It will also help to seek solution of the problems based on previous records.

Historical evidence subject to undergo two types of evaluation; *external* and *internal criticism*. *External criticism* refers to examination of the historical data sources (maps, letters, documents, inscriptions, artifacts) for their validity, genuineness, or authenticity. Once the validity of source is established, the historical researcher turns his or her attention to determine the accuracy of the statements contained within the documents or historical material. The process involved in making such a determination is called *internal criticism*. Historical research should not be confused with a review of the literature. One important difference between historical research and a literature review is that historical researchers often guided by specific hypotheses or questions. Historical research follow the basic steps of research process from selection of research question to dissemination of research findings.

Historical researcher collects the data with the help of interview, observation, seeking written documents, artifacts, relics, remains, reading documents, textbooks, encyclopedia, newspaper and journals, etc.

Definition

'It is a process of critical inquiry into past events, in order to produce an accurate description and interpretation of those events.' *(Wiersma, 2000)*

Steps of Historical Research

- *Formulate a research question:* Formulate a searchable question that is best approached with a historical research design
- *Specify types of data:* A research should specify what types of data are needs to address the research question
- *Determine quantum of data:* Historical research need a bunch of information to reach on a conclusion. A researcher should verify whether sufficient amount of data or information would be available or not.
- *Data collection:* Historian data collection is long and tiresome job. A researcher should explore all possible primary and secondary sources to collect significant information
- *Evaluate strengths' of data sources:* It is always appropriate to evaluate data sources to check their authenticity, genuineness and validity for anticipating objective results.
- *Data analysis:* Usually, historical research impute descriptive analysis to formulate the results.
- *Conclusion and interpretation:* Draw interpretive conclusions with respect to the original research question.

Strengths of Historical Research

- Historical research answer a research question easily and inexpensively
- Historical research is suitable to study the developmental of an organization or a particular problem
- Historical research flashlight on past and present trends of an event
- Historical research illuminate the solution of current problem based on the experience of earlier one.

Limitations of Historical Research

- Sometimes, it is difficult to race the source of information, especially records and artifacts
- Researcher do not have control over the influence of external variables on findings
- It is challenging for the researcher to interpret the information collected from primary and secondary sources
- There is a great chance of researcher bias in analysis and interpretation of data.

> **Box 7.36:** Example of Historical Research.
>
> Connolly and Gibson (2011) conducted a historical study on tuberculosis, race and children to describe the efforts of nurses at 20th century in pediatric TB prevention and treatment in one state, Virginia. Study findings reported that nurses played a leadership role in designing a template for children's care. They helped forge a system funded by a complicated, poorly coordinated, race- and class-based mix of public and private support that is now delivered through an idiosyncratic web of community, state, and federal programs. Ultimately, however, their legacy is a mixed one.

CASE STUDY

Case studies are one of the oldest types of research used in field of qualitative research. Much of what we know today about empirical world is the result of case study only. Case studies have been largely utilized by social sciences. However, now it is realized that case studies are especially important to practice oriented disciplines (such as nursing, medicine, education, management and public administration, etc.). Usually, qualitative studies are qualitative in nature but may contain combination of qualitative or quantitative information. *Interpretive paradigm* and *idiographic approach* are key elements of a case study. *Interpretive paradigm* refers to subjective experience of and meaning they have for an individual. *Idiographic approach* deals with an individual's perspective on the investigative situations, process and relations, etc.

Case study is a comprehensive description of one or a few participants to get detailed descriptions of the phenomenon under study. Participants for case study may be a single individual, family, an institution or a social unit. The main focus of case studies is typically on determining the dynamics of why an individual thinks, behaves, or reacts in a particular manner rather than on what his or her states, progress, or actions. Data are often collected to the person's present state, past experiences and situational factors relevant to the problem being examined.

In case study design, investigator explore and collect information with the help of interview, observations, and reading relevant documents, i.e. letters, memos, agendas, administrative documents, newspaper articles and from physical artefacts. Usually, case study limited to small sample size (usually 1-10).

Definitions

'A case study is a description and analysis of an individual matter or case [...] with the purpose to identify variables, structures, forms and orders of interaction between the participants in the situation (theoretical purpose), or, in order to assess the performance of work or progress in development (practical purpose).'
(Mesec 1998)

'[a] case study is a general term for the exploration of an individual, group or phenomenon".
(Sturman, 1997)

'An empirical inquiry that investigates a contemporary phenomenon with in real life context, especially when the boundaries between phenomenon and context are not clearly evident.'
(Yin, 2003)

'Case study is an in-depth exploration from multiple perspectives of the complexity and uniqueness of a particular project, policy, institution, program or system in a 'real life'.
(Simons, 2009)

> **Box 7.37:** Example of Case Study.
>
> Lioyd J, et al. (2015) in a qualitative case study focus on the importance of treatment outcomes as perceived by the informal carers of people caring schizophrenia patients. This qualitative study included 38 individuals and 8 couples who are person with schizophrenia/schizoaffective disorders. Carers described the importance of well-recognized outcomes in terms of safety, reduction of vulnerability to stress, several aspects of physical health, insight, respite from fear, distress or pain and socially acceptable behavior, etc.

Strengths of Case Study
- Case studies are useful for generating hypotheses, while other studies are more suitable for testing hypotheses or theory
- A case study can provide concrete context dependent experience that increases their research skills
- Case study enable a researcher to study a phenomenon of interest in detail
- Case studies are potential to achieve higher degree of conceptual validity and therefore, enable a researcher to present best concept about a problem under study
- Case study can provide a clearer picture of accounting practice in relation to its larger social context
- Case study is a wonderful approach to study a limited number of individual, groups or institutions
- A detailed account of information often produced in case studies not only help to explore the phenomenon but also disclose complexities of real life situations.

Limitations of Case Study
- Generalization of the findings upon a single case is never possible; therefore, case study cannot contribute to scientific development
- Case study is not a suitable approach to study cause effect relationship
- There is no formal guidelines for analysis and interpretation of findings, therefore, every researcher has their own way to present the findings
- Case study is a labor intensive, expensive and time-consuming research approach.

ACTION RESEARCH

Kurt Lewin (1946), a social scientist first used the word action research to study the intergroup relations and minority problem in United States. Action research is one form of emancipatory research. It is been widely used in social sciences to alleviate social problems and to increase understanding of the process involved. Action research as a means of investigating nursing is comparatively new innovation. Therefore, the popularity of action research in nursing is still questionable. However, Green Wood (1984) suggests that action research approach is ideal for the investigation of nursing problem as nursing is a practice rather than an academic discipline (Table 7.3).

In present scenario, action research gained popularity in health care setting and nursing as well. In action research, practitioner can choose to research their own practice or an outsider researcher can engaged to help them identify problem, seek and implement practical solutions and systematically monitor and reflect on the process and outcomes of changes.

Action research is somewhat synonymous to qualitative research and use interview and observation as a method of data collection.

Table 7.3: Action research typology.

Features	Experimental	Organizational	Professionalizing	Empowering
Educative basis	Re-education	Re-education or training	Reflexive practice	Consciousness raising
	Enhancing social science or administrative control and social change towards consensus	Enhancing managerial control and organisational change towards consensus	Enhancing professional control and individuals' ability to control work situation	Enhancing user control and shifting balance of power; structural change towards pluralism
	Inferring relationship between behavior and output; identifying causal factors in group dynamics	Overcoming resistance to change or restructuring balance of power between managers and workers	Empowering professional groups; advocacy on behalf of patients or clients	Empowering oppressed groups
	Social scientific bias, researcher focused	Managerial bias or client focused	Practitioner focused	User or practitioner focused
Individual in groups	Closed group, controlled, selection made by researcher for purposes of measurement, inferring relationship between cause and effect	Work groups or mixed groups of managers and workers, or both	Professional(s) or (interdisciplinary) professional group, or negotiated team boundaries	Fluid groupings, self-selecting or natural boundary or open/closed by negotiation
	Fixed membership	Selected membership	Shifting membership	Fluid membership
Problem focus	Problem emerges from the interaction of social science theory and social problems	Problem defined by most powerful group; some negotiation with users	Problem defined by professional in group; some negotiation with users	Emerging and negotiated definition of problem by less powerful group(s)
	Problems relevant for social science or management interests	Problem relevant for management/social science interests	Problem emerges from professional practice or experience	Problem emerges from members' practice or experience
	Success defined in terms of social sciences	Success defined by sponsors	Contested, professionally determined definitions of success	Competing definitions of success accepted and expected

Contd...

Contd...

Features	Experimental	Organizational	Professionalizing	Empowering
Improvement	Toward controlled outcome and consensual definition of improvement	Towards tangible outcome and consensus definition of improvement	Towards improvement in practice defined by professionals and on behalf of users	Towards negotiated outcomes and pluralist definitions of improvement: account taken of vested interest
Research relationships, degree of collaboration	Experimenter or respondents	Consultant or researcher, respondent or participants	Practitioner, or researcher or collaborators	Practitioner researcher or coresearchers or co-change agents
	Outside researcher as expert or research funding	Client pays an outside consultant—"they who pay the piper call the tune"	Outside resources or internally generated, or both	Outside resources or internally generated, or both
	Differentiated roles	Differential roles	Merged roles	Shared roles

Source: Hart and Bond.

Definitions

Action research methodology is a systematic research process that can be articulated by the researcher, involving data collection and analysis as well as reflection and discussion with co-researchers or others for the purpose of making change in a situation overtime.

'It is action which is intentionally researched and modified leading to the next stage of action which is then again intentionally examined for further change and soon as part of their search itself'. *(Wadsworth Y, 1998)*

'Essentially, action research is concerned with generating knowledge about a social system, while, at the same time, attempting to change it'. *(Meyer, 2001:173)*

Elements of Action Research

Action research is a style of research rather than a specific method. Most definitions of action research include following as key characteristics of an action research:

- *Participatory character:* Participation is fundamental to action research—it is an approach which demands that participants perceive the need to change and are willing to play an active part in the research and the change process. All research requires willing subjects, but the level of commitment required in an action research study goes beyond simply agreeing to answer questions or be observed.
- *Democratic impulse:* "Democracy" in action research usually requires participants to be seen as equals. The researcher works as a facilitator of change, consulting with participants not only on the action process but also on how it will be evaluated. One benefit of this is that it can make the research process and outcomes more meaningful to practitioners, by rooting them in the reality of day-to-day practice.
- *Simultaneous contribution to social sciences and social changes:* There is increasing concern about the "theory-practice" gap in clinical practice; practitioners have to rely on

their intuition and experience since traditional scientific knowledge—for example, the results of randomized controlled trials—often does not seem to fit the uniqueness of the situation. Action research is seen as one way of dealing with this because, by drawing on practitioners' intuition and experience, it can generate findings that are meaningful and useful to them.

Box 7.38: Example of Action Research.

Siebens K, et al. (2012) use action research to develop and implement a critical pathway for patient with chest pain. The process follows identification of population and assignment of a coordinator. A multidisciplinary workgroup for pathway development was prepared. The pathway was developed in 4 phases: (1) Evaluation of current process of care for patients with chest pain, (2) Searching evidence of medicine and practice in other hospitals, (3) Optimization of the process, and (4) Preparation of final draft. Later on, the draft was used to triage different categories of patients, orders and protocols preparation, revision of medical records and in development of admission and discharge brochures for patients.

Strengths of Action Research
- Action research helpful to change rather than simply to test hypotheses or to provide an explanation
- Action research helps to change the behavior of those taking part and empower them
- Action research can be used in hospital setting to facilitate closer partnership between staff and users
- Action research is particularly suited to identifying problems in clinical practice and helpful to develop potential solution.

Limitation of Action Research
Action research reduces the generalizability of findings.

DELPHI TECHNIQUE

Delphi technique is another form of research approach used to gain consensus an issue of common interest. It is used as a series of questionnaire or rounds to collect information on the issue until the expert consensus is reached. The fundamental assumption of Delphi technique is that group opines is always better than an individual view.

Delphi technique based on novel and contemporary television program called, *Kaun Banega Crorpati* (KBC), where audience effectively act as group of expert to reach on a final decision. Delphi technique believed that group opinions are always valid and reliable in comparison to individual one. Delphi technique particularly helpful to deal the issue of priority setting in research, role clarification, defining vague concepts and identification of core competencies (Fig. 7.4). Advantages limitations of Delphi technique are discussed in Table 7.4.

Definitions
'Delphi technique is an interactive process designed to combine expert opinions in to group consensus.' *(Lynn, et al. 1998)*

'Delphi is a method for the systematic collection and aggregation of informal judgement from group of experts on specific question and issues.' *(Reid, et al. 1998)*

144 Nursing Research and Statistics

> **Box 7.39:** Crux of Delphi Technique.
> - Use of expert to obtain information
> - Exert do not face others control personal bias and prejudices
> - Use of multiple rounds to meet specific requirement
> - Use of multiple rounds (2–3) which include summary of the previous rounds reach to experts
> - Systematic analysis of suggestion and opinions of experts
> - Anonymity of suggestion and opinions

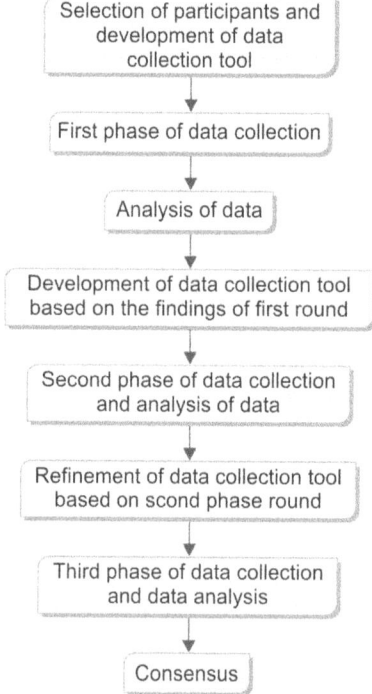

Fig. 7.4: The Delphi approach.

Table 7.4: Advantages and limitations of Delphi technique.

Advantages	Limitations
Inexpensive to use	No formal guidelines
Universal technique	True anonymity is questionable
Simple and easy to use	Lack of rigorous methodology
No restriction to choose experts globally	Lack of response of experts
Confidentiality in experts' response	Lack of interest of participants/experts
Group opinions are better than individual one	No scientific evidence for validity and reliability
Avoids 'groupthink'	Time consuming

REVIEW QUESTIONS AND ANSWER

Long and Short Answer Questions

1. Mention the characteristics of a qualitative research design. *(TNMGRMU, MSc N-2001)*
2. Explain qualitative research design with suitable example. *(AIIMS, MSc N-2009)*
3. Define research design; classify the various types of research design and discuss in detail true experimental designs. *(PGI, MSc N-2012)*
4. Explain quasi-experimental research approach. *(PGI, MSc N-2008)*
5. What are the advantages and disadvantage of experimental research? *(BFUHS, MSc N-2003)*
6. Discuss the different types of survey studies. *(RGUHS, MSc N-2017)*
7. Explain the characteristics of experimental research with examples. *(RGUHS, MSc N-2006)*
8. Explain phenomenology. *(PGI, MSc N-2011)*
9. Write in detail about historical research. *(TNMGRMU, MSc N-2006)*
10. Elaborate on case study and action research. *(KUHAS, MSc N-2012)*

Multiple Choice Questions

1. It is a blueprint of a study which facilitate where, how and what data to be collected from the participants is called:
   a. Research approach
   b. Research design
   c. Conceptual framework
   d. Hypothesis

2. It is a types of design which help to test the effect of independent variable on dependent variables is called as:
   a. Experimental design
   b. Exploratory design
   c. Descriptive design
   d. Comparative design

3. Which of the following are salient features of a true experimental research design?
   a. Manipulation
   b. Control
   c. Randomization
   d. All of the above

4. It is a threat to internal validity refers to the extent to which low or high scores of an instrument move towards the sample mean at the second time administration of the instrument.
   a. Maturation effects
   b. Statistical regression effects
   c. Experimenter effects
   d. Instrumentation effects

5. It is a threat to internal validity which occur when research participants behaved in different way because they are aware of presence of researcher or by being observed by someone:
   a. History
   b. Hawthorne effects
   c. Testing effects
   d. Reactive measurement effects

6. It is the process of doing something to study subjects (independent variable) to see the desired effect on outcome variable in experimental research is called as:
   a. Manipulation
   b. Control
   c. Randomization
   d. Testing

7. It is a types of experimental research design in which treatment administered on experimental group and only post-test performed to see the desired effect of treatment on an experimental group?
   a. True experimental
   b. Quasi-experimental
   c. Post-test only design
   d. Time series design

8. Cross over design involves the exposure of the same subjects to more than one experimental treatment. This design also known as:
   a. Solomon four group
   b. Factorial design
   c. Randomized block design
   d. Repeated measure design

9. Carry over effect is a classical demerits attached to which of the following research design?
   a. Solomon four group
   b. Repeated measure/crossover design
   c. Factorial design
   d. Randomized block design

10. This is an experimental study in which one of the salient feature, either randomization or control, is missing is called as:
    a. True experimental
    b. Quasi-experimental
    c. Pre-experimental
    d. Time series design

11. Which of the following is weakest design in experimental research?
    a. True experimental design
    b. Clinical trials design
    c. Quasi-experimental design
    d. Pre-experimental design

12. A design in which a researcher selects a case and go to past/history to study the present outcomes is called:
    a. Retrospective design
    b. Prospective design
    c. Analytical design
    d. Epidemiological design

13. Which of the following design allow a researcher to collect data from different groups of people who are at different stage in their experience of the phenomena at same time?
    a. Longitudinal design
    b. Cross-sectional design
    c. Time series design
    d. Survey design

14. Which of the following research deign is appropriate to develop tool, intervention, guidelines and clinical technique?
    a. Meta-synthesis
    b. Secondary analysis
    c. Methodological study
    d. Evaluative studies

15. Which of the following qualitative study deal with the live experience of participants?
    a. Phenomenology
    b. Grounded theory
    c. Case study
    d. Ethnography

16. This a types of qualitative study which focus on study of culture and its impact on experience of people and their views is called as:
    a. Phenomenology
    b. Grounded theory
    c. Case study
    d. Ethnography

Answer Key

1.	2.	3.	4.	5.	6.	7.	8.	9.	10.	11.	12.	13.	14.	15.	16.
b.	a.	d.	b.	b.	a.	c.	d.	b.	b.	d.	a.	b.	c.	a.	d.

SUGGESTED READING

1. Aggarwal A, Sheikh S, Pallagatti S, Bansal N, Goyal G. Comparison of knowledge, attitude and behavior of dental and nursing students towards HIV/AIDS. Journal of Medicine and Medical Sciences. 2012;3(8): 537-45.
2. Bandana, Walia I, Saini SK. Development of audit tool: A methodological study for auditing the family health records. Nursing and Midwifery Research Journal. 2009;5(4):166-75.
3. Bennett KL1, Ohrmundt C, Maloni JA. Preventing intravasation in women undergoing hysteroscopic procedures. AORN Journal. 1996;64(5):792-9.
4. Birk M, Santamaria N, Thompson S, Amerena J. A clinical trails of the effectiveness of water as conductive medium in electrocardiography. Australian Journal of Advanced Nursing. 1993;10(2): 10-3.
5. Blink P, Wood M. Advanced design in nursing. Thousand Oaks: Sage Publications; 1998.
6. Burns N, Grove SK. The practice of nursing research: conduct, critique, and utilization, 5th edition. St Louis: Elsevier; 2005.
7. Burns N, Grove SK. Understanding nursing research. Philadelphia: Saunders; 2003.
8. Campbell D, Stanley J. Experimental and quasi-experimental designs for research. Chicago, IL: Rand-McNally; 1963.
9. Cassol H, Pétré B, Degrange S, et al. Qualitative thematic analysis of the phenomenology of near-death experiences. PLoS One. 2018;13(2):e0193001.
10. Charmaz K. Constructing grounded theory. A practical guide through qualitative analysis. London: SAGE; 2006.
11. Cheng HG, Phillips MR. Secondary analysis of existing data: opportunities and implementation. Shanghai Archives of Psychiatry. 2014;26(6):371-5.
12. Cimiotti JP, Marmur ES, Nesin M, et al. Adverse reactions associated with an alcohol based hand antiseptic among nurses in a neonatal intensive care unit. AJIC. 2003;31(1):43-8.
13. Connolly CA, Gibson ME. The 'White Plague' and color: Children, race, and tuberculosis in Virginia 1900-1935. Journal of Pediatric Nursing. 2011;26:230-8.
14. Creswell JW. Qualitative inquiry and research design: Choosing among the five approaches. Thousand Oaks, CA: Sage publications, Inc; 2013.
15. Creswell JW. The strength and weakness of research designs involving quantitative measures. J Res Nurs. 2005;10(5):571-82.
16. Crossman A. "Critical Theory." About.com Sociology; 2013.
17. Darvishi N, Farhadi M, Haghtalab T, et al. Alcohol-related risk of Suicidal Ideation, Suicide Attempt, and Completed Suicide: A Meta-Analysis. PLoS One. 2015;10(5):e0126870.
18. Denzin N. The research act in sociology. London: Butterworths; 1970.
19. Denzin NK, Lincoln YS. Handbook of qualitative research, Newbury Park: Sage Publications; 1984.

20. Dey I. Grounding Grounded Theory. Guidelines for Qualitative Inquiry. Bingley: Emerald Group; 2008.
21. DiMattio MJ, Tulman L. A longitudinal study of functional status and correlates following coronary artery graft surgery in women. Nurs Res. 2003;52(2):98-107.
22. Dorathy YB. Fundamentals of nursing research, 3rd edition. Sudbury: Jones and Bartlett Publishers; 2003.
23. Fain J. Reading, understanding, and analyzing nursing research. Philadelphia, PA: FA Davis Company; 2009.
24. Fawcet J, Garity J. Evaluating research for evidence-based nursing practice. FA Davis Company. 2008; pp. 92-105.
25. Foley G, Timonen V. Using grounded theory method to capture and analyze health care experiences. HSR: Health Services Research. 2015;50(4):1195-210.
26. Garbossa A, Maldaner E, Mortari DM, Biasi J, Leguisamo CP. Effect of physiotherpautic instructions on anxiety of CABG patients. Rev Bras Cir Cardiovasc. 2009;24(3):359-66.
27. Gilson L. Health policy and systems research: a methodology reader alliance for health policy and systems research, World Health Organization. 2012;443-67.
28. Glaser BG, Strauss AL. The discovery of grounded theory: strategies for qualitative research. Piscataway, NJ: Transaction Publishers; 2009.
29. Gupta SN, Gupta N. Evaluation of revised national tuberculosis control program, district Kangra, Himachal Pradesh, India, 2007. Lung India. 2011;28:163-8.
30. Hart E, Bond M. Action research for health and social care: a guide to practice. Buckingham: Open University Press; 1995.
31. Heidegger M. Being and time. New York: Harper (Original work published 1927); 1962.
32. Hughes CC. Ethnography: What's in a word–Process? Product? Promise? Qualitative Health Research. 1992;2(4):439-50.
33. Husserl E. The idea of phenomenology. The Hague, Netherlands: Martinus Nijhoff; 1970.
34. Ibrahim N, Amit N, Suen MWY. Psychological factors as predictors of suicidal ideation among adolescents in Malaysia. Plos One. 2014; 9(10): e110670.https://doi.org/10.1371/journal.pone.0110670
35. Kothari RC. Research methodology, New Delhi: Wiley Eastern Ltd; 1985.
36. Kumar R, Kaur S, Reddemma K. Family needs of caregivers of stroke survivors. Adv Practice Nurs. 2016;2:120.
37. Kumar R, Nancy. Stress and coping strategies among nursing students. Nursing and Midwifery Research Journal. 2011;7(4):141-51.
38. Kumar R. Academic climate, academic stress and self-esteem among baccalaureate nursing students. Nursing and Midwifery Research Journal.2018;14(2):53-61.
39. LeSeure P, Chongkham-Ang S. The experience of caregivers living with cancer patients: a systematic review and meta-synthesis. J Pers Med. 2015;5(4):406-39.
40. Lincoln YS, Guba EG. Naturalistic inquiry. Beverly Hills, CA: Sage publications, Inc; 1985.
41. Lloyd J, Lloyd H, Fitzpatrick R, et al. Treatment outcomes in schizophrenia: qualitative study of the views of family carers. BMC Psychiatry. 2017;17(1):266.
42. LoBiondo-Wood G, Haber J. Nursing research: Methods, critical appraisal, and utilization, 5th edition. St Louis: Mosby; 2002.
43. LoBiondo-Wood G and Haber J. Nursing research: Methods and critical appraisal for evidenced based practice, 8th edition. St Louis, MO: Elsevier; 2014.

44. Marcin JP, Rutan F, Rapetti PM, et al. Nurse staffing and unplanned extubation in pediatric intensive care unit. Pediatr Crit Care Med. 2005;6(3):254-7.
45. Mesec B. Uvod v kvalitativno raziskovanje v socialnem delu. Ljubljana: Visoka šola za socialno delo, 1998.
46. Meyer J. Action research. In: Fulop N. et al. (Eds). Studying the organisation and delivery of health services: research methods. London, Routledge. 2001:172-87.
47. Meyer J. Qualitative research in health care: Using qualitative methods in health related action research. BMJ. 2000;320;178-81.
48. Parahoo K. Nuring Research: principles, process, issues. London: Macmillan; 1997.
49. Patten SB, Wang JL, Williams JVA, Currie S, Beck CA, Maxwell CJ, et al. Descriptive epidemiology of major depression in Canada. Can J Psychiatry. 2006;51(2):84-90.
50. Ploeg J. Identifying the best research design to fit the question. Part 2: Qualitative designs. Evidence-Based Nursing. 1999;2:36-7.
51. Polit DF, Beck CT. Essential of Nursing Research: methods, appraisal, and utilization, 5th edition. Philadelphia: Lippincott; 2001.
52. Polit DF, Beck CT. Essential of nursing research: methods, appraisal and utilization, 6th edition. Philadelphia: Lippincott Williams Wilkins; 2006.
53. Powers BA, Knapp TR. A dictionary of nursing theory and research. London: Sage Publications; 1990.
54. Reeves S, Kuper A, Hodges BD. Qualitative research methodologies: ethnography. BMJ. 2008;337:512-4.
55. Reeves S, Peller J, Goldman J, Kitto S. Ethnography in qualitative educational research: AMEE Guide No. 80. Med Teach. 2013;35:e1365-e79.
56. Rubin A, Babbie E. Essential research methods in social work, 2nd edition. Cengage Learning; 2009.
57. Sawaengdee K, Tangcharoensathien V, Theerawit T, et al. Thai nurse cohort study: Cohort profile and key findings. BMC Nursing. 2016;15(1):2-12.
58. Schram TH. Conceptualizing qualitative inquiry: mindwork for fieldwork in education and social sciences. Upper Saddle River, NJ: Merrill Prentice Hall; 2003.
59. Seabrook MA. Clinical students' initial reports of the educational climate in a single medical school. Med Educ. 2004;38(6):659-69.
60. Seers K, Crichton N. Quantitative research: Designs relevant to nursing and health care. NT Res. 2005;6(1):487-500.
61. Shadish WR, Cook TD, Campbell DT. Experimental and quasi-experimental designs for generalized casual inference. New York: Houghton Mifflin Company; 2002.
62. Simons H. Case study research in practice. London: SAGE; 2009.
63. Smith DG. Hermeneutic inquiry: the hermeneutic imagination and pedagogic text. In: E Short (Ed), Forms of curriculum inquiry (pp. 187-209). New York: Sunny Press; 1991.
64. Sparrow S, Robinson J. Action Research: an appropriate design for research in nursing? Educational Action Research. 1994;2(3):347-35.
65. Spradley JP. Participant Observation. New York: Holt, Rinehart and Winston; 1980.
66. Starman AB. The case study as a type of qualitative research. Journal of Contemporary Educational Studies. 2013;1:28-43.

67. Stepehnson TJ, Setchell KD, Kendall CW, Jenkins DJ, Anderson JW, Fanli P. Effect of soy protein rich diet on renal function in young adult with insulin dependent diabetes mellitus. Clin Nephrol. 2005;64(1):1-11.
68. Strauss AL, Corbin J. Basics of Qualitative Research. Techniques and Procedures for Developing Grounded Theory, 2nd edition. Thousand Oaks, CA: Sage; 1998.
69. Sturman A. Case study methods. In: JP Keeves (ed). Educational research, methodology and measurement: an international handbook, 2nd edition. Oxford: Pergamon. 1997; pp. 61-6.
70. Taylor BJ. Research in nursing and health care: Evidence of practice. Cengage Learning, Australia. 2006:185-95.
71. Van Kaam A. Existential foundations of psychology, Pittsburgh, PA: Duquesne University Press; 1996.
72. Van Manen M. Researching lived experience: human sciences for an action sensitive pedagogy, 2nd edition. London, Canada: the Althouse Press; 1997.
73. Wadsworth Y. What is participatory Action Research? Action Research International, Paper 2. 1998. Available online: http://www.aral.com.au/ari/pywadsworth98.html.
74. Wiersma W. Research methods in education: An introduction. Boston, MA: Allyn and Bacon; 2000.
75. WIndartik E, Zakiyah A, Effect of yoga exercise on blood pressure reduction in elderly. International conference on public heath, Indonesia.2018;78.
76. Yada H, Xi Lu, Hisamitsu Omori, et al. Exploratory study of factors influencing Job-related stress in Japanese psychiatric nurses. Nursing Research and Practice. 2015;1-7.
77. Yin RK. Case study research: design and methods, 3rd edition. London: SAGE Publications Ltd; 2003.

Sample and Sampling Techniques

INTRODUCTION

Sampling in the educational research is generally conducted in order to permit detailed study of part, rather than the whole of a population. The information derived from the obtained sample is employed to develop useful generalization about the population. This generalization based on one or more characteristic related to population or may be on the strength of the relationship between some characteristics within population.

The selection of sample provides many advantages compared to study whole population. For example, reduced cost associated with gathering and analysis the data, reduced requirement for trained personals to conduct research, improved speed of data collection and reporting and summarization and improve the accuracy in field work and data preparation.

SAMPLING TERMS

In any educational research, it is important to have precise description of the narrow elements of sampling. These definitions will helps and provide clear guidelines to include the derived elements of the population.

Population

Population is the entire aggregation of cases in which investigator is interested. In order to prepare a suitable description of population, it is essential to distinguish between the population on which result are generalized and fulfill the eligibility criteria (the target population) and the population which is ideally available for investigation (the accessible population) to make generalization.

For example: A target population may involves all the patients' with cerebrovascular accident (CVAs) in Punjab state but accessible population might only consists of all CVA patients joined with stroke associations for health tips in order to overcome residual effects of CVA. Researcher usually collect sample from accessible population and generalize the findings to target population.

Sample

A sample is a 'subgroup of population'. It has also been described as a representative 'taste' of a group. The sample should be representative in the sense that each sampled unit will represent the characteristics of known number of units in the population.

Representative Sample

A sample is often described as being representative if certain percentages of sample characteristics are similar to corresponding population. The population characteristics selected for these comparisons are referred to as '*Marker variables*'. These variables usually selected from those demographic variables that are readily available for both population and sample. However, there is no objective rule for selecting marker variables. Further, there is no agreed benchmark for assessing the degree of representative of sample for given population.

The most popular marker variables in the field of education are sociodemographic factors associated with subjects (gender, age, education, socioeconomic status, etc.).

Sampling

It is systematic process of selecting a small portion or subsets of the population to represent the entire population. The sample method involves taking representative selection of the population and collecting the data as research information. The standard definition of sampling always includes the ability of the researcher to select a portion of the population that is truly representative of said population. It is well known that appropriate sampling method allow researcher to reduce research costs, helps to conduct research more efficiently (speed), have greater flexibility and provides greater accuracy, etc.

Strata

It is very difficult to conduct and study whole population at a time. So, it is better to divide population in two or more than two subgroup or strata. A stratum (singular) is mutually exclusive segment of population which made on the basis of one or more characteristics of population. For instance, suppose our population is all staff nurses working in Punjab. This population can be divided into two groups on the basis of gender; male and female. Alternatively the above said population can be divided into three subgroups by taking age; younger than 25 years, 26–30 years and >31 years of age, etc.

Element

An individual unit of a population is called an *element*. An element can be a person, event, behavior or any other single unit under study.

Generalization

It is process of expression of finding from sample to the larger similar population. For instance assessing stress level among 500 randomly selected BSc (N) 3rd year students and implicating result on all BSc (N) 3rd year students in a particular state.

Sampling Frame

It is list of all the elements and subjects in the population from which the sample will be taken. In accessible population, to enhance the opportunity for selection in the sample, every person in the population must be identified. For instance, the investigator may collect the cumulative records of BSc (N) students for assessing level of anxiety in a selected nursing college.

Sampling Bias

It is over and under representation of sample characteristics. The sampling bias can be from researcher side or attributed by some external factors.

Sampling Error

This is statistically calculated variation from one sample to another sample drawing from same population. The selected samples may be varying in characteristics to other samples and population as well. Selecting large sample size from homogenous population may decrease sampling error.

Sampling Mortality/Attrition

It is withdrawal or loss of subjects from a study. Many factors are responsible for sample mortality like inadequate information by researchers, migration, work related problem and house hold problem, etc. In a well-designed study sample attrition should not be more than 20%.

Sampling Plan

It is formal plan which specify sampling method, techniques, size and procedure to collect sample. It outlines the strategies used to obtain a sample for a study and should increases representativeness and decrease bias.

SAMPLING CRITERIA

Sampling criteria also known as *eligibility criteria*. This includes *exclusion (delimitations) and inclusion criteria*. The inclusion criteria specify the population characteristics. The characteristics of population and sample must be congruent. The exclusion criteria help to delimit the selection of sample. The exclusion criteria/delimitation defines attributes that the sample does not possess. Examples of inclusion or eligibility criteria and exclusion criteria or delimitation include the following: gender, age, marital status, socioeconomic status, religion, ethnicity, level of education, age of children, heath status and diagnosis. The degree of congruence between the criteria and population is evaluated to assess the representativeness of the sample.

Box 8.1: Example of Inclusion Criteria.

Research statement: 'A study on caregivers burden of stroke survivors in selected rural community district Rishikesh, Uttarakhand'.
The inclusion criteria of the study are:
- Age equal or more than 18 years
- Staying with patient since at least 12 months
- Caring the patient for more than one month
- Able to communicate verbally in English and Hindi
- Willing to participate and sign a consent form

Inclusion and exclusion criteria should have rationale, presumably related to contaminating effect on the dependent variables.

> **Box 8.2:** Example of Exclusion Criteria.
>
> **Research statement:** 'A study on depression and quality of life in caregivers of individual with mental illness'.
> **Exclusion criteria:** The study exclude:
> - Paid caregivers involve in care of patient
> - Caregivers diagnosed with physical or psychiatric illness
> - Caregivers involve in care of other patients simultaneously

IMPORTANCE OF SAMPLING IN RESEARCH

Sampling is very complex and technical task in research. The opportunity to study the entire population of people, places and things is an endeavor that most researchers do not have the time and/or money to undertake. The idea of gathering data from a population is one that has been used successfully over in years and is called *censes*. For most researchers collecting data from an entire population is almost impossible because of the amount of people, places, or things within population.

The sampling serve many purposes in research, including followings:

- *Economical:* A well-designed sampling techniques will help to save lot of time, money and other expenditure related to selection of sample.
- *Convenient to select sample:* It is convenient to use sampling to collect data from small proportion of population than studying whole population. Selecting whole population is troublesome and not feasible in terms of time, money, machine and man, etc.
- *Efficiency (speed):* The suitable sampling technique will improve the speed of data collection and reduce the wastage of time. Sampling will help to generate faster result, which is another important step of research.
- *Greater accuracy and precision of data:* Selecting whole population will be difficult to handle then handling the information of a small portion of the population (sample). It is easier to maintain quality of data with small samples investigation rather than selecting the whole population. For example, collecting data on adjustment problems among baccalaureate nursing students from 1,000 populations is much more easy, accurate and precise than studying 10,000 nursing students.
- *Better organization:* Dealing with the whole population will be difficult to organize resources like time, money, printing facilities, vehicles, etc. Sampling will help to overcome the problem of disorganization of resources and help organization of the project.
- *Better rapport:* It is challenging task for a researcher to maintain rapport with whole population. Selecting representative sample will help the researcher to maintain one to one rapport and seek objective informations, which is one of the important objective of research.

CHARACTERISTICS OF A GOOD SAMPLE

A good sample should bear following essential characteristics:

- *Representative:* A good sample should be ideal representative in almost all characteristics to population. Representative samples will help the researcher to generalize the findings over whole similar population.

- *Adequate in size:* The sample size should be analyzed before proceeding to the study. Appropriate sample size estimation will save lot of time, money and other research related expenses.
- *Free from bias/error:* The sample should be free from any type of subjective (researcher) or environmental bias.
- *Complete in all aspects:* The selected sample should complete in all the characteristics of a researcher interest. Sample should not be incomplete in any dimensions of the need of study.

TYPES OF SAMPLING TECHNIQUES

Sampling is a procedure wherein a fraction of the data is taken from a large set of data, and the inference drawn from the sample is extended to whole group. The researcher initial task is to formulate a rational justification for the use of sampling in research.

In educational research many sampling method/techniques are used. The sampling techniques broadly classified under following headings (Fig. 8.1):
1. Probability sampling techniques.
2. Non-probability sampling techniques.

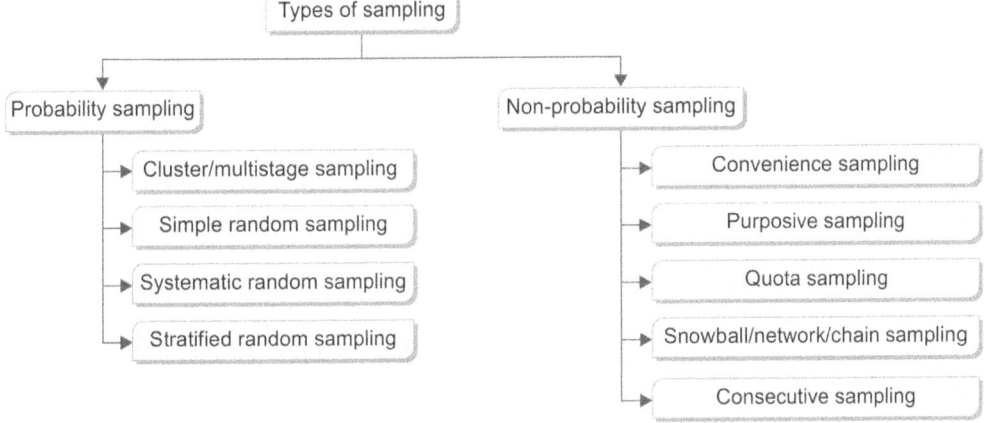

Fig. 8.1: Type of sampling techniques.

PROBABILITY SAMPLING TECHNIQUES

Probability sampling technique is works on principle of probability where each sample has an equal and independent chance to select in a research study. Probability sampling technique decreases the subjective bias and, hence, increase the representativeness of the sample in the study. In this sampling technique, researcher must guarantee that every sample has an equal chance for selection in a given study.

Types of Probability Sampling Techniques

Probability sampling techniques are further classified under following four subtypes:
1. Simple random sampling
2. Stratified random sampling

3. Systematic random sampling
4. Cluster/multistage sampling

Simple Random Sampling

It is most basic and frequently used probability sampling design. This sampling technique allows equal opportunities/independent choice for selection of each subject in study.

Types of Simple Random Sampling

The sample can be drawn in two possible methods:
1. *Simple random sampling with replacement*: It is a method of selection of sample (n) from accessible population (N) in such a way that at one stage of selection, removing samples have same chance of being selected.
2. *Simple random sampling without replacement*: It is method of drawing sample in which researcher draw the sample (n) from the accessible population (N) one by one and at each stage chances for selection of sample will be reduced.

Methods of Simple Random Sampling

- *Lottery method:* Random selection can be accomplished in a variety of ways. The way of selection depends on size of population. In case of small population size, names can be written on a piece of paper, which are then placed in a container, hat and bowl, mixed well to draw adequate size of samples.
- *Table of random numbers:* Once the sampling frame has been developed and numbers are assigned consecutively. A table of random number will be developed to draw desired number of sample size. To draw the sample from random table, researcher blindly put the finger/pencil on anyone number then move the finger/pencil up/down or right and left to select desired number of samples. The sample selected randomly is not subjected to researcher bias. Still, drawing samples by using random table will not give 100% guarantee for random selection of samples.
- *Computer table:* In this method, a random number of table is created with the help of computer software to draw a desired number of samples for study. It is similar but advanced method of creating a table of random number with the help of computer software to minimize bias in random selection of samples. A sample of table of random number is given in Table 8.1.

Table 8.1: Table of random numbers.

1	3	12	15	27	13	14	19	22	25
5	29	42	52	89	74	65	62	59	23
8	26	45	54	77	79	56	23	87	21
2	24	40	58	76	83	66	57	64	73
60	31	38	42	86	9	75	81	24	27
88	35	39	44	82	7	55	63	84	60
53	34	32	61	72	11	85	22	58	83
55	49	43	46	78	8	67	59	84	25
90	41	36	51	88	6	80	65	63	71

Strengths of Simple Random Sampling
- Simple random sampling tends to give more representative sample
- It will reduce the chances of researcher/subjective bias in sample selection
- It is helpful to draw sample from a large population
- The probability of selection of non-representative sample decreases as the size of the sample increases
- In simple random sampling, selection of sample is independent and every sample has an equal chance for their selection. However, the chances of being selected are not independent in systematic random sampling technique
- It is generally easier than other probability sampling techniques (multistage sampling) to recruit the sample
- Use of statistical procedure to analyzes and compute errors is easy in simple random sampling as compared to their counterparts.

Limitations of Simple Random Sampling
- Simple random sampling will not give 100% guarantee that randomly selected sample will be true representative of population. Sometimes, representation can be purely a function of chance
- It is inefficient, time consuming and laborious method to collect sample, i.e. collecting list of whole sample, assigning number and developing a sampling frame, etc.
- In case of use of computer table, the computer can be programmed to select sample automatically
- A researcher need to computer friendly to generate computer table for sample selection
- Simple random sampling is not appropriate for a small group population
- Simple random sampling has large sampling errors and less precision than stratified sampling technique.

Stratified Random Sampling

Stratified sampling select the sample from population subgroups (strata) that are homogeneous (represent similar characteristics). The strata formation may be based on any characteristics of the population (i.e. age, gender, level of education, religion, etc). A research may fix ten appropriate numbers of sample from each strata to improve the representativeness in the sample selection. The sampling technique helps to draw small size and more representative samples. In stratified sampling, whole population divided into some sub-population (strata) and the samples are selected randomly from each strata.

Types of Stratified Random Sampling
Stratified sampling technique is classified based on proportion selected from each strata. Stratified random sampling has following subtypes:
- *Proportionate stratified random sampling:* In proportionate stratified random sampling, researcher select a pre-specified and equal percentage (portion) of sample from each strata, e.g. there are five stratas with a population of 50, 100, 150, 200, and 250. The researcher decided 5% sample from each strata. So, proportion of sample will be 10, 20, 30, 40, 50 from each strata respectively.
- *Disproportionate stratified random sampling:* In disproportionate sampling techniques, the sample drawn from each strata is not in equal proportion. The decided sample size is

vary from strata to strata, e.g. there are three stratas with a population of 1000, 2000, 3000 and researcher taken 300, 500 and 800 samples respectively from each strata. So, here exact proportion of samples is not drawn from each strata.

Steps of Stratified Sampling Technique
- Define the target population
- Identify stratification variable(s) and determine number of strata to be used
- Develop a sampling frame that include information on the stratification variable(s) for each element in the target population
- Divide the sampling frame into strata based on the stratification variable(s)
- Fix the sample size for each strata
- Select the desired number of sample from each strata.

Strengths of Stratified Random Sampling
- Stratified random sampling give small and more representative sample
- It is a good approach to study a large proportion of population
- Stratified sampling is inexpensive in terms of money, efforts and time
- Stratified sampling techniques helpful not only to estimate population parameter but also to make within stratum inference and comparison across strata
- Stratified sampling technique yield smaller sampling errors than simple random sampling technique.

Limitations of Stratified Random Sampling
- A researcher should have prior knowledge about size of strata to select a fix proportion of sample
- This sampling is only helpful to study large population size. A researcher has to use different sampling technique to study a small size population
- Stratified sampling technique requires more efforts to prepare strata, implement sampling and analysis of the data
- Misclassification of population elements into strata may increases variability and hence, increase sampling errors.

Systematic Random Sampling

Systematic random sampling is very helpful to draw a sample from an ordered list of population. This involves the selection of every kth sample from list of population.

Box 8.3: Example to Calculate Sampling Interval.

For example, we have a list of 1500 nursing students studying at selected colleges of nursing North India and we are trying to take a sample of 100 students.
Then, sampling interval = 1500/100 = 15
Hence, every 15th student from list will be taken as a sample for the said study.
Sampling size interval calculation:

$$k = \frac{\text{Population size (N)}}{\text{Desired sample size (n)}}$$

To calculate sampling interval, a researcher divides the population (N) by the size of the desired sample size (n).

Ideally, a researcher should include first sample in the element list as a starting sample.

Steps of Systematic Random Sampling
Generally, a researcher should follow following given steps to select samples by using systematic sampling technique:
- Define target population
- Determine desired sample size (n)
- Develop sampling frame for target population
- Evaluate sampling frame strength and weakness, i.e. under coverage, over coverage, variability, clustering, etc.
- Determine number of elements (N)
- Calculate sampling interval (N/n)
- Randomly select number of sample starting from '1'.

Types of Systematic Random Sampling
Systematic sampling technique can be done by following:
- *Linear systematic sampling:* It is most frequently used technique in systematic sampling technique. It follows the basic seven steps of systematic random sampling to choose a sample.
- *Circular systematic sampling:* It is subtype of linear sampling technique. Here, researcher selects a random number between '1' and 'N' rather than between '1' and 'i'.
- *Repeated systematic sampling:* A researcher go for selection of several smaller systematic samples rather than start with one random sample. However, this expensive and more time-consuming sampling among all systematic sampling.

Strengths of Systematic Random Sampling
- Systematic random sampling provides more efficient and convenient result
- It is a easy, time efficient and appropriate approach for manual selection for sample
- In case of homogeneous population, a more representative sample can be expected.

Limitations of Systematic Random Sampling
- A researcher can expect representative sample from large, uniform distributed population
- It does not give equal opportunity for sample selection, hence, bias is possible
- Researcher need to have a complete list of element to calculate sample interval. So, it is laborious and time consuming.

Cluster/Multistage Sampling

Cluster or multistage sampling is an appropriate option to choose sample from a large geographical distributed population. This is successive in nature and proceed from large to small sample. The first stage sampling unit consists of large units or cluster followed by small sampling units in second and so on. Cluster sampling involves random selection of population elements from each cluster. Researcher has to prepare a list of states, cities, institution and select a random sample from each unit.

Steps of Cluster Sampling
- Define the target population
- Determine desired sample size
- Develop sampling frame of clusters of population

- Select desired number of clusters randomly
- Select the number of samples from each cluster randomly.

Box 8.4: Example of Cluster Sampling.

Problem statement: 'A study to assess stress level among baccalaureate nursing students in North India'.
Steps under cluster sampling are as follows:
- Define baccalaureate nursing students (i.e. 50,000)
- Define desired number of sample size (i.e. 1000 students)
- Develop sampling frame of clusters (i.e. 50 districts)
- Select desired number of clusters randomly (i.e. 10 districts)
- From the selected district (10 districts), select desired number of nursing students through random sampling (i.e. 1000 nursing students)

Strengths of Cluster Sampling
- This technique is an appropriate and useful to study large and wide scattered population
- This technique helpful to develop insight of different region/zone of studied population
- It is quick and easy to study large scattered population.

Limitations of Cluster Sampling
- This sampling technique will give least representative sample as the samples taken from cluster are representative to concerned cluster only
- In case of increase number of clusters, the sampling error will be more from cluster to cluster.

NON-PROBABILITY SAMPLING

Non-probability sampling is less likely produce accurate and representative samples. Here, sample does not get an equal and independent chance of being selected for the study. Despite this weakness, nursing and other educational research using non-probability sampling in most.

The downside of the non-probability sampling method is that an unknown proportion of the entire population has not sampled. Therefore, the result of non-probability sampling techniques cannot be generalizing to entire population.

Types of Non-probability Sampling

Non-probability sampling has following subtypes:
1. Convenience sampling (accidental sampling)
2. Snowball/network/chain sampling
3. Quota sampling
4. Purposive or judgmental sampling
5. Consecutive/total enumeration.

Convenience Sampling

Convenience sampling (incidental or accidental) is the most preferred sampling chosen in nursing and other social sciences. This sampling allows the researcher to choose most readily and convenient available group of participants for the sample. This sampling technique reduce lot of effort and hard work of a researcher in selection of sample. However, convenience sampling is not a good choice for sample selection from a heterogeneous population. For example, a law student sitting on road side distribute questionnaires to know the public opinions about provision of capital punishment for rape accused.

Strengths of Convenience Sampling
- Convenience sampling is easy, cheapest, and least time consuming
- Convenience sampling helpful to draw desired number of samples from big population
- It is an appropriate sampling design to draw sample from homogeneous population.

Limitations of Convenience Sampling
- This sampling design is not appropriate choice to draw sample from heterogeneous population
- Convenience sampling is more bound to researcher' bias
- This is considered weak sampling approach because of not using any method to select sample.

Snowball Sampling

Snowball (network) sampling is an appropriate approach to study the population difficult to locate (i.e. substance abusers, commercial sex workers and alcohol abusers, etc). This approach use friends or colleagues or social media tend to have common features, habits or characteristics.

In this type of sampling early sample (very few in numbers) are asked to identify and refers other sample who fulfill the eligibility criteria.

Snowball sampling start with a small size of sample (1-2) and continue till study objectives will not fulfilled. The sampling makes a chain or network of sample; therefore, known as chain/network sampling, e.g. a researcher interested to know the extent of substance abuse in a particular district. For this particular condition, snowball sampling is choice of sampling techniques to locate substance abusers.

Types of Snowball Sampling
Snowball sampling can be done by using following methods:
- *Linear/single chain snowball sampling:* In this type, the early sample refer or register only one next sample for study and at the end of completion a single chain will be formed.

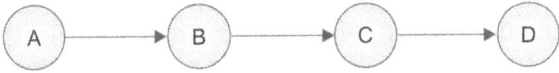

- *Exponential nondiscriminative snowball sampling:* In this subtype, initial/early sample is requested to refer/register at least two next samples for the study. Later on these two samples will register more samples and the chain will keep continuing till the sample size will not completed. Therefore, researcher use this sampling technique when sample size is very rare or limited to some specific subgroup.

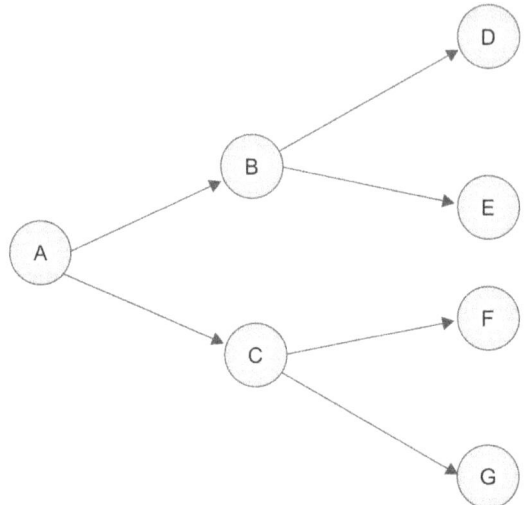

- *Exponential discriminative snowball sampling:* It is similar to nondiscriminative sampling where one subject/sample will register at least two samples and out of these two registered subjects, at least one will active further and refers two more subjects and again in these two subject one will active, for further subject registration.

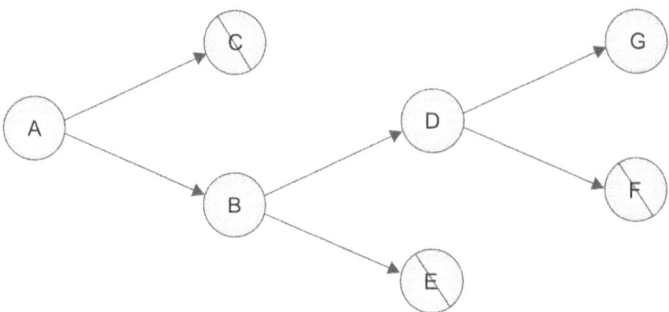

Strengths of Snowball Sampling
- It is easy, economic and convenient method to identify and recruit the difficult population
- The chain process helps researcher to locate extreme and rare case or phenomenon.

Limitations of Snowball Sampling
- This sampling gives less representative samples
- It does not give guarantee that recruitment of initial sample will help to reach next subjects, i.e. people belong to specific area will give reference of those area people only
- Sometimes, it is difficult to complete desired sample size by using snowball sampling as initial registered samples fail to register new samples.

Quota Sampling

Quota sampling is an another form of non-probability sampling approach in which a research use prior knowledge about the population under study to improve the representativeness.

A quota sample take into accounts different proportion (strata) of a defined population. A researcher create quota based on the knowledge of population and variables of interest (i.e. age, gender, socioeconomic status, marital status, etc.). In other ways, we can say that quota sampling is a derived version of stratified sampling without randomization of the subjects.

For example, researcher would like to study attitude of BSc Nursing students (1000) towards people with mental illness. We also know that male and female students or students studying in higher class have different attitude towards people with mental illness. Then, we can guide the selection of sample using quota sampling (Table 8.2).

Quota sampling can be disproportionate (Table 8.2) or proportionate (Table 8.3) in nature.

Table 8.2: Number and percentage of students in strata (gender).

Strata	Population	Quota sample
Male	100 (10%)	30 (30%)
Female	900 (90%)	630 (70%)
Total	1000 (100%)	660 (100%)

Table 8.3: Number and percentage of students in strata (course).

Strata	Population	Quota sample
BSc 1st year	200	50 (25%)
BSc 2nd year	200	50 (25%)
BSc 3rd year	200	50 (25%)
BSc 4th year	200	50 (25%)

Strengths of Quota Sampling
- Quota sampling approach is easy, inexpensive and time efficient
- It is an appropriate approach to study a large size population
- It is helpful to draw a representative samples from a homogeneous population
- A researcher should prefer quota sampling over convenience sampling for better representative sample.

Limitations of Quota Sampling
- Researcher bias is more frequent in quota sampling
- It is not a suitable approach to draw a representative sample from heterogeneous population and hence generalization is questionable.

Purposive Sampling

In purposive sampling, researcher decide the purpose for what he want informants to serve, and he go out to find someone. Purposive or purposeful sampling is the researcher's judgmental and conscious selection of participants and other sources of information for the study. Purposive sampling used for any unit of analysis, such as individual, families or community doing or practicing a particular activities or work. It is also called as *theoretical or judgmental sampling.*

Purposive sampling requires investigators to make judgment regarding the selection of participants. This is often based upon factors such as participant's knowledge, experience and role.

> **Box 8.5:** Example of Purposive Sampling.
>
> Kumar R, et al. (2015) conducted a study to identify needs, burden, coping and quality of life among stroke caregivers. The 100 subjects were selected using purposive sampling technique using inclusion criteria of age more than 18 years, blood relative and unpaid family members involves in direct care most of times

Consecutive/Total Enumeration Sampling

Consecutive sampling is a form of convenience sampling. Prospective study, which usually does not have sampling frame in beginning prefer consecutive sampling. This sampling technique involves all the samples meet inclusion criteria for a study over a period. This sampling technique has advantage to select all accessible subjects that make a better representation for the selected population. Further, this sampling approach is better in comparison to convenience sampling especially for a long sampling duration to deal seasonal and time related biases. This is a good approach for *'rolling enrollment'* into an accessible population.

> **Box 8.6:** Example of Consecutive Sampling.
>
> - Kumar R, et al. (2011) conducted a study to determine stress and coping strategies used by nursing students. Total enumeration technique was adopted and 180 nursing students were included in the:
> - Kassa E, et al (2016) conducted a study to see the effect of anti-tuberculosis drugs on hematological profiles of tuberculosis patients attending at University of Gondar Hospital, Northwest Ethiopia. He used a consecutive sampling technique to recruit 168 new TB patients

Strengths of Consecutive Sampling

- Consecutive sampling is an appropriate approach especially when the data collection period is sufficiently long
- It is comparatively easy and straightforward way to enroll the subjects
- Less opportunity for subjective bias in sample selection.

Limitations of Consecutive Sampling

There may be variation in selecting of sample over a different time/period of interval.

> **Box 8.7:** Reason for Use of Non-probability Sampling (Tappen, 2011).
>
> - Limitation on resources (limited fund and time to develop an accurate sampling plan)
> - Accessibility (inability to identify potential subjects)
> - Limited number of subjects (rare condition or events, where all subjects have to be selected for study)
> - Subject availability (e.g. high-risk group, youth like drug abusers)
> - Nonresponse or decline to participation in research
> - Experimental mortality or attrition (loss of subject from experimental group)

FACTORS AFFECTING SAMPLING/SAMPLE SIZE

- *Nature of research design:* Sample size and technique is vary from one research design to another. Preferably, a RCT need a small sample size than a survey design. Size of sample also varies in quantitative and qualitative research approach. Quantitative research approach needs large sample size than qualitative research.
- *Sampling method:* Probability sampling technique needs small sample size as compared to non-probability sampling technique.

- *Homogeneity of population:* Sample size varies in homogenous and heterogeneous population. In case of homogenous population, a smaller sample size can be works. A small number of selected samples from a homogenous population will represent most of the characteristics of population.
- *Availability of resources:* Selection of sample size depends on availability of resources like time, money, machine, manpower, etc. Therefore, researcher should think on resources before deciding sample size.
- *Effect size:* In experimental research study effect size should calculated for drawing sample. Effect size can be defined as degree of strength of relationship between independent and dependent variables. Effect size helps to decide/calculate accurate sample size in experimental studies.
- *Population characteristics:* Population characteristics also influence the sample size and technique. A large and heterogeneous population need to have large sample size in comparison to their counterparts. A small size may be a true representative for a group of homogeneous population. Further, a researcher should also look for attrition rate before deciding the sample size, a higher attrition rate tend to choose large sample size. A large sample should be preferred from vulnerable population by considering the availability of sample. For example, in case of higher attrition (sampling mortality), large sample size should be decided for research. Researcher should also keep in mind availability of adequate sample size while taking vulnerable population (older age, children, laborer, prisoner, pregnant mother, etc.) for the study.

SAMPLING PROCESS IN QUANTITATIVE RESEARCH

It is crucial to understand the steps and formal process of sampling in clinical studies. A well-framed sampling frame and sampling technique enable a researcher to draw empirical conclusion and helps in generalization of the research finding over target population. This section describe the basic steps involves in sampling process (Fig. 8.2).

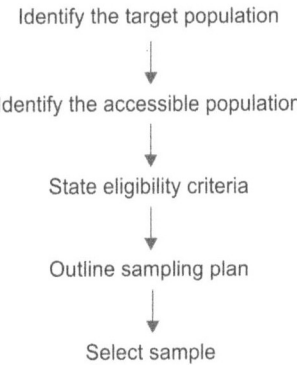

Fig. 8.2: Sampling process.

- *Identify the population:* Knowledge about target and accessible population is important to access a representative sample in a study.
- *Specify eligibility criteria:* The specific and strict criteria about characteristic of population help to exclude potential participants.

- *Specify the sampling plan:* Plan method of drawing sample, sample size and choose large sample to represent population characteristics.
- *Recruit the sample:* Recruit the participants according to the plan and exclusion and inclusion criteria after getting appropriate permission from concerned authority.

PROBLEMS IN SAMPLING

Sampling in research is economic in various aspects and make the research process convenient for a researcher. However, there are many drawbacks attached to sampling. A common problems are discussed here:
- *Sample representativeness:* Selection of representative sample is very difficult task for a researcher. It is difficult to select representative sample from a heterogeneous population.
- *Sample size analysis problem:* Estimating an adequate size of sample for research study is a challenge for a researcher. Sometimes, the population parameters are unavailable to calculate the desired sample size (i.e. effect size, SD, precision level, etc).
- *Lack of resources:* Lack of sufficient resource for nursing research is a big barrier to select a desired sample size for nursing studies. Therefore, lack of resources will impede the good quality of research in nursing.
- *Lack of knowledge of sampling process:* A researcher should have good knowledge and experience about different attributes of sampling and sampling process, i.e. sampling types, techniques, sample size analysis, process of random sampling, etc. Conducting research with superficial knowledge of sampling process will ultimately effect the worth and credibility of study.
- *Lack of support:* A research is a coordinate and group work. A high quality research work is the result of cooperation of experts such as administrator, statistician, writer, editor and supporting colleagues. Similarly, clinical research need cooperation of different category of personnels. Lack of support may hinder the selection of appropriate sample size.
- *Sampling bias (Sampling error/variation):* It is always impossible for a researcher to study all the population elements. Therefore, the concept of sampling has been followed. The bias that can occur while selecting sample is known as sampling/selection bias. Bias may be in the form of over representation or under representation of population characteristics (Polit and Beck, 2012). The variation can be two types, (1) Systemic variation and (2) Random variation (Burns and Grove, 2011). Systematic variation is a continuous bias of selection sample whose representative value is differs from population. Systematic variation increases when the sampling frame is poorly designed. Systematic bias is more harmful and limits the generalization of study findings. Random bias/variation is difference in value of selection of different subject at different time interval. As sample size increases, random variations decreases, and representativeness improve.

SAMPLE SIZE CALCULATION

Calculation of exact sample size is an important part of research design. It is very important to understand that different research design need different method of sample size calculation and one formula cannot be used in all designs. The sample size calculations for most frequently used study designs are given as follows:

Sample Size for Cross-sectional/Survey Designs

Cross-sectional studies are conducted to describe a phenomenon or variables in a defined population. Calculation of sample size for qualitative and quantitative variables is explained here:

Qualitative Variables

For example, a researcher is interested in knowing proportion of adult (18–40 years) suffering with hypertension (blood pressure >140 mm Hg) in a population. Researcher set 5% precision and at 95% confidence interval (5% of type 1 error).

Now, researcher found that previous study indicates that only 10% population have hypertension, he fix 5% precision and type I error of 5%. Therefore, if we substitute the value in above formula, it will give a value of 138. Hence, the calculated sample size will be 138 for the study.

$$\text{Sample size} = \frac{Z_{1-\alpha/2} \, p(1-p)}{d^2}$$

Here,

$Z_{1-\alpha/2}$ = Standard normal variate
p = Expected proportion in population based on previous studies or pilot testing
d = Level of precision decided by the researcher

$$\text{Sample size} = \frac{1.96^2 \times 0.10 \, (1-0.10)}{0.0025} = 138$$

Quantitative Variables

Suppose same researcher interest to know the average diastolic blood pressure of adults of the same area, then below formula can be used to calculate sample size;

For example, a researcher is interested in knowing the average diastolic blood pressure in adult age group (19–40 years) in a population. Researcher set 5% precision and at 95% confidence interval (5% of type 1 error) with a standard deviation 20 in previous studies, then below formula can be used to determine sample size.

$$\text{Sample size} = \frac{Z_{1-\alpha/2}^2 \, SD^2}{d^2}$$

Here,

$Z_{1-\alpha/2}$ = Standard normal variate
SD = Standard deviation, decided by previous study or through pilot study on similar variables
d = Absolute error or precision

$$\text{Sample size} = \frac{1.96^2 \times 25 \times 25}{(5)^2} = 61$$

Hence, the calculated sample size is 61 for the study

Sample Size for Case Control Studies

Case control studies are aims to compare known cases of disease with controls (without disease) regarding exposure to the risk factor under study. Following formula can be used to estimate sample size in case control studies.

For example, a researcher is interested to know the effect of cigarette smoking on lung cancer with a power of 80% and assuming expected proportion 40% and 20% in case and controls respectively and he want to have equal number of case and control.

$$\text{Sample size} = \frac{r+1}{r} \frac{(p^*)(1-p)(Z_\beta - Z_{\alpha/2})^2}{(p_1 - p_2)^2}$$

Here,

r = Ratio of case to control is 1 for equal number of ratio

p^* = Average population exposed = $\dfrac{\text{Proportion of exposed population} + \text{Proportion of control exposed}}{2}$

Z_β = Standard normal variate (0.84 for 80% variate and 1.28 for 90% variate)

$Z_{\alpha/2}$ = Standard normal variate for level of significance (previous study), 1.96 at 0.05 level of significance

$p_1 - p_2$ = Effect size, difference in population between cases (p_1) to control (p_2)

For substitution the values in above formula, $p^* = \dfrac{0.40 + 0.20}{2} = 0.30$

$$\text{Sample size} = \frac{2(0.30)(1-0.30)(0.84+1.96)^2}{(0.40+0.30)^2} = 329$$

Therefore, the calculated sample size is 329 for the above study.

Sample Size for Experimental Studies

In this type of research design researcher want to be see the effect of independent variables (cause) on dependent variables (effect). When the variables are quantitative like height, weight and blood pressure than following formula used to determine sample size,

$$\text{Sample size} = \frac{2SD^2(Z_{\alpha/2} + Z_\beta)^2}{d^2}$$

Here,

SD = Standard deviation (it can be calculated after pilot study or can be taken from previous related studies)

$Z_{\alpha/2} = Z_{0.05/2} = 1.96$ (Type I error at 0.95 level)

$Z_\beta = Z_{\beta 0.20} = 0.842$ (80% power, from Z table)

d = Effect size (difference between means of experimental and control groups)

For example, a researcher interested to test the new antihypertensive drug in comparison to placebo among hypertensive patients. Here, researchers trying to see the effect of antihypertensive medications on improvement on blood pressure, so he will select two or more than two groups. One group will be given antihypertensive drugs (experimental) and another group will keep refrain (control) from medications. He fixed that a difference of 15 mm Hg in blood pressure will be significant between experimental and control group. Let us assume that standard deviation is 20 mm Hg with 80% power and 5% level of significance. Use of above formula to calculate sample size is as below;

$$\text{Sample size} = \frac{2(20)^2 (1.96+0.84)^2}{(15)^2}$$

$$\text{Sample size} = \frac{(2\times 400)(1.96+0.84)^2}{225} = 28$$

Therefore, the calculated sample size for the study is 28.

POWER ANALYSIS

It is most favored and scientific method of sample size analysis in experimental or clinical trials studies. A researcher must have knowledge of following element of power analysis before its application.

- *Effect size:* This is referring to difference between means of experimental and control group (quantitative data) or proportion of incidents in two groups (in qualitative data). This should be determined before the study begins or can be taken from previous studies on similar concept.
- *Standard deviation:* Standard deviation refers to variability with in-group. Information on standard deviation is only required in case of quantitative information. Standard deviation can be calculated by pilot study or can be taken from previous studies on same concept.
- *Type I error:* This is level of significance, usually fix at the beginning of the study (5% = p = .05). However, it can be increased or decreased.
- *Power:* Power refers to probability of findings an effect. It usually kept 80% to 99%.
- *Attrition rate:* A researcher should also keep attrition rate in mind before final sample size estimation. The precise calculation of attrition rate helps to compensate effect of normal sample size. The final sample size should be as per the expected attrition in the study.

SAMPLE SIZE FOR ANIMAL STUDIES

Sample size in animal studies can be computed by using two formulas. The most commonly used method is the using same formula used for sample size calculation in experimental studies. With this method researcher can face some problem like getting SD and effect size from previous studies. In this condition, another formula can be used known *'resource equation method'*.

In this method E value has to be calculated based on decided sample size. The range of E value falls between 10 and 20. In case of E values <10, then more animals to be added in decided sample size and if E value >10, than sample size can be reduced.

E = Total number of animals − Total number of group

> **Box 8.8:** Sample Size Calculation in Animal Study.
>
> For example, in an animal study, researcher formed 5 groups of animals having 10 animals in each group for different interventions.
> So, total number of animals = 5 × 10 = 50
> Number of groups = 5
> So, E = 50 – 5 = 45
> The calculated sample size is more than >20. So, animals from each group can be decreased for study.

Although, this is very old method for sample size analysis in animal research and should be used if sample size calculation cannot be done by power analysis.

REVIEW QUESTIONS AND ANSWER

Long and Short Answer Questions

1. Describe sampling process in detail. (KUHAS, MSc N-2002)
2. Write in detail about the factors influencing sampling and the various sampling techniques. (AIIMS, MSc N-2001)
3. Discuss random sampling. (RGUHS, MSc N-2000)
4. Elaborate on probability sampling methods. (PGI, MSc N-2000)
5. What are sampling errors? Explain in detail. (TNMGRMU, MSc N-2000)
6. What is sampling? and What is its importance in nursing research? (AIIMS, MSc N-2008)
7. How to calculate sample size? Explain in detail. (PGI, MSc N-2000)
8. What are the characteristics and features of good sample? (BFUHS, MSc N-2000)

Multiple Choice Questions

1. Which one of the following is the main problem with using non-probability sampling techniques?
   a. Expensive
   b. Human errors (subjectivity)
   c. Not representative to whole population
   d. Practical problem in implementation

2. Which of the following is an example of non-probability sampling techniques used to study a rare group or population?
   a. Convenience sampling
   b. Snowball sampling
   c. Purposive sampling
   d. Quota sampling

3. Which of the following is an example of probability sampling technique used in research?
   a. Simple random sampling
   b. Snowball sampling
   c. Purposive sampling
   d. Quota sampling

4. Which of the following sampling technique is most appropriate to select sample when a researcher is well known about population characteristics in advance?
   a. Stratified random sampling
   b. Systematic random sampling
   c. Quota sampling
   d. Network sampling

5. This sampling technique has advantage to select sample from large geographical distributed population and successive from large to small simple.
   a. Cluster sampling
   b. Quota sampling
   c. Convenience sampling
   d. Simple random sampling

6. Which of the following non-probability sampling is considered weak among sampling techniques?
   a. Convenience sampling
   b. Snowball sampling
   c. Purposive sampling
   d. Quota sampling

7. It is commonly use sampling design in which a researcher uses his judgement and select the participants consciously who can serve the purpose of the study is called as:
   a. Simple random sampling
   b. Snowball sampling
   c. Purposive sampling
   d. Quota sampling

8. It is a process of selecting small group from of participants from a larger group is termed as:
   a. Sampling
   b. Cross matching
   c. Triangulation
   d. Trimming

9. A sampling technique in which each sample has equal and independent chance of selection is termed as:
   a. Non-probability sampling
   b. Probability sampling
   c. Biased sampling
   d. Stratified sampling

10. A sample which begin with a random number and then precedes with every Kth element from the population is termed as:
    a. Simple random sampling
    b. Stratified random sampling
    c. Systematic random sampling
    d. Quota sampling

Answer Key

1.	2.	3.	4.	5.	6.	7.	8.	9.	10.
b.	b.	a.	a.	a.	a.	c.	a.	b.	c.

SUGGESTED READING

1. Burn N, Grove SK. The practice of nursing research: Appraisal, synthesis and generation of evidence, 6th edition. St Louis: Elsevier; 2009.
2. Charan J, Biswas T. How to calculate sample size in different design in medical research? Ind J Psychol Med. 2013;35(2):121-6.
3. Charan J, Kantharia ND. How to calculate sample size in animal studies? J Pharmacol Pharmacother. 2013;4(4): 303-6.
4. Festing MF, Altman DG. Guidelines for designed statistical analysis of experiment using laboratory animal, Institute for laboratory animal research. 2002;43:244-58.
5. Houser J. Nursing Research: Reading, using, and creative evidence. USA: Jones and Bartlett Learning; 2008.
6. Kasiulevicius V, Sapoka PV, Filipaviciute R. Sample size calculation in epidemiological studies. Gerontology. 2006;7:225-31.
7. Kassa E, Enawgaw B, Gelaw A, Gelaw B. Effect of anti-tuberculosis drugs on hematological profiles of tuberculosis patients attending at University of Gondar Hospital, Northwest Ethiopia. BMC Hematology. 2016;16:1.
8. Kothari CR. Research methodology-methods and techniques. Wiley Eaetern Limited; 1991.
9. Kulbir SS. Methodology of research in education. Sterling Publishers Private Limited; 1992.

10. Kumar R, Kaur S, Reddemma K. Need, burden, coping and quality of life in stroke caregivers: A pilot survey. J Nur Mid Resear. 2015;11(2):57-67.
11. Kumar R, Nancy. Stress and coping among nursing students. J Nur Mid Resear.2011;7(4):141-51.
12. Patra P. Sample size in clinical research, the number we need. Int J Med Sci Public Health. 2012;1:35-9.
13. Polit DF, Beck CT. Nursing research generating and assessing evidence for nursing practice, 8th edition. Philadelphia: Lippincott William and Wilkins; 2008.
14. Punita E. Sampling in quantitative research. Ind J Contin Nur Edu. 2014;15(1):48-54.
15. Shah H. How to calculate sample size in animal studies. Natl J Physiolo Pharma Pharmacol. 2011;1:35-9.
16. Sharma SK. Nursing research and statistics. India: Saunders-Elsevier; 2011.
17. Singh AK. Tests measurement and research methods in behavioral sciences. India: Bharti Bhawan; 2013.
18. Tappen RM. Advanced nursing research: From theory to practice. Sudbury: Jones and Bartlett Learning; 2011.

Data Collection Methods in Research

Chapter 9

INTRODUCTION

After all planning is done, approvals have been obtained, and participants are being recruited, it is time to begin collecting data. The type of data you decide to collect and how you go about collecting it will have a great impact on its value in the analysis, reporting and application phase of your research study. Therefore, which data collection method to use would depend upon the research goals and the advantages and disadvantages of each method. In order to collect data, the researcher should be able to access the data that needs to be collected for the study.

PURPOSES OF DATA COLLECTION

Data are collected to serve many purposes, sometimes data are collected to test hypotheses, testing effectiveness of intervention in nursing and medical field, identifying needs of particular group, describe incidents and prevalence or distribution of a particular disease in a particular geographic area, and to find out sample characteristics, etc. The purposes of data collection can be explained as given below:

- *Needs identification:* Data are collected to identify needs of a particular individual, group, family, community and a particular group of people. For example, in nursing data are collected for different kinds of needs identification like identification of needs related to legal and ethical issues in field of psychiatric nursing or needs of staff nurses working in ICUs regarding ventilator care, and need of caregivers taking care of patient at home, etc.
- *Hypothesis testing:* Data collection leads to hypothesis testing in experimental studies, i.e. testing hypothesis regarding effect of soya milk protein diet on renal function improvement.
- *Distribution of disease pattern:* Descriptive, cross-sectional and epidemiological studies conducted to find the incidence and prevalence of a disease in a particular region or locality, i.e. incidence of epilepsy in urban region of district Amritsar, Punjab.
- *Sample characteristics identification:* Basic research collects data to find out the socio-demographics pattern and different characteristic of people residing in a particular geographic region. For example, study on socioeconomic status, education level, nutrition pattern and occupation styles of people residing at a rural community, New Delhi.
- *Bias and barriers identification:* Sometimes, researcher collect data to identify the possible barriers and potential bias in upcoming research project. Data collection will help to take anticipated measures to overcome these bias and barriers.

TYPES OF DATA

Research depends on different types of data to fulfill above mentioned purposes. Researcher collects data according to types of research approach, i.e. quantitative and qualitative approach. Following types of data can be collected in research:
- *Quantitative data:* Quantitative research collects data in numerical or quantitative format. The collection of quantitative data is challenging and complex task but tabulation, analysis and interpretation are hurdle free. The quantitative research uses well designed and formal structured instruments to collect data, i.e. rating scale, questionnaire, structured interview and checklist, etc.
- *Qualitative data:* Narrative and descriptive data are collected in qualitative research. The data are collected with the help of semi-structured interview, in-depth conversation, focus group interview, joint interview and observation methods. The researcher also uses research instrument in qualitative studies. Data collection is an easy task in qualitative study.

SOURCES OF DATA

The design of the research project specifies both; the data that are needed (type of data) and how data to be obtained (methods). The first step in the data-collection process is to look for source of data. Researchers need to consider the sources on which to base and confirm their research and findings. Researcher has a choice between primary and secondary sources and selection of source or both. Researcher should give preference to primary sources over secondary sources for collecting data in research.

Primary Sources

These are first hand informations collected by researcher. Information collected from primary sources are more objective and empirical in nature. Primary sources enable the researcher to get as close as possible to what actually happened during an event or time period. Primary sources are either created during the time period being studied or produced at later date by participant or eye witness of the event (as in the case of memoirs). Primary sources may be in their original format or may have been reproduced later in a different format, including translated, transcribed or printed documents, book, microfilms collection, videos, and internet archives, so long as later version is an authentic and accurate 'word for word' rendering of the original.

Box 9.1: Example of Primary Sources.

Letters, personal papers, diaries, journal, paintings, photographs, memoirs, advertisements, posters, banners, original maps, oral histories, news footages, vital records, newspaper articles, minutes of meetings, mail survey, questionnaire, etc.

Secondary Sources

These are second hand information (sometime third and fourth hand) collected by researcher after the event has been occurred or over. Secondary sources are source of data that consists of summarization of or commentary about primary data, such as writing or life experiences by someone other than the person who produced the data or lived through the experiences. Secondary sources are analogs to human conversation. If I tell you something, I am your primary source. If you tell someone else what I told you, you are the secondary sources for my words.

> **Box 9.2:** Example of Secondary Sources.
>
> Official statistics, content analysis, historical methods, informatics, mass media products, letters and web information, etc.

DATA COLLECTION PLAN

Data collection is nothing more than planning for and obtaining useful information on key quality characteristics. However, simply collecting data does not ensure that you will obtain accurate, relevant and specific enough information. The key issue is not: how do we collect data? Rather is: how do we obtain useful data? Data collection plan is mandatory to collect data in uniform and consistent pattern. The elements of data collection plan should be clear, unambiguous and operationally defined to get useful data. Data collection planning have variety of benefits:

- Well-developed data collection plan helps to gather accurate and empirical information
- It prevents errors and involvement of external variables involvement in data collection plan
- It saves time and money that otherwise might be spent on repeated or failed attempts to collect useful data
- Directions for data collection.

Essential of Data Collection

The data collection process begins with answering following questions. These are also known as 5 Ws of data collection:

1. **What** data is to be collected? Type of data, number of variables, needs for data collection, type of selected statistical computation or tests, etc.
2. **How** data will be collected? Instruments to collect the relevant data, i.e. questionnaire, interview, rating scale, and checklist, etc.
3. **Who** will collect data? It is concerned with investigator or co-investigator who is going to collect data, in case of multiple data collectors, the training part should be kept in mind to ensure consistency and accuracy in data collection.
4. From **Where** data will be collected? Data setting should be explained and defined properly to avoid any confusion and ambiguity, i.e. individual, family, school, college, wards, department, and community, etc.
5. **When** the data collection will be collected? Timing of data collection should be preplanned and defined properly. Many factors define the time of data collection in research. For example, in cross-sectional study at one point of time, and longitudinal study at different point of time, etc.

> **Box 9.3:** Essential of Data Collection (5 W's).
>
> 1. **What:** What information is to be collected
> 2. **How:** Use of instruments and devices
> 3. **Who:** Investigator or person who collect data
> 4. **Where:** Place where data to be collected
> 5. **When:** Timing of data collection

Development of Data Collection Plan

A formal data collection plan needs lot of efforts, expert advice, guidance and experience. A researcher should keep certain points in mind while developing a data collection plan. Some of the important instructions are given as follows:

- *Easy to follow:* A data collection plan should be easy to follow for researcher and participant under investigation. Using a flexible plan is another good idea while preparing a data collection plan. However, a researcher should see the feasibility of data collection plan for his own work.
- *Pre-test the plan:* It is always good to pretest the data collection plan for its feasibility in terms of time, effort, implementation for hurdle free use in research work. Therefore, a pilot study is necessary before moving to the main study.
- *Training to data collectors:* A researcher should deliver a training to data collectors to ensure the consistency in data collection. An appropriate training will also help to prepare the data collectors for easy use of data collection plan. Further, it will also make the data collectors clear about the steps and any doubts or related quarry.
- *Focus on objective information:* A data collection plan should prepare to collect only empirical information. A robust data collection plan will help to provide first-hand information.
- *Critical assessment of plan:* A data collection plan should be critically evaluated before proceeding for final phase. It should be thoroughly review for its strengths and weakness to follow while data collection.
- *Maintain a record:* A data collection plan should mention the recording and reporting of information to prevent uneventful loss of data or information. A researcher should also make ensure to record the information timely without undue loss.

DATA COLLECTION METHODS

Data collection is a crucial component of a research process. A researcher should use valid and reliable instrument to collect data. There are numerous methods by which data may be collected for research and administrative purposes. Whenever, using two or more methods or measures for data collection, researcher must carefully consider and document the order in which data are collected. Researcher use data collection method, techniques and tool synonymously in research but actually they are different in origin and use. A detail of the data collection methods is given here (Fig. 9.1 and Table 9.1).

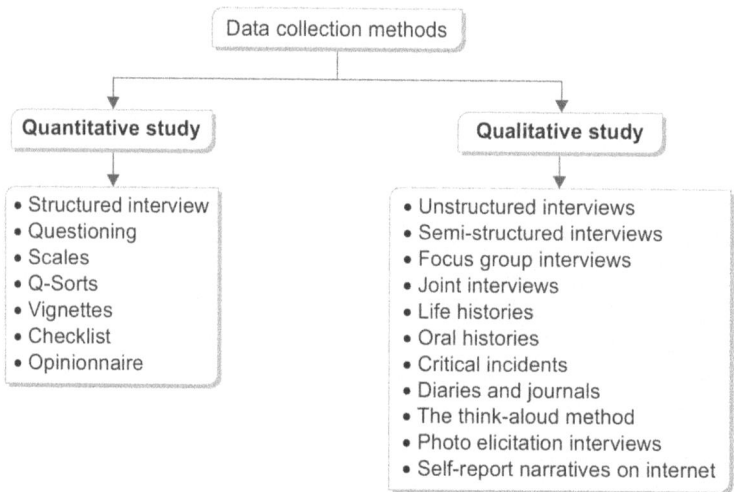

Fig. 9.1: Data collection methods.

- *Data collection method*: Steps and strategies to collect, tabulate and analyze data, i.e. self-report method, observation method, etc.
- *Techniques of data collection*: Specific tools of a method, i.e. paper and pencil techniques for self-reported method.
- *Instrument/tool for data collection*: Specific measures to collect information on a particular construct, i.e. questionnaire and rating scale, etc.

Table 9.1: Data collection tools/methods and techniques.

Data collection methods/techniques	Tools
Questioning	• Questionnaire • Structured interview • Rating scale • Checklist/inventory

Measurement	• Physical measurement
	   – Physical measurement, i.e. temperature
	   – Chemical measurement, i.e. hormone and sugar level
	   – Microbiological measurement, i.e. bacterial count
	• Psychological measurement, i.e. IQ testing

Interview	• Interview (structured and unstructured) • Opinionnaire
Observation	• Observation checklist • Rating scale • Anecdote records
Other methods	• Record analysis (content analysis) • Q-sort techniques • Vignettes • Projective techniques

Selection of Data Collection Methods

A valid and reliable method of data collection will help to collect objective information. Selection of data collection methods depend on many aspects of research study such as, type of study, variables, sample characteristics, hypothesis testing, availability of resources, researcher knowledge and experience, time duration of study, resources and manpower, purpose of study, and need of data, etc. Many factors may influence the selection of method of data collection including followings:

- *Type of research study:* Research study will direct the selection of data collection instrument, i.e. quantitative study will use structured and formal instrument while qualitative studies use unstructured interview method to collect data.
- *Variables under study:* Variable under study will also influence the selection of data collection method, i.e. to collect information regarding children behavior, observation method will be best suited.
- *Hypothesis testing:* Numerical information is required to test a hypotheses. However, a narrative information is more appropriate to collect information in qualitative study to develop theory.

- *Availability of resources:* Selection of method of data collection will be depend on availability of resources. Freely access to resources may help a researcher to choose interview as a method of data collection. However, a researcher should go for questionnaire as a method of data collection for limited resources and supply.
- *Sample characteristics:* Data collection methods will depend on characteristic of the research subjects. In case of illiterate subjects, interview method will be best suited rather than using questionnaire for the same subjects.
- *Researcher experience:* Researcher knowledge and experience will also influence selection of data collection method. Selecting interview will need more expertise and experience rather than using questionnaire which merely need presence of researcher.
- *Time duration:* Researcher should keep in mind the time duration of the study. Questionnaire can be best measure to collect data within a very short period of time in place of interview and observation method.

QUESTIONNAIRE

Questionnaire is developed by **Fransis Galton.** It is commonly used self-report method for collecting data in quantitative study. It is one of the inexpensive and easy methods of data collection.

The instrument sometime called questionnaire or self-administered questionnaire (SAQ), when subjects having instruction to complete the questionnaire on their own. A researcher will play a passive role in administration and data collection through questionnaire.

A questionnaire is a systematically developed series of questions prepared by investigators to fill or complete by participants in order to collect required information on construct under study.

Types of Questionnaire

A different types of questionnaires are available to collect the information. A research can choose anyone suitable for data collection.
- Open Ended Questionnaire: Open ended questionnaire allow subjects to express their own thought, ideas, feeling, etc. The question 'how did you react when you witnessed bloodshed first time?'. In this type of method subjects are asked to give their free and frank opinion regarding construct under study. Researcher plays a passive role in recording response of the subjects.

Box 9.4: Example of Open Ended Question.

1. What do you understand by mean of quality of life?
2. What is your opinions on quality of nursing education?

- Closed Ended (Fixed Alternative) Questionnaire: In fixed response alternative, respondents give or choose a answer from given alternatives which is most closely to their ideas, feeling and thoughts. The alternative question can be following types:
  - *Dichotomous question:* In this type of questionnaire respondents has to select choice of response between two alternatives, i.e. male and female, yes or no, etc. Dichotomous questionnaire are useful to collect exact and factual information for particular attribute.

> **Box 9.5: Example of Close Ended Question.**
>
> Q. 1: Have you ever visited Delhi?
> Ans: a. Yes
> b. No
> Q. 2: Did you ever check your weight?
> Ans: a. Yes
> b. No

- *Multiple choice questions:* Respondent has to choose most relevant or correct response from 3 or more than 3 alternatives. Researcher should not keep the alternatives less than three or more than seven in numbers.

> **Box 9.6: Example of Multiple Choice Question.**
>
> Q. 1: Which of the following is most common cause of HIV/AIDS?
> Ans: 1. Sharing clothes
> 2. Sharing toilets
> 3. Sharing utensils
> 4. Unprotected sexual intercourse

- *Rank order questions:* Respondent should rank the given alternatives along a continuum, i.e. extremely important to not at all important.

> **Box 9.7: Example of Rank Order Question.**
>
> Q. 1: Arrange following given attributes on importance continuum in your life (from most important to least important):
> 1. Money
> 2. Family
> 3. Carrier
> 4. Self-satisfaction
> 5. Self-esteem

- *Rating questions:* Respondents ask to evaluate a particular construct/phenomena along an ordered continuum. Questions are on bipolar dimension where each end point represent extreme opposite view regarding investigated concepts. The number of rating along the continuum is often in odd number like 3, 5, 7 and so on. The continuum consists 0 to 10 rating and will be considered a 11 point rating scale.

> **Box 9.8: Example of Rating Question**
>
> Q. 1: Rate your job satisfaction on a scale ranging 0 means 'extremely unsatisfied' to 10 means 'fully satisfied':
>
> 0   1   2   3   4   5   6   7   8   9   10
> Extremely   Fully
> Unsatisfied   Satisfied

- *Checklist:* Checklist includes a list of question against which some response pattern will be assigned. It is two dimension in format in which a set of questions in one dimension and their responses will be on opposite dimension. Checklist is easy to fill, tabulate and analysis rather than other types of self-report methods (Table 9.2).

Table 9.2: Sample format of checklist (steps of conducting ECT).

Instruction: Place tick (√) mark in given option

S. No.	Steps of ECT	Yes	No	Remarks
1.	Explain procedure			
2.	Prepare patient			
3.	Wash hands			
4.	Collect necessary equipment			
5.	Prepare tray for ECT			
6.	Check the ECT machine			
7.	Place patient in supine position			
8.	Place tongue depressor			
9.	Administer 100% oxygen			
10.	Administer ECT			

- *Cafeteria questions:* It is one form of multiple choice questionnaire in which respondents should select the alternative which one is most suitable for their view, ideas and belief.

> **Box 9.9:** Example of Cafeteria Question.
>
> Q. 1: Which statement most close to you view regarding Indian government?
> 1. I am not interested in politics
> 2. Politics ruin the country
> 3. Politics is worthless job
> 4. Politics help the country to grow

- *Contingency questions:* It is also known as *lead questionnaire* in which respondent asked further question in case they are able to answer the pervious question.

> **Box 9.10:** Example of Contingency Question.
>
> Q. 1: Are you married?
> 1. Yes
> 2. No
> If yes, mention year of marriage……………………

- *Matrix questions:* It is another type of questionnaire in which multiple questions and their concerned responses are given to respondent in matrix format.
  Example question. Which is your favorite animal? (1—Most like animal, 5—Most hate animal)

Animals	1	2	3	4	5
Cat					
Dog					
Lion					
Leopard					
Horse					

- *Importance questions:* It is type of rating scale in which respondent rate a question along the continuum of importance. It could be 3 point or 5 point rating scale.

> **Box 9.11:** Example of Importance Question.
>
> Q. 1: Eating green leafy vegetables daily is
> 1. Very important (4)
> 2. Important to some extent (3)
> 3. Not so important (2)
> 4. Not important (1)

- *Single item indicator questionnaire:* A questionnaire made up of just one item sometimes is referred to as a single item indicator.

> **Box 9.12:** Example of Single Item Indicator Question.
>
> Q. 1: In general, how satisfied are you with your life?
> 1. Very dissatisfied
> 2. Dissatisfied
> 3. Satisfied
> 4. Very satisfied

Steps of Construction of Self-report Methods

Self-report is the most common method used for data collection in quantitative information. A different approaches and steps are mentioned in literature to develop a self-report method. However, these following steps may be used as supplementary to develop a self-report method. These steps are describing the systematic way of developing a structured questionnaire and may be followed to develop other self-report method as well.

- *Selection of construct/concept:* The researcher should select researchable construct, phenomena or concept that is going to be explored. The selected construct must be specific enough to investigate in a research such as stress level, quality of life and pain perception, etc.
- *Selection a pool of items:* The next step is to develop a pool of items related to selected construct. Developing pool of items need lot of experience, knowledge, review of literature, expert advice, higher authority guidance and population experience, etc.
- *Deciding number of items and response alternatives:* Researcher should work on needed number of a sample of items that can cover all aspects of given construct and response alternatives carefully to assess the construct in depth. Appropriate selection of response alternative will help a researcher to assess the construct from different angles such as questionnaire on knowledge on ethical issues in medical sciences will consist items related to ethics terminology, torts, law, and act, etc.
- *Wording of questionnaire:* Use of simple, clear and subject friendly language will help as researcher to explore the topic in detail. A researcher should avoid use of technical jargon and abbreviation while preparing a self-report method. Further, the language of questionnaire should be according to level of participants, i.e. using local language translated questionnaire for local community people.
- *Organization of questionnaire:*
  - *Introduction and instructions:* This is beginning part of a self-report or questionnaire. A standardized question need specific instruction how to fill and what to fill. Further, it is important to note down the purpose of the questionnaire along with instruction.

- *Personal data:* It consists of information regarding age, gender, education, etc.
- *Background data*: Family income, occupation, living environment whether urban or rural, etc.
- *Main body:* This is main part of questionnaire consist items related to the construct/variable under study.
- *Acknowledgment for participants:* A few words of thanks and cooperation for participants should be mentioned at the end of questionnaire.

- *Administration of questionnaire on pilot project:* Once the questionnaire is ready, it should be tested for feasibility, practicability and other issues. Pilot study play an important role in pre-testing of the questionnaire.
- *Evaluation of psychometric properties:* The questionnaire psychometric properties (validity and reliability) should be checked by taking expert opinions from concerned experts in field or by using appropriate statistical formula (KR_{20}, Cronback's alpha, and Coefficient correlation, etc.).
- *Preparation of final draft:* Once all things will be checked, corrected and modified, the final draft of the questionnaire should be prepared for using in research study.

Methods of Questionnaires Administration

The questionnaire can be administered by using following methods:
- *Self-administration (Face to Face Method):* Investigator can administer questionnaire on one to one basis. This method of administration leads high response rate (>60%) than other methods of administration.
- *Computer-Assisted Method:* Internet-based technology such as the World Wide Web (web) is fast becoming accessible to large segments of society. Use of computer in data collection is quite popular nowadays. Computer-assisted method can help in numerous ways. A researcher can use telephonic, web-based and mail to send the questionnaire to the study participants.
  - *Email questionnaire:* A word or pdf file can mail to participants through mail. Participants can respond on the same file or can attach the scan copy of questionnaire after filing it. However, the response rate is low as compare to face-to-face method.
  - *Telephonic questionnaire:* Investigator convey instructions on phone to participants to fill the questionnaire. This method ensure high speed, easy, and high response rate. However, it is recommended to use telephonic questionnaire for short survey.
  - *Web-based questionnaire:* This is another computer-assisted method of sending questionnaire in which investigator has to send a link on mail address of respondent. The respondent has to click on that link that will go to questionnaire and then respondent have to fill and submit it via same mail to investigator. The web-based questionnaire and mailing questionnaire are easy to respond. However, limitations of these methods lies in high cost, need of computer, computer literacy and electricity problem, etc. Therefore, the investigators should keep in mind all the issues before using computer-assisted method of administration of questionnaire.

Essentials of a Good Questionnaire

Preparation of a questionnaire is an art a researcher should know. Preparation an ideal questionnaire need special talent, experience and knowledge of education pedagogy. However, an effective questionnaire must meet certain requirements as given below:

- *A cover letter:* An ideal questionnaire must accompany a cover letter with certain details like name of the investigator, working place, qualification, contact details and purpose of survey, etc.
- *Do not overcrowd questionnaire:* The questionnaire should have limited number of questions to catch the attention of the respondents.
- *Use a large, clear print:* Questionnaire can be made user-friendly by making use of a large and clear print. Too small print makes it difficult to read.
- *Provide clear instructions:* Specific instruction regarding response filling should be provided in the beginning of the questionnaire.
- *Do not split question across page:* Responded find it difficult if a question split over two pages; especially in respect of response categories for a closed question.
- *Pre-code all questions:* Pre-coding allow the participants to simply circle the answer.
- *Easy language:* The questionnaire should be developed in easy and understandable language.
- *Short questions:* The questions should be short as much as possible.
- *Logical flow:* A logical flow in the questions and section must exist. For example, a questionnaire developed to assess knowledge regarding HIV/AIDS among urban population should consist, questions on introduction, risk factors, sign symptoms, management, etc.
- *Avoid duplications:* A good questionnaire should avoid duplication of the questions.
- *Provide blue print:* In case of self-developed or standard questionnaire, a blue print should accompany the questionnaire to get an overview of variables under study.
- *End the questionnaire in a proper way:* Respondents should be thanked for their participation.
- *Avoid leading question:* A questionnaire should not contain leading question. It is easy for a subject to hit the right response for these types of questions. A question such as," Do you think that Indian politics is ruin the country" is not neutral.
- *Interpersonal wording of question:* A careful use of interpersonal wording of question sometimes helpful to encourage honest response and decrease embarrassment to a participant. To understand this point, mind the following two questions with which respondent was asked to rate quality of nursing care:
    1. I am not happy with quality of nursing care I received during my hospitalization.
    2. I am personally feel bad about quality of nursing care during my hospitalization. Here, a participant may feel more comfortable to answer the question with less personally worded.

Strengths of Questionnaire

- Questionnaire is an effective method to study a large group of population in short span of time
- It is inexpensive, rapid and easy way to collect information
- Face to face questionnaire control the respondent bias
- Questionnaire method ensure high response rate as compared to other methods of data collection
- Questionnaire method is much more less costly, require less time and energy to the investigator.

Limitations of Questionnaire
- Questionnaire only focus on superficial information and therefore not an appropriate choice to explore a topic in detail
- It will not give freedom to participant to choose the right response (forced choice category)
- In case of lengthy questionnaire, printing cost will be a concern
- Questionnaire can only feasible to literate people. It is not a good choice to study illiterate, blind and deaf population
- Subjects' non-verbal cues cannot be recorded
- Sometime, participants may miss or omit the question and provide incomplete information.

RATING SCALE

Rating scale is another self-report method to collect data in quantitative research. Rating scale provides numeric score to rate an attribute along a continuum. Rating scale can be used to measure attitude, belief, value, needs, desire, demands, pain and comfort level, etc. It is a form of closed or fixed alternative questions in which a pool of close ended questions are grouped together.

Rating scale for individual may be completed by the person being evaluated (self-rating) or by some significant other such as a parent, spouse, supervisor or social worker, etc. Sometimes a client and a significant other are asked to complete the same rating scale, to provide us with two different views about a concept.

Types of Rating Scale
1. Likert scale
2. Semantic differential scale
3. Visual analogs scale
4. Graphic rating scale.

Likert Scale

Likert scale is most widely used form of attitude measurement, named after the psychologist Rensis Likert. Likert scale is a series of five to seven response for each item, ranging from strongly agree to strongly disagree. It is recommended to include approximate number of positive or negative items in a Likert scale to get a fair degree of agreement or disagreement toward a construct. It is considered '*balance*' with equal number of positive and negative items.

For a five point rating scale, score on each item generally range from 1 to 5. A score of 5 usually given to "*strongly agree*", 4 to "*agree*", 3 to "*uncertain*", 2 to "*disagree*" and finally 1 to "*strongly disagree*". It is recommended to reverse the negative items before proceeding to the final analysis. "*Strongly agree*" response to negative item would receive a score of 1 rather than 5. At the end, total score is determined by summing up individual items score. Therefore, this scale is called *Summated rating scale*.

Uses of Likert Scale
- It is used to measure value, belief, feeling, practices, and attitude towards a particular attribute.
- It helps to quantify the subjective phenomena and opinions towards a particular construct like attitude and stigma towards mental illness, etc.

Table 9.3: Example of Likert scale.

Instruction: Please put (√) in appropriate column

S. No	Statement	Strongly Agree (5)	Agree (4)	Uncertain (3)	Disagree (2)	Strongly Disagree (1)
1.	Mental illness are results of devil spirit, black magic or sin of past birth					
2.	Marriage can cure mental illness					
3.	Mental illness are contagious in nature					
4.	Mental illness once occurs will not cure					

Tips for Preparing Likert Scale

- Collect a large pool of item by reviewing relevant literature or with discussion to experts
- Try to take a balance of negative and positive items to get a fair agreement for an attribute under study
- It always good to convert reverse score for negative items before proceeding final analysis
- The items used in scale should be brief and concise for ease of understanding
- Use of simple, unambiguous and clear language make the scale interesting to read and respond to subjects.

Table 9.4: Reverse scoring in Likert scale.

Statement	Strongly agree	Agree	Neutral	Disagree	Strongly disagree
Positive statement	(5)	(4)	(3)	(2)	(1)
Negative statement	(1)	(2)	(3)	(4)	(5)

Strengths of Likert Scale

- It is en expensive and cost-effective method to collect information from a widely distributed population
- Likert scale is easy to develop because of limited number of items
- Likert scale is only method to assess attitude, belief, value and perception towards a particular construct
- It is easy for a researcher to administer the scale for a large population at a time.

Limitations of Likert Scale

- Sometimes, a researcher find it difficult to generate adequate amount of items pool for a scale
- Likert scale is not an appropriate choice for illiterate and mentally challenged population
- In Likert scale, participants feel forced to respond to items for a given construct
- Likert scale findings only describe a phenomenon but unable to answer cause for same.

Semantic Differential Scale

Charles Osgood, Suci and Tannenbaum (1957) first used semantic differential scale to measure connotative and denotative meaning attached to a concept. He asked respondent to choose where his/her position lies on a scale between two bipolar words or range of words or numbers ranging across a bipolar position (i.e. genius, excellent, intelligent, average, dull and mad). So, on the basis of above explanation it can be said that semantic differential scale is a rating scale used to measure the connotative meaning attached to object, concept, events, etc.

The semantic differential scale is made up of one or more items that are rated on a series of bipolar adjective scales. It is used to measure the meaning of each item to the respondent. Each item may be considered a separate concept or may be a component of a concept. Questionnaire may include one or more of three dimensions of semantic differential scale. The three dimensions, with examples of bipolar adjectives used to rate them, are:

The scale consists polar adjective (opposite meaning terms) at each end. Charles Osgood and his associates identified three major dimension of semantic differential scale: **Evaluation** (i.e. good/bad, effective/ineffective), **potency** (strong/weak, small/range) and **activity** (fast/slow, active/passive). Though, it is not compulsory to take all three dimensions related items in a scale. Items related to any adjective can be taken to explore underline construct in an instrument. These dimensions can be arranged in a rating scale as follows:

Box 9.13: Dimension of Semantic Differential Scale.

- **Evaluative**—good–bad, kind–cruel, beautiful–ugly
- **Potency**—hard–soft, heavy–light, strong–weak
- **Activity**—active–passive, fast–slow, hot–cold

Semantic differential scale is 7 points rating scale used to measure psychometric traits. The participants are asked to rate a concept on 7 points scale. 7 points rating scale ranging from one extreme dimension to another.

Box 9.14: Example of Semantic Differential Scale.

Instruction: Please place a mark (X) on the space that indicate what nursing means to you.

Nursing profession is:

Risky	:	:	:	:		Not risky
Respected	:	:	:	:		Not respected
Good	:	:	:	:		Bad
Satisfactory	:	:	:	:		Not satisfactory
Hard work	:	:	:	:		Easy work
Important	:	:	:	:		Not important
Busy	:	:	:	:		Not busy
Interesting	:	:	:	:		Not interesting
Female oriented	:	:	:	:		Male oriented

Uses of Semantic Differential Scale

Semantic differential scale is helpful in following areas:
- It helps to decide the acceptance of a product in the market
- It is only approach to measure psychological traits such as personality and behavior, etc.

- It is used in different kind of survey like job satisfaction, employees appraisal survey, etc.
- Sometimes, semantic differential scale used to predict election poll.

Limitations of Semantic Differential Scale
- In semantic differential scale, a researcher may feel difficult to collect a pool of adjacent item to measure a concept
- It does not allow the participants for their frank response. It is a forced choice method.

Visual Analog Scale

Visual analog scale (VAS) is another psychosocial measure to assess subjective experience like pain, sleep, fatigue, comfort level, alertness, drowsiness, anxiety, and dyspena, etc. Visual analog scale measures depth and intensity of subjective feelings and sensation that are believed to range across a continuum of value and cannot be measured directly. For example, the amount and intensity of pain can range from worst or extreme pain to no pain on a continuum (Fig. 9.2).

Operationally, VAS is a 100 mm length horizontal or vertical line, each end labeled as the extreme limits of a sensation. However, graphic and nonverbal visual analog scale also available to measure certain clinical conditions like face pain scale for infants (Fig. 9.3).

For example, VAS for pain rating consists no pain at left hand and worst or extreme pain in right hand.

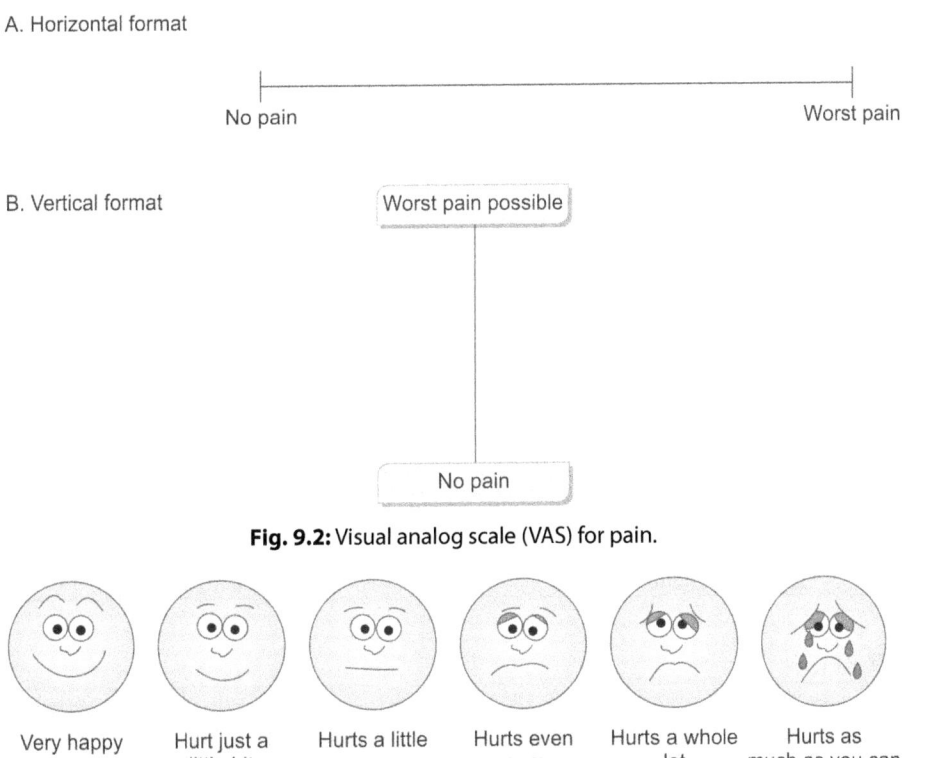

Fig. 9.2: Visual analog scale (VAS) for pain.

Fig. 9.3: Face pain scale for infant.

Uses and Strengths of Visual Analog Scale
- Visual analog scale used to measure certain subjective phenomenon such as pain, anxiety, drowsiness, and sleep, etc.
- The findings of visual analog scale help a clinician to choose right drug and determine dose for same
- It helps to track the progress or improvement of patients' condition in clinical area
- Scale can be administered verbally or in writing and thus are useful for all population.

Limitations of Visual Analog Scale
- The scale measure the subjective experience of a phenomenon and hence, chance of bias are more in findings
- Generalization of findings is another limitation of visual analog scale.

Box 9.15: Example of Visual Analog Scale.

Meek R, et al. (2009) use visual analog scale (VAS) in an undifferentiated emergency department population to calculate minimum significant difference in VAS rating of nausea severity in the population

---

Graphic Rating Scale

This is most widely used scale to measure performance or behavior in quantitative or qualitative ways. The quantitative scale move from 1 (poor) to 5 (excellent) while qualitative adjacent range from poor, average, good, excellent and outstanding to describe numbers or rating. Graphic rating scale can be used by peer or superior to rate their colleagues or subordinate. Overall score will be calculated by summing up the total score together and divide it by the total number of items. Items left or not rated should be excluded from total numbers of items.

Strengths of Graphic Rating Scale
- The graphic rating scale is easy to construct and use
- It is an appropriate method to measure the employees performance to be gathered over a period of time.

Limitation of Graphic Rating Scale

Graphic rating scale lack specificity and promote halo effect.

Box 9.16: Example of Graphic Rating Scale.

The BLS team Leader assigned the role to team members

1   2   3   4   5   6

Ineffective   Effective

CHECKLIST

Checklist is the most common method of data collection used in health care setting. Checklist is easy to fill and only concerned with the absence and presence of the event, attribute, practice, skills, steps or behavior, etc. Checklist can be self-reported or observed one. In self-reported checklist, participant has to fill the absence or presence of traits, while in observed checklist, observer has to record the incident and fill their presence and absence accordingly. For example, investigator give a checklist to staff nurses and asked to fill the steps of hand-washing they follow in clinical setting (self-reported). In observed checklist case, investigator himself observe the staff nurses for hand-washing steps and then record the absence and presence of steps in the checklist (Table 9.5).

Checklists are constructed by breaking a performance and the quality of a product, which specifies the presence or absence of an event or phenomena which is then 'checked' by a rater/observer.

Table 9.5: Example of checklist.

	Instruction: Place tick(√) mark in given option			
S. No.	Steps of ECT	Yes	No	Remarks
1.	Explain procedure			
2.	Prepare patient			
3.	Wash hands			
4.	Collect necessary equipment			
5.	Prepare tray for ECT			
6.	Check the ECT machine			
7.	Place patient in supine position			
8.	Place tongue depressor			
9.	Administer 100% oxygen			
10.	Administer ECT			

Guidelines of Constructing a Good Checklist

Although preparation of checklist is quite easy and comfortable job for a researcher. However, it is always good to follow certain rules for preparation of a good checklist.
- Write clear instructions to participants to fill the checklist
- Divide the construct (topic under study) into pieces to develop ample number of items
- A good checklist is free from double negative and barred statements
- A checklist should not include technical jargon, and abbreviations
- Select a pool of items which are mutually exclusive and exhaustive in nature.

Strengths of Checklist
- Checklist is easy to develop and economical to use
- Checklist facilitate ease of data collection
- Observation checklist help to focus on more empirical findings.

Limitations of Checklist
- Checklist only provide a superficial knowledge about a construct
- Self-reported checklist has more chances of bias
- Use of checklist in qualitative study is limited
- Checklist only answer about presence and absence of the phenomenon but does not answer why the phenomenon absent or present.

INTERVIEW METHOD

Interview is most widely used method of data collection in quantitative and qualitative research. In interviews method, researcher and participant sit face to face to provide information on given concepts. Interview schedule is an oral questionnaire that is read to the respondents by a researcher.

Interview is a two way systematic conversations between an investigator and an informant initiated for obtaining information relevant to underlying construct. Interviewer not only collects information from respondent, but also records non-verbal behavior of a participant and environmental conditions.

Interview is a systematic way of talking and listening to people and collecting data through conversation. The respondents are primary source of data and interviewing is a way to collect data as well as gain knowledge from individual regarding underlying attributes.

Types of Interviews

Following types of interviews are commonly used in quantitative and qualitative research studies:

- *Structured Interviews:* It is most common form of interview used in qualitative research. It is also known as standard interview. In this type of interview, interviewer ask same question to all participants in similar manner. This process will ensure consistency in asking question and response as well. The strength of structured interview lies in that it has greater control over the question, format of interview and respondents. Researcher may use an interview guide to direct the interview process. Consequently, there is a common ground for collected information which makes tabulation, analyses and interpretation easy.
- *Semi-structured Interviews:* This form of interview is commonly used in qualitative research. It is also known as non-standardized interview. An interviewer may have list of theme, concept, issue and questions to be covered in the interview schedule and he is free to cask anything related to these in his own way. An interview guide may also used to sought supplementary information from participants. Unstructured interview give opportunity to probe the participants for concerned problems or issues. However, the role of researcher is active in unstructured interview then structured interview, where researcher only has to ask relevant information but cannot probe the subject to provide supplementary information related to underlying construct.
- *Unstructured Interviews:* It is nondirective and flexible method of collecting information. There is no detail formal interview guideline or interview guide. In unstructured interview, each interview is different in nature. Participants are encouraged to speak more and more to give as much as details they can share related to the construct. The investigator does not need any formal training to conduct unstructured interview. The interviewer asks the question that interviewee has to furnish with their own knowledge and experience. The tabulation, analysis and interpretation are most challenging task in unstructured interview. The limitation of unstructured interview lies in the thing that it will be time consuming as interviewer does not have any formal guidelines to conduct interview. The strength of unstructured interview is that supplementary information regarding other relevant issues can be sought simultaneously.

- *Focused Group Discussion (FGD):* Focus group interview commonly used in qualitative research. Focus group involves a group of 6-12 members who gathered together to discuss a problem in their own way. The interviewer direct or guide the interview according to interview guide. The role of interviewer is as moderator in focus group interview. Selecting a homogenous group is more preferable to improve group dynamics and get more related themes on underlying construct. The strength of focus group interview lies in the statement that researcher can give and gain informations to/from all participants at a time (economic in time and money). Further, it is also important to select a comfortable setting for conducting focus group interview. It should be free from temple, hospital and other religious places to get more accurate findings.
- *Joint Interviews:* Joint interview is common in qualitative studies. In joint interview two or more than two people interviewed/questioned simultaneously to develop a consensus on a issue from different perspective. The only difference between focus group and joint interview is that, in joint interview participants know each other but in focus group participants are not so familiar to each other. For example, experiences of parents of a mentally challenged child, and experience of caregivers of stroke patients, etc.

Guidelines for Preparing a Qualitative Interview (Unstructured and Semi-structured)

Pattern of qualitative interview is vary from one interviewer to another. Each interviewer has their own way of questioning and may not match to another. However, Kvale (1996) has suggested nine different types of questions a interviewer should cover in his interview. Details of these questions are provided here.

1. *Introducing question:* 'Please tell me about your interest in bird watching'; 'Have you even seen a mouse?' 'Why did you go to National Park?'
2. *Follow-up questions:* Getting the interviewee to elaborate his/her answer, such as could you say some more about that? What do you mean by that.....?; even 'Yeeeees?'
3. *Probing questions:* Following up what has been said through direct questioning.
4. *Specifying questions:* 'What did you do then?' How did he react what you said?
5. *Direct questions:* 'Do you have your opinion on the lethal control of large carnivores in Norway?' 'Are you happy with the way you and your husband were treated while visiting the Park's interpretation center?' Such questions perhaps best left until towards the end of interview, in order not to influence the direction of the interview too much.
6. *Indirect questions:* 'What do people a round were thinking of the way park ranger treat local people living in the park?' Perhaps followed up by 'Is that the way you feel too?' In order to get at the individual's own view.
7. *Structuring questions:* 'I would now like to move on to a different topic?'
8. *Silence*: Allow pauses to signal that you want to give the interviewee the opportunity to reflect and amplify the answer.
9. *Interpreting questions:* 'Do you mean that your opinions has changed because of the recent conservational actions?' 'Is it fair to say that what you are suggesting is that you do not mind having wolves in the area where you live, but when they are causing damage you should be compensated?'

Guidelines for Interviews Preparation

Conducting interview needs lot of preparation to collect relevant, accurate and unbiased information regarding underlying issue. Researcher has to select a comfortable environment and prepare participants simultaneously. A researcher may take many measures to prepare environment and participants including followings:

Preparation of Environment
- Ask participants about their choice of interview setting
- A setting free from cultural and religious issues (i.e. temple, hospital) is appropriate to get bias free findings
- Ensure the basic supply at interview venue such as water and air, etc.
- Choose a setting which is free from natural climate problems such as extreme temperature, traffic noise, etc.

Preparation of Participants
- Participants should explained the purpose, needs of questioning, and anticipated benefits of study
- Anonymity, privacy and confidentiality should be assured
- Participants may get nervous by seeing their responses are written, therefore, a researcher should explain the purpose of writing or recording their responses
- If researcher using any recording devices, it should make familiar to participants
- Researcher should explain tentative time duration of interview and provide full autonomy concepts to participants
- Leave contact information to participant to contact or answer any queries related to interview in future
- Give opportunity to clarify any doubts related to underlying issues.

Box 9.17: Tips for Conducting Interviews.

- Interviewer should be qualified and trained properly to conduct interview
- Interviewer should carry interview guide to avoid wastage of resources (time, money) and collect necessary relevant information
- Interviewer should use simple, clear and understandable language
- The dress up sense of interviewer should be according to population or geographic region for developing easy rapport
- Interviewer should be gentle, polite, sensitive and unconventional in nature
- Try to focus on relevant information rather than wasting time in discussing unnecessary information
- Take permission before asking personal questions to avoid any emotional trauma to participant
- Do not force the patient to give information on any topic or issue, encouragement can be used a tool to collect information
- Make a brief note of information simultaneously to avoid forgetful problem

---

Guidelines for Conducting Interviews

Bryman (2001) and McNamara (2006) prepared a draft of guidelines to facilitate interview.
- It is important to explain the purpose of interview to interviewee before proceeding to interview

- Interview should be recorded for detail analysis. It is suggested that one hour recorded interview takes around 5-6 hours to transcribe
- An interviewer should announce tentative time duration to make him comfortable for his participation
- Maintain a reasonable flow of question during interview to encourage participation of interviewee. Asking random questions may not be a good idea to get in-depth information
- Interviewees often came from different social and educational background; therefore, it is necessary to use a language that is understandable and comfortable for everyone attending interview
- It is always good to collect a background information (i.e. age, gender, educational status, area of living, etc.) in the beginning to develop rapport and understand the level of interviewees
- Finish the interview with a note of thank for their cooperation and give opportunity and time to resolve their quarries, if any
- At the end of interview, make a summary of interview, process, setting, level of cooperation of participants, nervousness felt by participants, and any new ideas emerged during interview, etc. Ask for participants feedback to improve upon the shortcoming for future interview.

Interviewing Process

Researcher may use several methods to conduct an interview. However, selection of interviews method depends on characteristics of participants, nature of study, and availability of resources. Face to face interview, telephonic interview, and computer-assisted interview are common interviewing methods used by a researcher.
- *Face to face interviews:* It is most common method to conduct an interview in which interviewer and interviewee sit face to face and conversation will take place. It has high response rate and have good control over respondent with less chances of bias.
- *Telephonic interviews:* In telephonic interview, interviewer will ask question on telephone to interviewee. It is economic means for small sample size, specific information and short interview schedule. Telephonic interview limitations lie in lack of cooperation of participants and non-availability of electricity and technical resources. With small sample, telephonic interview have higher response rate.
- *Computer-assisted interviews:* It is conducting interview with the help of small portable computer. It is costly and ineffective in case of devices and other resources are not available. Participants' computer illiteracy and unfamiliarity also make this method less useful than face to face interview and telephonic interview.

Strengths of Interviews
- Interview, facilitate in-depth exploration of the topic and hence, provide a detail information
- Interview method offer great deal of control over respondents
- It is hardly possible poor respondents to leave a question unanswered or to give an answer 'don't know'
- It is appropriate method in terms of high response rate
- Interview is a suitable method for illiterate and challenged population
- A well-planned interview able to furnish supplementary information.

Limitations of Interviews
- Interview is not an appropriate measure to study a wide scattered population
- A poorly planned interview schedule and guide may furnish inconsistent and biased information
- In case of lack of training to interviewers, interview bias may creep in
- Use of recording devices is an another challenge for a interviewer
- Tabulation, analysis and interpretations of findings from an unstructured interview is an obsolete challenge for an interviewer.

The Problems with Interviews
Interviews is a natural and socially-accepted method of collecting data in various situations. Although interviewing is relatively a simple methodology to utilize; interviewing challenges are enough for calling researchers' attention. An interviewer may face following problems in interviewing (Table 9.6).
- Presence of interviewer may change the natural way of responding of the participants (Hawthorne effect)
- Sometimes, only one participant represent a group of people and 360 degree opinions is not possible to explore the problem under investigation
- An interviewer may also face the problem of sample mortality in interview
- Sometimes, interviewer may lose train of thoughts and irrelevant discussion may start. This problem is quite common in unstructured interviews
- Interviewer may have to spend lot of time in writing and recording response, therefore interviewing is a time consuming method of data collection
- Sometimes, interviewer may not enough qualify to resolve the quarries raised by the participants.

Table 9.6: Interview and questionnaire: A comparison.

Interview	Questionnaire
Costly due to time intensive nature	Less costly-slower data collection method
Longer and more complex questions are possible	Limited in length and complexity
High response rate	Often associated with poor response rate
Can adapt to include visual material like flash card	Exclude the less literate and those who may have disability, e.g. dyslexia and blind
Provides additional opportunity to clarify questions and responses	No opportunity to explain question and answer or to probe for more detail information on a construct
Interviewee is not anonymous	Respondent cannot be connected to their responses. As a result more honest responses may be provided
Can be subject to bias-acquiescence and social desirability bias if not carefully prepared	Respondents have more time to weigh the issue carefully before responding less prone to acquiescence
Enables researcher to ensure data are being collected from correct sample	Researcher cannot ensure the target person completed questionnaire. For example, a questionnaire aimed to explore the views of patient may be completed by a caregiver

OBSERVATION METHOD

Observation is one of the most common and oldest method of collecting data. Observation is the process of systematic watching and recording the behavior of participants in their natural setting. This process enable researcher to record the behavior pattern, functions, actions and interactions. Observation is an important method to record the behavior which cannot be record and measured by using other methods such as behavior of children, and psychiatric patients, etc.

Elements of Observation

Observation is a systematic description of events, behavior, and artifacts in their natural setting chosen for the study. An observer should answer following before choosing observation as a method of data collection in research:
1. *Who will observe?* Someone to observe, i.e. observer.
2. *What should be observed?* Something going to be observed, i.e. incident, event, behavior, competency and skills, etc.
3. *How should observations be recorded?* The device which will be used to observe behavior like video recording device, camera, etc.
4. *What procedure should be used to try to assure the accuracy of observation?* A well-developed observation schedule should be there with timing, duration, special measure, participants details, and steps of recording incident, etc.
5. *Nature of relationship.* What relationship should exist between the observer and the observed and how can such relationship be established?

Phenomena Amenable to Observation

Observation is helpful to record number of incidents, events, characteristics including following:
1. *Verbal communication and behavior:* Linguistics behavior, content, structure of conversation and entire process of social interaction, etc.
2. *Nonverbal communication behavior:* Facial expression, touch, posture, gesture, body movement, manner of speaking, etc.
3. *Skill attainment and performance:* Medical and nursing procedure, their steps, competency and skills, etc.
4. *Environmental characteristics/attributes:* The environmental features like sanitation, temperature, noise source, pollution, humidity can also be recorded.
5. *Characteristic and condition of individual:* Observation method also used to record attributes, behavior, status, expression, emotion, physical and psychological aspects of an individual or group.

The Observer-Observed Relationship

Observer can interact with participants in an observation setting to varying degree. The relationship between observer and observed has significant important in true recording of an event.

On the basis of participation of observer in observation process, observation can be divided in following types:
1. *No concealment and participant:* Observer make no alteration in the social setting, Observer does not make observation covertly and subjects are aware of the presence of the researcher but not to underlying motive. This observation have following drawbacks.

- *Hawthorne effect* (subjects' awareness of being observed). Presence of observer may change actual behavior of the subjects.
- Interaction between the observed and observer may alter the behavior of participants.

2. *Concealment and participant:* Researcher observes subject's behavior in their natural setting but adopts a passive role while observing subjects. Researcher observes and records observation with minimum intervention. It has following disadvantages:
   - *Reactive measurement effect:* Presence of observer intent to change the behavior of the participants is known as reactive measurement effect.
3. *Concealment and non-participant:* Researcher makes observation from the periphery of a social setting in such a way that he is present but does not interact with others (also called *lurking*). Observer does not make his intentions known to the group, nor does he make any effort to participate. It helps to collect great deal of information. This type of observation have following demerits:
   - If observer is not nearby, difficulty in hearing can lead to misunderstanding.
   - Question of ethical issue–lack of dignity in data collection because the observed are neither aware of the observer nor being informed.
4. *No concealment and non-participant:* Extremely valuable for interventional nursing studies. Participants are aware about observer's presence and underlying motive as well. Use of this kind of observation have following limitations:
   - Information can be biased as subjects are known to observer presence as well as intention of research.

Types of Observation Methods

Observation is a useful and economic method to collect information related to specific as well as general phenomenon. A structured, specific and detailed observation schedule is required to collect in-depth information about a particular attribute under observation. Structured observations not only help to collect or record accurate information but also prevent errors and bias in recording observation. Following observation method can be used to collect information.

1. Structured Observation: It is excellent method of data collection or recording specific behavior, phenomena, incident and events. Structured observation will consists a formal developed observation schedule or protocol for recording attributes like when to observe, who will be observe, how long single observation will run, steps of observation, device which will be used to record, etc. It is challenging and time consuming task to develop a structured observation schedule. Observer may record the incident as whole (molar approach) or in parts (molecular approach).
   - *Molar approach:* Observer want to observe large unit of behavior or incident, i.e. study of verbal and nonverbal behavior pattern of manic patient.
   - *Molecular approach:* Observer record a specific part of incident or phenomena i.e. nonverbal behavior of schizophrenic patient.

   Methods in structured observation: Observer use well-designed and formal instrument to record specific behavior pattern or phenomenon, i.e. checklist, rating scale and category system.

- *Category system:* It is used to record qualitative behavior pattern in qualitative as well quantitative studies. Category system is designed to record specific behavior pattern in defined category. While developing category system, researcher should keep in mind that category should be independent or mutually exclusive and exhaustive in nature.
- *Rating scale:* Rating scale used to rate an individual phenomenon along a continuum of scale. A rating scale enable a researcher to differentiate one phenomenon to another on a good or bad parameter.
- *Checklist:* Checklist is an another widely used method to record the presence or absence of the behavior. Structured questionnaire used checklist to record specific behavior or vent in natural setting.

2. Unstructured Observation: Unstructured observation is common to record information which is not specific enough but can supplement main information. Unstructured observation consist a loosely developed observation protocol or schedule. The researcher has to involve with participants to collect information (participant observation).

Methods in unstructured observation: Observation information recorded either in daily notes (logbook) or field notes, but photographs and video recording can supplement the information.

- *Logbook:* It is daily record of information, event, conversation and activities in field setting. Logbook only list out activities in chronological orders. It is descriptive illustration of activities. Logbook can be use to trace the information.
- *Field notes:* Flied notes are detailed description of activities described in logbook. It is broader and interpreted in nature. Field notes need more efforts to write and interpret the activities. Field notes are lengthy and detail and can be written while observing the phenomena or after completing the observation. Field notes can be descriptive or reflective in nature.

Sampling in Structured Observation

Structured observation is well-planned process to collect and record information/phenomena. In structured observation, observer should determine time duration, specific behavior, number of observation in observation schedule to record accurate observation. Observer decides on type of sampling to make the observation more specific and accurate.

- *Time sampling:* Observer has to define time limit to observe a particular event or behavior like 5 minutes every day for consequent 30 days.
- *Event sampling:* Researcher has to decide to select specific event of a phenomena related to research question. Researcher should have strong knowledge and experience of time of occurrence of events, duration of event like reactions of child after intramuscular injection.

Development of Observation Schedule

A structured observation is a well planned and systematic way to collect unbiased finding for an observation. Therefore, it is essential to follow a structured schedule to avoid any haphazard way of recording findings and make the observation complete. A structured observation schedule may be developed by going through following steps:

1. *Selection of behavior/phenomenon:* An observer should specify the behavior or event going to be observed. A clear delineation of event or behavior help to focus an observer on the target.

2. *Specifying behavior/phenomena:* Phenomenon under observation should be specified to observe and collect specific information, i.e. only nonverbal behavior of interaction between nurse and patient.
3. *Training observer:* An observer should be given adequate training to record a event or behavior completely. In case of multiple observers, a consistent and structured plan of training should be developed.
4. *Quantifying observation:* Observed behavior should be quantify in terms of time, duration, hours and frequency, etc.
5. *Record behavior/observation:* Behavior under observation should be recorded adequately and according to structured plan.

Strengths of Observation Method

- It is one of the important techniques to record the behavior and phenomenon which cannot be recorded by any other method like behavior of mentally retarded children
- Observation method enable a researcher to utilize maximum information collected through observation. However, it is difficult to utilize all information collected through self-report methods
- Observation method use recording device which makes the information reproducible anytime and anywhere
- Observation provide depth and variety of information to study an event from different angles.

Limitations of Observation Method

- Observation is a time consuming and expensive in terms of time and money
- Observer need training to observe a phenomenon, therefore, an observer has to take extra efforts to train himself or data collectors
- Observation depends on the use of recording devices. An observer need to train to operate recording device. Maintenance of device is an another challenge for a researcher
- In concealed observation, lack of consent may creep ethical problems
- In participant observation, observer may get involved with participants that may lead to loss of objectivity in observation
- Observation limitations lies in many biases like error of leniency, error of severity, halo effect, reactive measurement effect, central tendency effect, and assimilatory bias, etc.

BIOPHYSIOLOGICAL METHODS

Biophysiological measures are very common in healthcare setting and healthcare research. This trend is come due to increased technological advancement in healthcare setting for diagnostic as well as therapeutic purposes. Bio-physiological measures includes, but not limited to blood pressure, temperature, blood sugar, heart rate, weight measurement, etc. The only advantage of bio-physiological measures line in empirical and bias free information that is more objective than any other methods of data collection.

Types of Biophysiological Methods

Biophysiological measurement can take place inside (*in-vivo*) or outside (*in-vitro*) of human body. *In-vivo* measures directly performed inside the living organism. Example includes body temperature, blood pressure and oxygen saturation, etc.

Data Collection Methods in Research

An *in-vitro* measurement, by contrast, is performed outside the body of an organism. Example includes blood sugar, sodium and potassium level. *In-vitro* measurement data are gathered by extracting body material from organism and submitting it for laboratory analysis.

In-vitro Measurement

In-vitro measurement performed outside with the help of laboratory analyzer. *In-vitro* measurement further classified in following two headings.

a. Physiological Measurement
- Physical measurement: Height and weight, etc.
- Chemical measurement: Hemoglobin level, hormones analysis, RFT, LFT, etc.
- Microbiological measurement: Bacterial culture and sensitivity tests.
- Cytological measurement: Tissue biopsy, autopsy, etc.
- Radiological measurement: X-ray, MRI, CT scan, and bone scan, etc.

b. Psychological Measurement

It mainly makes use of psychological test. Psychological tests are designed to measure only a specific psychological aspect of human behavior. These tests are standardized and objective description of behavior, quantified by numerical score, i.e. IQ testing.

In-vivo Measurement

In-vivo measures directly performed inside the living organism, e.g. body temperature, blood pressure and oxygen saturation, etc.

Purposes of Biophysiological Measurement

Use of biophysiological measures in quantitative nursing research is becoming popular nowadays. Many nursing studies using biophysiological measures both for creating dependent variables to see the outcomes. Following are the important purposes of biophysiological measures in nursing research.
- *To study basic biophysiologic process:* These study focus on studying normal physiology of a living organism (human or animal). These researches enable a researcher to differentiate normal process to abnormal in an organism.
- *To describe the physiological consequences of health care and nursing:* Biophysiological measures used in these study to describe the impact of standard procedure on physiological outcomes.
- *To evaluate nursing interventions:* Usually, these studies involves testing the new intervention or protocol and compare the effectiveness with the existing intervention or protocol.
- *To assess or compare clinical procedures:* The nursing studies use biophysiological measures to compare and assess two or more than two procedures for their efficacy and effectiveness. These researches helps to refine the existing one or design new intervention.

Strengths of Biophysiological Methods
- Biophysiological measures are accurate and provide quantitative numerical data that are comparatively easy to analyze
- They are objective measure of data collection because they are sensitive to change and can record relatively small changes.

Limitations of Biophysiological Methods
- Biophysiological measures are relatively expensive and data collector has to have the training to use the instrument
- Biophysiological instruments may be adversely affected by extreme climate condition such as extreme temperature
- These instruments may also have Hawthorne effect since the participants usually know that a test is being made
- Biophysiological measures are invasive in nature and there may be potential harm to study subjects.

RECORD ANALYSIS

Records are essential part of every organization, institution and department. It is part of daily work in office and department. Records are primary sources of information and serve important purpose by providing useful and pertinent information. Record could be best source of information if they are maintained adequately and completely. Historical research use records as primary source of information to collect data. Health care organization maintain different types of record like admission records, drug administration record, movement record, investigation report, discharge record, intake and output record, indent inventory and hand over record, etc.

Strength of Records
Records are primary sources of information that have many advantages over other methods of data collection:
- Records are primary and economical source of information as collection of information is inexpensive and less time consuming
- Records are free from bias in collecting information as information already being written and recorded
- Record provides all information at a time so it is inexpensive in nature
- Availability of large quantity of record makes the data collector to choose the best record for gaining information
- Record do not rely on recall of information so chances of forgetfulness can be avoided.

Limitations of Records
- Maintaining consistency is very big problem with record as different organization prepare record in their own manner and pattern
- Institutional permission is again big headache for researcher.
- Sometime institution will not allow external person to come and see their organization records
- Sometime records are kept deep and inside, gaining access is not possible for researcher
- Researcher lack of awareness regarding use of records, translating them in their own language is another problem
- No one sure about accuracy of records
- It is very difficult to know that in which conditions records are written or maintained
- Sometimes person who written or prepared record is missing or not available or died. In such cases it is not possible to interpret and translate some information for research purpose

- Incompleteness and inadequacy is another big problem with records
- Taking helps of people who are not a part of research activity will make interference in their usual work schedule.

> **Box 9.18:** Example of Record Analysis.
>
> Setz Vg, et al. (2009) evaluate the quality of nursing documentation on medical records. A retrospective descriptive approach was adopted to review 424 medical records of the patients from medical and surgical unit admitted between November 2006 to January 2007. The focus of review was on the demographic and background information, operation room, flow sheet, nursing progress note, nursing diagnoses order, nursing records, medical records, nursing documentations and discharge and death records.

Problems in Accessing Records

Although records have many advantages as well disadvantages also, but still record are commonly used for many purposes. A researcher may face some problem in accessing records including followings:

- Organization/authority do not want that their records are used for fear of misplacing or loss of paper from records
- Organization will refuse to give permission to access records
- Interpretations of records will be a another problem
- It is difficult to locate the records in case they are kept too inside or underground basement
- Sometime organization demand a copy of research project
- Maintain privacy, and confidentiality is a big issues in using records.

Guidelines for Using Records

Records can be available in both primary and secondary data format. It is researcher ability to check their validity and reliability before using records. Researcher may use following measures to check validity and reliability of records:

- *External criticism:* It is concerned to validity and authenticity of records, i.e. historical researcher can check the external criticism of a record, piece of paper or diary written by Kalpana by asking or checking; whether it is handwriting of Kalpana? Or paper of diary is of right age? It is concerned with validity of records.
- *Internal criticism:* It is concerned with accuracy of record and deals with written content of records. For measuring internal criticism, historical researcher may ask: whether records are written and maintained in unbiased condition or situation? It is concerned with reliability of the records.

Q-SORT

Q-sort is a measurement strategy first introduced by the psychologist William Stephenson (1953) as a self-report technique for determining the relative relevance to an individual subject of a set of declarative statements. This is common method used in psychology and social sciences. It can be used both in clinical as well as research setting for ranking the views by given items towards a particular variable. Q-sort is universal and can be applied in variety of settings. Q-sort consists a group of 50-100 cards that are sorted in 9-11 piles. The subject is given a deck of cared, one statement per card, and is asked to sort the card into several piles with ranking from 'most like me' to 'least like me'. The number of piles and number of cared to be placed in each piles are predetermined by the researcher (but not which cards) and usually chosen so as to form a normal or near normal distribution frequency curve. The difference between Q-sort and traditional Likert scale is that, in Q-sort certain constraints will be placed on the rater. Specifically there is predetermined number of items for each category out of them few items will be placed in extreme categories and many items in middle categories.

Box 9.19: Example of Q-sort.

A nurse researcher interested to know the various reason for joining nursing as a profession could prepare cards listing 16 reasons that might be given and ask each prospective nursing students to sort a deck of cards containing those reason into five piles, with one card to be placed in first pile (most compelling reason), four in the second pile, six in the third pile, four in fourth pile, and one in last pile (least compelling reason).

Strengths of Q–Sort
- It is helpful to know variety of subjective feeling, attitude, belief, values and opinion towards a particular attributes
- It is widely used in different sciences, i.e. medical, nursing, psychology, sociology, social sciences, etc.

VIGNETTES

Vignettes are the another self-report measure which provide a brief description of an event or situation to which participants are asked to react. This description could be fictitious or real.

The vignette is a tool used in social science research and has long history in disciplines such as anthropology and psychology. Though early nursing studies recognized the usefulness of vignettes. It is only more recently that it has received significant attention. Indeed, more textbook on nursing and healthcare research make little, if any, reference to the vignette in their content and index list.

'Simulation of real life event which can be used in research studies to elicit subjects' knowledge, attitude or opinions according to how they state they would behave in the hypothetical situation depicted.' *(Gould, 1996)*

'Vignette is a technique used in structured and in-depth interview as well as focus group, providing sketches of fictional (or fictionalized) scenario.' *(Bloor and Wood, 2006)*

Vignettes are inexpensive and economical means of soliciting information of individual regarding ideas, attitude, values, sensitive issue and respondents are invited to respond to these by using them as a means of reflecting or, as drawing from personal experience. A vignette can be in the form of cartoons, video recording or live events.

This method is widely used in examination and teaching as well. Vignettes can be open ended (participants are free to express our view for a situation) or close ended (participants are supposed to select the most relevant view from given alternatives of options) in nature.

Box 9.20: Example of Vignette.

Chan, et al. (2006) used videotaped vignettes to evaluate nursing practice model in the context of severe acute respiratory syndrome (SARS) epidemic in Hong Kong. In examination, students are given brief description of an event or case and their knowledge is tested by focused questions.

Steps of Constructing Vignettes

Researcher can use following steps to develop vignette (how to vignette):

- *Step 1:* Use the clustering technique or another technique that works for you to organize your ideas for each vignette. Begin with an event from social situation or personal sensitive issues that has meaning for participant. If using the clustering technique for organizing, then write the event at the center of the page and circle it. Then brainstorm other ideas related to that event, writing them in circles and connecting them with lines to the center word. Keep your ideas organized.
- *Step 2:* Write the first draft without thinking too much about words, structure or quality. Just as a camera takes a picture of what is there, vignette should photograph what is in participants' mind.
- *Step 3:* Reread vignette and add more information from participants—simile, metaphor, hyperbole, personification, imagery and allusion. Remember to underline and label each literary device you use.
- *Step 4:* Read vignette out loud to feel the rhythm of the language. Pay attention first to how well it expresses your ideas, then to how well it is written. Make necessary changes.
- *Step 5:* Proofread and edit each vignette using the proofreading and editing checklist.
- *Step 6:* Write the final draft of vignette.

Strength of Vignettes

- It is economic tool to elicit information regarding stigma, attitude and certain social problems
- It allow face to face contact and conversation with participants
- Vignettes enable a researcher to compare the attitude, and perception of one participants with other participant
- It helps to explore the sensitive topic in depth which cannot be explored by other means like sexual abuse
- Vignettes require minimal resources and easy to administer
- In vignettes, participants do not need to have in-depth knowledge of the topics but they can provide sufficient details to reduce unwarranted assumptions
- Vignette-based methodologies are frequently used to examine judgments and decision-making processes, including clinical judgments made by health professionals
- Vignette safeguard the subjects in ethical sense.

Limitations of Vignettes

- Vignettes are hypothetical in nature; in real situation, participants may react differently when they are asked to respond to situation
- Vignettes are subjective format of ideas and expression, no consistent pattern followed for response pattern, therefore tabulation, analysis and interpretation is difficult task for researcher
- Vignettes are suitable to study small sample size
- There is no formal guideline for analysis and interpretation and therefore, bias can creep in recording as well interpretations of vignettes.

PROJECTIVE TECHNIQUES

Projective technique is the use of vague, ambiguous, unstructured, stimulus, object or situation on which the subjects 'project' his/her personality, attitude, opinion, ideas, self- concept and self-expression. Projective techniques are used to identify the underlying motives, urges or intention. In projective technique, the responded under study unconsciously project his own attitude or feelings on the subject under study. Projective techniques help to discover the modes of perceiving his/her world and how he/she behave in it. Scope of projective techniques is increasing in psychology for personality assessment, clinical and psychoanalytic treatment.

Classification of Projective Techniques

Projective techniques classified on the basis of word response pattern of subject for particular stimulus.

1. Word Association Techniques: This is the most common projective technique used in research. The subjects are given a stimulus or situation to which they have to respond with the first word comes in their mind. The investigator correlates the response with given stimulus like investigators announce word 'fire' and subject may respond 'danger'. This technique commonly used to illicit inner conflict regarding particular construct.
2. Construction Projective Techniques: Construction projective techniques concerned with product or outcome of the subject for certain stimulus. Researcher asked to construct a story or a picture for a given stimuli or concept. Researcher can give stimulus in the form of a single picture or in ambiguous picture. The construction process requires more controlled and complex intellectual activity. Construction projective techniques categorized in following ways:
   - Thematic apperception test (TAT): The psychologist Henry Murray and his colleagues in 1935 developed this test. It consists of 20 pictures, all black and white, that are shown to a client. Then, the client is asked to tell a story about the person or people in the picture. Again, the story developed by the client is interpreted by the psychoanalyst, who looks for revealing statements and projection of the client's own problems into the people in the given picture.

     TAT further classified into three types of projective tests:
     a. *Sentence completion tests:* In the sentence completion test, the client is given a series of sentence beginnings, such as 'I wish my mother..' or almost every day I feel..... and asked to finish the sentence.
     b. *Draw-a-person test:* In the draw-a-person test, the client is asked to draw the named items in their own words.
     c. *House-tree-person test:* It is developed by John Buck, a psychologist, in 1948 to measure attributes of personality. Patient asked to draw a good house, tree and person (as good as possible), take as much time as needed. The test is then used to measure self-perception, outlook and attitude.
   - Rorschach inkblot technique: Hermann Rorschach (1921) invented this technique to describe personality, diagnose psychological disorder, and predict the type of behavior. There are ten inkblots, five in black ink on a white background and five in colored inks on a white background. These plates are standardized. Subject is presented these plates one by one and subject has to tell what he observes in these ink plates. He can give

many responses as he desires by observing from different angles to it. These responses are interpreted from various perspectives. The therapist assesses normal and abnormal personality traits by analyzing the responses of subjects.

3. **Completion Techniques:** In completion techniques, researcher gives the incomplete stimulus in the form of sentence or story, and participant asked to complete the given story with their own ideas and views. It needs complex creativity, intellectual skills and creative thought process to complete the given task. Completion techniques can be sentence completion and story completion.
4. **World Association Test:** Word association test was developed by Jung. It consists of hundred words. Mr X is instructed that he will be presented 100 words one by one and he has to respond to each word immediately in their own way. Time is noted for response. The response is also recorded simultaneously. During this procedure, verbal and non-verbal responses are also noted down. From these responses, various complexes and sensitive areas of his life are identified to understand his personality.
5. **Expressive Techniques:** These techniques allow the participant to express ourself regarding certain stimulus like music, specific paining or situation, etc.
6. **Choice Ordering Techniques:** The most common techniques in which subjects are asked to put a situation or concept of life on rating priority like 'very important' to 'not at all important'. The technique commonly used in quantitative research like using rating scale to collect data on various social and psychological issues.

■ VALIDITY AND RELIABILITY

Validity and reliability are quality indicators of a research study. A research findings should be judged based on rigor used in a study. Rigors refers to measures a researcher used in a study to enhance the quality of a research study. In quantitative research, rigors achieved through validity and reliability. Validity concern how extent a concept is accurately measured in a study. Reliability refers to accuracy and consistency of a research instrument used in a study. This section deal with validity and reliability element of a research study.

Validity

Validity is the extent to which an instrument measures the attributes of a concept accurately. The validity of an instrument concerns its ability to gather the data that it is intended to gather. The content of instrument is of prime importance in validity testing. If an instrument is expected to measure assertiveness, does it, in fact measure assertiveness? It is not difficult to say that validity is the most important characteristic of a research tool. The greater the validity of an instrument, the more confidence you can have that instrument will obtain data that will answer the research question or test the research hypotheses.

Definitions

'Validity refers to the degree to which an instrument measures what it suppose to measure.'
(Polit and Hungler)
'Validity describes the extent to which measures accurately represent the concept it claims to measure.'
(Punch, 1998)

Measures of Validity

There are two broad measures of validity—external and internal validity.
1. *External validity* refers to application of findings on whole population apart from study population (generalization) and for that representative sample should be collected from defined population.
2. *Internal validity* refers to strength of relationship between dependent and independent variables. It is a reason of outcome and helps to reduce other, often anticipated, reason for these outcomes.

Approaches to Internal Validity

Researcher basically use three internal validity approach namely *content validity, criterion validity* and *construct validity*.
- *Content validity:* It is a better way to test the measuring ability of an instrument. This is extent to which a research instrument accurately measures all aspects of a construct or variable under study. This category ensure whether the research instrument adequately cover all the content that can measure the whole variable in a study. In simple words, does your instrument cover all areas related to variable, or construct that was designed to measure. Content validity can be established by giving the instrument to experts of that area/field for their valuable suggestion, advise and judgment for supplementing or omitting items.

    Face validity is subset of content validity. In face validity, experts are asked for their opinions whether an instrument measure the intended concept or not. However, it is very rudimentary and subjective form of validity where experts confirm the validity by looking on an instrument. There is not mathematical formula to calculate face validity. This is considered external approach of validity.
- *Criterion validity:* It is a stronger form of validity established by comparing one instrument to other validated instrument (usually gold standard) on same construct. Criterion validity refers to the extent to which one instrument correlates with other instrument measure same construct at present time or predict subject's response in future. These two types of criterion validity are called *convergent* and *predictive validity*, respectively. However, where no other criterion measures exist, this kind of validity is not possible.
    - *Convergent validity:* Convergent validity means an instrument is highly correlated with another instrument measuring similar construct.
    - *Predictive validity:* Predictive validity concerned with the ability of an instrument to predict behavior or responses of a subject in future. Predictive validity refers that an instrument should have high correlation with future criterion. For example, a score high on self-esteem related to participation in cultural activities should predict the likelihood consistent participation in cultural events.
    - *Divergent validity:* Divergent validity refers that an instrument is poorly correlated with another instrument measure the different concept. For example, there should be low correlation between an instrument that measure depression and one that self-esteem.
- *Construct validity:* Construct validity refers to the extent to which one instrument correlate with other instrument measure similar construct. Construct validity is the broadest type of validity and can encompass both content and criterion validity. It is most challenging task for a researcher to establish construct validity of an instrument (Table 9.7).

Table 9.7: Types of instrument validity.

Types	Description	Examples
Content validity	Extent to which an instrument measure all aspects of a construct	Content validity Face validity
Construct validity	Extent to which a research tool (instrument) measure the proposed concept	Convergent Discriminant validity
Criterion validity	The extent to which a research tool is related to other tools that measure the same concept	Concurrent and Predictive validity

Measurement of Content Validity

The content validity of an instrument may be reported as percentage of agreement among the experts or as a *content validity index (CVI)*. The content validity index is derived from the rating of the content relevancy of the item on an instrument using 4 point ordinal rating scale, where 1 connotes an *'irrelevant item'* and 4 an *'extremely relevant'* item. The actual CVI is the proportion of items that received rating of 3 or 4 by the experts.

Popham's average congruency procedure is a special case approach using percentage of agreement among experts to estimate content validity. This approach is a measure of the average percentage of aggregation of all questionnaire items across all content validity experts.

Interpretation of Content Validity Coefficient

In general, the higher the validity coefficient, the more acceptable the estimate of validity. Validity coefficient can range from 0.00 to 1.00 or 0% to 100%. Coefficient of at least 0.70 or 70% are typically considered acceptable validity estimate. However, in the case of some approaches to estimating validity, such as discriminate validity, a very low coefficient may indicate a more acceptable estimate of validity.

Reliability

Reliability is another important feature of a research instrument. Reliability refers to the consistency and accuracy of an instrument. A test is considered reliable if researcher frequently gets the same reading at different time interval. A student completing an instrument meant to measure self-esteem should have approximately the same responses each time the test is completed. Although, it is not possible to calculate exact reliability of an instrument. However, a range of reliability can be calculated through different measures. It is observed that the people and instruments employed in a research study are consistent the way data is obtained and recorded from one subject to next, one data collector to next, and one data collection point to next.

Concept of Reliability

The concept of reliability can well understood with classical measurement theory (CMT). CMT said that the total score of an instrument is the combination of true score and random and systematic errors.

Classical measurement theory assesses the random measurement errors. The basic tenet of CMT evolved from the assumption that random error is an element that must be considered in all measurement. The underlying principle of this theory is that every observed score is composed of true score and an error score. The basic formula of CMT is represented in Box below.

Box 9.21: Classical Measurement Theory (CMT).

$$(X) = X_T + X_E (e)$$

Where,

X = Observed score (actual score obtained)
X_T = True variance (consistent, hypothetical stable or true score)
X_E = Measurement error (chance/random errors)

This equation simply indicates that every observed score that result from any measurement procedure is composed of two independent qualities: a *true score*; which represent the precise score that would be obtained if there were no random error of measurement; and a *error score*, which represent the contribution of random measurement error that happens to be present at the time of measurement.

For example, a student nurse attempt to take pulse rate of a patient for 1 minute and misread the second hand on her watch. She count the patient's pulse rate for 64 sec in place of 60 sec, thereby increasing the actual pulse rate of 82 (hypothetical true score) to 88 (observed score). According to CMT, the error in this instance is +6 beats, since this is the discrepancy between the patient true pulse and observed pulse (Fig. 9.4).

$$O = T + E, \quad 88 = 82 + 6$$

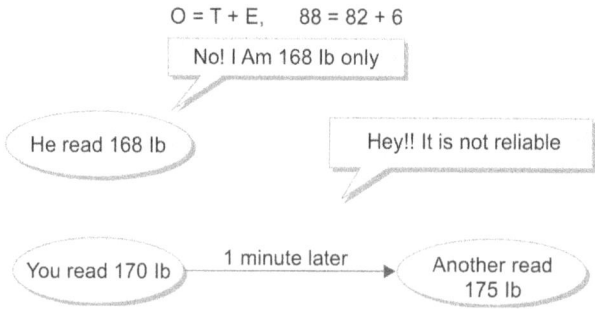

Fig. 9.4: Concept of reliability.

Imaging, having a research assistant who rates an infant as calm and easily quitted on day but rates the same infant as irritable and difficult to quiet the next day despite no change in the infant: or having a sphygmomanometer that report a blood pressure of 140/80 on a person on day and 120/75 the next day without any change in the person's actual (true) blood pressure. These discrepancies are obliviously not acceptable. On the basis of *classical measurement theory*, it is evident that observed score (X) had too much error (e) in addition to the true score, making these instruments very unreliable.

Elements of Reliability

The main aspects of the reliability which are considered important in quantitative research include:
1. Stability
2. Equivalence
3. Internal consistency.

Stability

It is the extent of instrument to which similar score will be obtained at separate occasion. Stability measures the effect of extraneous variables on different time interval. Researcher makes ensure that research instrument is consistent in providing same result at different time interval.

Test-retest method is used to measures stability of an instrument. In test-retest method, researcher administer same test to same population at two different time interval. Both score of test will be compared to compute reliability coefficient. Coefficient correlation will be computed to test reliability coefficient. The value of coefficient correlation will be taken as reliability coefficient. Higher value of coefficient correlation indicates higher reliability and vice versa.

Steps of computing coefficient correlation
- Administration of a well-designed instrument to same population at two different points of interval.
- Compute coefficient correlation by using Pearson's Product Moment Coefficient Correlation formula.
- Reliability coefficient range from -1 to 00 to +1, where, 1.00 indicates perfect reliability and zero indicates no reliability. A value between 0.70 to 0.90 considered acceptable level of reliability for an instrument.

Equivalence

It is concerned to the extent to which two or more observers, raters or coders show higher level of consensus/agreement for an instrument. Higher level of agreement or consensus between observers indicates low level of measurement errors and higher reliability. Observation method follows equivalence approach for computing reliability (Fig. 9.5).

Inter-rater or interobserver reliability can be assessed by using interclass correlation (ICC) (continuous variables) or Cohen's Kappa (categorical variables) as mentioned (Table 9.8).

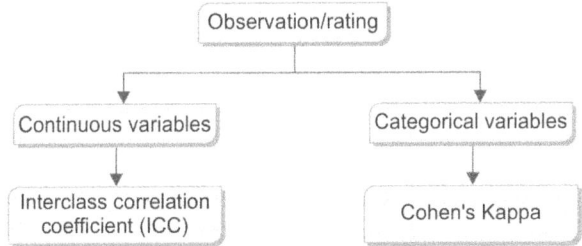

Fig. 9.5: Measures of equivalence.

Table 9.8: Level of Aggrement in Cohen Kappa.

Cohen's Kappa (κ)	Interpretation
< 0	No agreement
0.0–0.20	Slight agreement
0.21–0.40	Fair agreement
0.41–0.60	Moderate agreement
0.61–0.80	Good/substantial agreement
0.81–1.00	Perfect/very good agreement

Interclass coefficient correlation (ICC) can also calculate by below mention formula:

$$ICC = \frac{MS_{Bet\,S} - MS_{with\,in\,S}}{MS_{Bet\,S + (\kappa - 1)}\,MS_{with\,in\,S}}$$

Internal Consistency

Internal consistency (homogeneity) address the extent to which all items on an instrument measure the same variable. This type of reliability is appropriate only when the instrument is examining only one concept or construct at a time.

This reliability concerned with the pool of items used to measure the construct under study. For example, an instrument proposed to measure depression is expected that all items of the instrument should measure depression (Table 9.9).

Table 9.9: Attributes of reliability.

Type	Description	Examples
Internal consistency	The extent to which all the items on a scale measures the same construct	Split-half, KR_{20}, Cronbach's alpha, Spearman-Brown prophecy formula
Equivalence	Consistency among responses of multiple uses of an instrument, or among alternate form of an instrument	Cohen's kappa, Interclass correlation Coefficient
Stability	The consistency of results using an instrument with repeated testing	Test-retest, Alternate form reliability

Measures to Assess Internal Consistency

A number of statistical methods are used to measure internal consistency of an instrument. Selection of statistical method depends on types of alternatives response, number of items and types of an instrument (questionnaire or rating scale). Split-half reliability, Kuder Richardson coefficient, Cronbach's α and item-to-total correlation are most widely used methods to measures internal consistency of an instrument.

- *Split half-method or odd-even reliability:* In split-half method, the instrument is divided on two equal half (either taking odd or even items). These both parts of an instrument administer to same subjects and score separately. Correlation are calculated comparing the score of both halves. Strong correlations refers higher reliability while poor correlation refers the instrument may not reliable. A researcher should deal with the problem of homogeneity and heterogeneity of two half of instrument before computing reliability.

$$r_{xy} = \frac{\sum(X - \bar{X})(Y - \bar{Y})}{\sqrt{\left[\sum(X - \bar{X})^2\right]\left[\sum(Y - \bar{Y})^2\right]}}$$

Where,
r_{xy} = the correlation coefficient for variable X and Y
X = an individual score for variable X
Y = an individual score for variable Y
Σ = sum of
$\bar{X}$ = the mean score for variable X
$\bar{Y}$ = the mean score for variable Y

- **Kuder Richardson formula (KR$_{20}$, 1937, 1939):** Kr$_{20}$ is more complicated and accurate version of split-half method. In this method, average of all possible split-half combinations is taken and a correlation is computed between 0 to 1 is generated. Kr$_{20}$ can only computed to dichotomous response questions such as yes, no, 0 or 1.
  KR$_{20}$ can be calculated by given formula

  $$KR_{20} = \left[\frac{n}{(n-1)}\right] \times \left[1 - \frac{(\Sigma pq)}{Var}\right]$$

  Where,

  KR$_{20}$ = estimated reliability of the full length test
  n = number of item
  Var = variance of the whole test (standard deviation squared)
  Σpq = sum of the product of pq for all n items
  p = proportion of people passing the item
  q = proportion of people failing the items (or 1-p)

- **Spearman-Brown prophecy formula:** Spearman-Brown prophecy formula was given by C Spearman and W Brown in 1910. The Spearman-Brown prophecy formula (SB formula) is used to calculate the reliability when the number of items in a questionnaire changed. It provide a rough estimate in change of reliability of test if the number of items in an instrument were decreased or increased.

  $$r_{kk} = \frac{K(r_{11})}{[1+(k-1)r_{11}]}$$

  Where,

  r_{kk} = reliability of the test k times as long as the original test
  r_{11} = reliability of original test
  k = factor by which the length of the test is changed

- **Cronbach's alpha or coefficient alpha (Cronbach, 1951):** Lee Cronbach (1951), proposed the concept of Cronbach alpha (earlier known as coefficient alpha) from earlier version of KR$_{20}$, Cronbach alpha provides an estimate of reliability from all possible dimensions of split half correlations. In simple, this reliability coefficient tell us the degree to which the items are interrelated. Coefficient alpha is appropriate reliability measures for test items that allow for a range of responses. For example, on a 5-point agreement scale (strongly agree, agree, uncertain, disagree, strongly disagree). However, coefficient alpha can also be used for dichotomous score items.

  $$(\alpha) = \left[\frac{n}{(n-1)}\right] \times \left[\frac{Var_t - \Sigma Var_i}{Var_t}\right]$$

  Where,

  α = estimated reliability of the full length test
  n = number of items
  Var_t = variation of the whole test
  ΣVar_i = sum of the variance of all n items

- *Item-total correlations:* Item-total correlation is another measure of internal consistency. An item-total correlation is the correlation between a particular item and the total items of an instrument. It is also recommended to delete the item with a correlated item-total correlation of < 0.3 or high inter-item correlation (>0.8).

Box 9.22: Bivariate Correlations.

Item	Item 1	Item 2	Item 3	Item 4	Item 5
Item 1	1.00				
Item 2	0.89	1.00			
Item 3	0.78	0.84	1.00		
Item 4	0.97	0.81	0.84	1.00	
Item 5	0.82	0.79	0.83	0.87	1.00

.89 + .78 + .97 + .82 + .84 + .81 + .79 + .84 + .83 + .87 = 8.44/10 = .84

Interpretation of Reliability Coefficient

In general, higher the reliability coefficient, the more reliable an instrument is. Reliability coefficient can range from 0.00 to 1.00 or 0% to 100%. A reliability coefficient of at least 0.70 or 70% is considered acceptable for an instrument to be reliable. It is again said that Cronbach's alpha can actually take any value between minus infinity and +1. A researcher should keep in mind that negative alpha are reflective of very bad measuring instrument as far as internal consistency is concerned.

Factors Affecting Reliability

Various things affect the reliability of an instrument and a good researcher should keep in mind all these factors while selecting a research instrument.

- *Length of instrument (number of items):* Number of items in an instrument has great influence on reliability. Increase number of heterogeneous items in an instrument will increase the reliability. However, if the instrument is not reliable, to increase the number of items does not make the scale reliable.
- *Random error:* Reliability of measurement method is directly influenced by random error. There is an inverse relationship between amount of random error introduced into measurement and the reliability of the measurement.
- *Training of observer:* In case of observation method, reliability can be improved by greater precision in defining or explaining the underlying construct for observer or rater by providing consistent training. However, training is the best method to attain higher reliability in observational studies.
- *Number of observation:* The number of observation is directly proportional to reliability. This make intuitive sense, since multiple observation allow the rater to rate a underlying construct several times, leading more consistent estimate of construct.
- *Time:* In some research studies, a wide gap between two evaluations has an impact on reliability. Such as long gap between pretest and post-test in experimental study may reduce the reliability.

- *Language of items in scale:* A scale should consist items without linguistic problems and arranged appropriately. Items consist double meaning or negative connotation should be avoid to enhance reliability.
- *Group homogeneity:* Group homogeneity is another factor may affect reliability. A more homogenous group increase the reliability coefficient of an instrument.
- *Duration of the scale:* A scale should be administer with sufficient time to respond. The time must be enough for respondents to answer all the items. The insufficiency of time decrease the reliability of the scale.
- *Objectivity in scoring:* Objective scoring enhance the reliability index of an instrument. Researcher's subjectivity involvement in scoring reduce the reliability of an instrument.
- *Extreme climate condition:* Extreme climate condition such as extreme temperature, heat and lack of basic supply to respondents reduce the reliability.
- *Instruction for participants:* Explanation must be clear to respondents in the beginning of the scale so that all the respondents' will understand the same things. The aim of the scale must be clear to the respondents.
- *Difficulty index of scale:* Difficulty level of items in the scale may also influence the reliability coefficient. The reliability of the scale with very easy and difficult items will be low.

CULTURAL EQUIVALENCE OF AN INSTRUMENT

In nursing, there is a growing interest in cross-cultural studies, which have demanded greater concern about the quality and suitability of adapted and validated for use in different context. However, it has been noticed that adaptation process used in nursing is inadequate and merely translation of the instrument that is limited to back translation (semantic equivalence between two instruments) only.

Flaherty et al. (1988) identified five separate types of cross cultural equivalence of an instrument:

1. *Content equivalence* refers to the relevance of each item to the culture of interest.
2. *Semantic equivalence* refers to the extent to which the connotative meaning of each item is the same in the original culture and the culture for which the instrument being translated.
3. *Technical equivalence* refers to the extent to which the way the data were collected such as interview or questionnaire is similar in each culture.
4. *Criterion equivalence* refers to extent to which the interpretation of the data is similar across the culture.
5. *Conceptual equivalence* refers to the extent to which the researcher is able to measure the same middle range theory concept in each culture.

However, using literal translation results in misinterpretation of the words. In translation, a researcher go beyond finding the equivalent denotative meaning of the items used in the original version to capture their connotative. However, translation is the one-step of adaptation process of an instrument. An ideal adaption process should follows given steps:

1. *Instrument translation into new language:* This is preliminary stage concerning to translation of an instrument from the source language to target language. This is a complicated process and requires tremendous care to assure consistency in the new version. A literal translation does not produce desired product. It is been recommended to choose to independent and bilingual translators to adapt the item into new language. One translator for language proficiency and other should be construct expert.

2. *Synthesis of translated version:* A researcher should have at least two version of translated instrument. Researcher summarizes both the version of instrument in terms of semantic, idiomatic, conceptual, linguistic and contextual aspects. This process will help to devise a single version of new instrument. Experts in the area help to identify inappropriate choice and resolve it. The translated version of instrument should be judged for each item. Throughout this process, author and team of experts compare the comparability between translated and original version instrument.
3. *Evaluation of synthesized version by experts:* A team of experts evaluates the translated version of instrument on psychological domains. Experts' ass structure, layout, instruction for participants, scope and adequacy of expression contained in the items.
4. *Evaluation by target population:* This process aims on assessment of instructions, the response scale, and appropriateness of items for target population. The instrument administered to target population and asked to report items appropriateness, clarity or any ambiguity.
5. *Back-translation:* Back translation works as additional quality control check. Back translation refers to translating the synthesized and revised version of the instrument into the source language. It aims to evaluate the extent to which the translated version reflects the item content of the original version. This is considered final stage and after this tool must be ready to use. A minimum of two translators should involve in back-translation process. Back-translation aims to identify words that are not clear to target population or to report conceptual or inconsistency errors in the final version of instrument.
6. *Pilot study:* Before bringing new instrument in uses, researcher must perform pilot study. It is testing of final translated version of instrument to a similar but small size population to check clarity of items, meaning or any other difficulties. A more than one pilot testing may be required before reaching to the final version of an instrument. However, modifications suggested in the pilot study should be implemented with the help of experts.

PILOT STUDY/FEASIBILITY STUDY

Pilot stud is a crucial and essential element in a research project. The term 'pilot study' refers to mini version of a full-scale study (also called 'feasibility study'), as well or specific pre-testing of a particular research instrument such as interview or questionnaire. Pilot study conducted to identify the potential problem areas and deficiencies into research instruments and protocols before using in the main study. Therefore, pilot study serve as guide to develop a research plan rather than of being a test of the already developed plan. However, conducting pilot study does not guarantee success in the main study, but it does increase the likelihood.

Definitions

'Small study to test research protocol, data collection instruments, sample recruitment strategies and other researcher techniques in preparation for a larger study.' *(Stewart PW)*

'A pilot or preliminary study is a small scale of complete survey or a pre-test for a particular research instrument such as questionnaire or interview guide.' *(Polit & Beck, 2006)*

'Pilot study is a small scale rehearsal of main study to test the feasibility of proposed research process/protocol.' *(Kumar R, 2018)*

Importance of Pilot Study
Pilot study in a research project serve following important purposes:
- It helps to determine the feasibility of main study and identify the weakness in each section of the study
- Pilot study helps to determine appropriateness, comprehensiveness and relevancy of the research instrument(s)
- Pilot study test appropriateness of the data collection techniques (face-to-face interview or questionnaire and so on)
- It helps to study the data collection process in terms of time duration, willingness of the subjects and availability of the subject, etc.
- To obtain preliminary data for primary outcomes measures, in order to calculate the adequate sample size.
- To determine adequacy of data analysis process and use of statistical tests
- To determine the psychometric properties of research instrument (validity, reliability, difficulty or discriminative index, etc.).

REVIEW QUESTIONS AND ANSWER

Long and Short Answer Questions
1. How will you establish validity and reliability of the tools? *(BFUHS, MSc N-2011)*
2. Write in detail the methods of data collection approaches. *(AIIMS, MSc N-2013)*
3. Elaborate the means of ensuring the quality in data collection. *(BFUHS, MSc N-2006)*
4. Write in detail about questionnaires. *(RGUHS, MSc N-2001)*
5. What are the criteria's for selecting an instrument? *(PGI, MSc N-2012)*
6. Explain the steps in tool construction. *(KUHAS, MSc N-2012)*
7. Explain in detail about pilot study. *(TNMGRMU, MSc N-2007)*
8. Explain in detail the importance of pilot study. *(TNMGRMU, MSc N-2000)*

Multiple Choice Questions
1. Which types of validity of an instrument is determined by comparing it to Gold standard?
   a. Construct validity
   b. Content validity
   c. Face validity
   d. Criterion validity

2. Cronbach's alpha measures of reliability indicates which of the following characteristics of a research tool?
   a. Stability
   b. Internal consistency
   c. Interrater reliability
   d. Equivalence reliability

3. The degree to which an instrument measures what it is intended to measures is called as:
   a. Reliability
   b. Validity
   c. Sensitivity
   d. Objectivity

4. It is a method of data collection in which several rounds of questionnaires are mailed to an expert team, focusing on their opinions or judgement concerning a specific construct is called as:
   a. Systematic review
   b. Delphi technique
   c. Meta-analysis
   d. Meta-synthesis

5. The degree to which all items in an instrument measure the same construct is termed as:
   a. Internal consistency
   b. Homogeneity
   c. Stability
   d. Equivalence

6. Which of the following data collection method is most objective and provide empirical information?
   a. Self-report
   b. Observation
   c. Interview
   d. Biophysiological methods

7. Which of the following procedure used to confirm the stability index of a research instrument?
   a. Inter-rater reliability
   b. Cronbach's alpha
   c. Internal consistency
   d. Test-retest method

8. Which of the following sequence is correct for data collection in research?
   a. Inform, contact, consent, collect
   b. Contact, inform, collect, consent
   c. Contact, consent, inform, collect
   d. Contact, inform, consent, collect

9. Which of the following is a statistical measure of inter-rater reliability?
   a. Cohen's Kappa
   b. Cronbach's alpha
   c. Kuder-Richardson coefficient
   d. Pearson correlation coefficient

10. Open ended question provide primarily which of the following types of data?
    a. Qualitative data
    b. Confirmatory data
    c. Predictive data
    d. None of the above

11. Which of the following term is most synonymous to repeatability, stability, consistency and precision?
    a. Validity
    b. Reliability
    c. Specificity
    d. Objectivity

Answer Key

1.	2.	3.	4.	5.	6.	7.	8.	9.	10.	11.
d.	b.	b.	b.	b.	d.	d.	d.	a.	a.	b.

SUGGESTED READING

1. Beaton DE, Bombardier C, Guillemin F, et al. Guidelines for the process of crosscultural adaptation of self-report measures. Spine. 2000;25(24):3186-91.
2. Bhaduri A. Method of data collection. Nursing research society of India workshop proceedings; 1998.
3. Bloor M, Wood F. Keywords in qualitative methods: Vocabulary of research concept. London: Sage Publication; 2006.
4. Borsa JC, Damasio BF, Banderia DR. Cross-cultural adaptation and validation of psychological instrument: Some consideration. Paideia. 2012;2:53:423-32.
5. Bryman A. Social research method. Oxford University Press: New York: Oxford University Press; 2001. p. 540.
6. Burn N, Grove SK. The practice of nursing research: Appraisal, synthesis and generation of evidence, 6th edition. St Louis: Elsevier; 2009.

7. Chan EA, Chung JWY, Wong TK, et al. An evaluation of nursing practice model in the context of the severe respiratory distress syndrome (SARS) in Hong Kong: A preliminary study example of videotaped vignettes. Journal of Clinical Nursing. 2008;15:661-70.
8. Corbetta P. Social research theory, method and techniques. London Sage Publications; 2003. p. 336.
9. Crumbaugh JC. The meaning of projective techniques. In: Crumbaugh JC, Grace J, Hutzell RR, Whidon MF, Cooper EC (Eds). A primer of projective techniques of psychological assessment. San Diego: Libra; 1990.
10. Dewson B, Trap RG. Basic and clinical biostatistics, 3rd edition. Mc-Graw Hill Company; 2000.
11. Garrett EH. Statistics in Psychology and Education. New York: Longmans Green and Company; 1926.
12. Gjersing L, Caplehorn JRM, Clausen T. Cross-cultural adaptation of research instruments: Language, setting, time and statistical considerations. BMC Medical Research Methodology. 2010;10:13. doi:10.1186/1471-2288-10-13.
13. Gould D. Using vignettes to collect data for nursing research studies: How valid are the findings? Journal of Clinical Nursing. 1996;15;4:207-12.
14. Hambleton RK, Patsula L. Adapting tests for use in multiple languages and cultures. Social Indicators Research. 1998;45(1-3):153-71. doi:10.1023/A:1006941729637.
15. Hambleton RK. Guidelines for adapting educational and psychological tests: A progress report. European Journal of Psychological Assessment. 1994;10(3):229-44.
16. Hambleton RK. Issues, designs, and technical guidelines for adapting tests into multiple languages and cultures. In: Hambleton RK, Merenda PF, Spielberger CD (Eds). Adapting educational and psychological tests for cross-cultural assessment. Mahwah, NJ: Lawrence Erlbaum; 2005. pp. 3-38.
17. Houser J. Nursing research: Reading, using, and creative evidence. USA: Jones and Bartlett Learning; 2008.
18. Janda LH. Psychological testing: Theory and application. Boston: Allyn and Bacon; 1998.
19. Kline P. Personality: Measurement and theory. London: Hutchinson; 1983.
20. Kothari CR. Research methodology—methods and techniques, New Delhi: New Age Publication; 2004.
21. Kvale S. Interview: An introduction to qualitative research interviewing, Thousand Oaks. London: SAGE Publication; 1996. p. 326.
22. Lancaster G. Research methods in management. Burlington: Elsevier; 2007.
23. McNamara C. Field guide to consulting and organizational development: A collaborative and system approach to performance, change and learning. Minneapolis: Authenticity consulting, LLC. 2006. p. 499.
24. Meek R, Epi MC, Kelly AM, et al. Use of the visual analog scale to rate ad monitor severity of nausea in the emergency department. Academic emergency medicine. 2009;16(12):1304-10.
25. Norma GR, Vleuten C, Newble DI. International handbook of research in medical education. Springer Science and Business Media; 2002.
26. Olsen W. Data collection-Key data base and methods in social research. London: Sage Publication; 2011.
27. Pawar M. Data collecting methods and experience—A guide for social researchers, USA: New Dawn Press Group; 2004.
28. Polit DF, Beck CT. Essentials of nursing research: Methods, appraisal, and utilization, 6th edition. Philadelphia: Lippincott Williams & Wilkins; 2006. p. 65.

29. Polit DF, Beck CT. Nursing research generating and assessing evidence for nursing practice, 8th edition. Philadelphia: Lippincott William and Wilkins; 2008.
30. Polit DF, Beck CT. Nursing research generating and assessing evidence for nursing practice, 8th edition. Philadelphia: Lippincott William and Wilkins; 2012.
31. Pratt BF, Loizos P. Choosing research method—Data collection for development workers. UK: Oxfam; 1992.
32. Punch M. Introduction to social research: Quantitative and qualitative approaches. London: Sage Publication; 1998.
33. Rahman N. Caregiver sensitivity to conflict: the use of vignette methodology. Journal of Elder Abuse and Neglect. 1996;8:35-47.
34. Setz VG, D' Innocenzo M. Evaluation of the quality of nursing documentations through the review of patient medical records. Acta Paul Enferm. 2009;22(3):313-7.
35. Singh AK. Tests measurement and research methods in behavioral sciences. India: Bharti Bhawan Publication (P and D); 2013.
36. Stewart PW. Small or pilot study, GCRC protocols which propose "pilot studies". Cincinnati Children's Hospital Medical Center. [HTML]
37. Weller SC, Romney AK. Systematic data collection. London: Sage Publications; 1988.

Chapter 10

Data Analysis and Interpretation

INTRODUCTION

Data analysis is an important steps of a research process to make the information more meaningful and understandable to others. To avoid misinterpretation of the data, plans for final analysis and interpretation should be made prior to data collection. It is the responsibility of the researcher to organize every piece of information systematically to make it more meaningful. Nurse researchers should be more careful in collection, organization, analysis and interpretation of data.

Data analysis requires technical skills, judgment skill and intensive knowledge about the data to be analyzed. Analysis can be done either manually or with the help of computer. If the number of respondents is small, then manual analysis can be done. Manual analysis is extremely time consuming. For computer analysis, knowledge of computer and statistics is needed to create a data file and to apply statistical test for analysis and interpretation of the data.

Statistical methods describe appropriately the characteristics of mass of data and gives meaning to the raw data. To proceed the statistical analysis of a quantitative research, you will need to be able to do the followings:
- Identify the statistical analysis to be performed
- Determine whether they are appropriate and matched the research design and question/hypotheses/purpose of the study
- Judge whether the level of measurement match the statistical test
- Judge whether the interpretation of the statistical analysis made sense
- Evaluate not only the statistical significance of the findings but also the clinical significance of the findings.

STATISTICAL PROCEDURES

Statistical procedures can be divided into two major categories:
1. Descriptive statistics
2. Inferential statistics

DESCRIPTIVE STATISTICS

Descriptive statistics includes statistical procedures that are used to describe the population/sample we are studying. It includes frequencies, measure of central tendency (mean, median, mode), and measure of variability (standard deviation, variance and range). A researcher should have basic knowledge of frequency distribution and scale of measurement before use of descriptive statistics.

LEVELS OF MEASUREMENT

Level of measurement is otherwise called scales of measurement. There are four types of measurement scales:
1. Nominal scale
2. Ordinal scale
3. Interval scale
4. Ratio scale

As one moves up the level (nominal to ratio), the level of precision of the measurement increases. Further each level subsumes the characteristics of all of the levels below it and also adds to a new quality (All four levels of scales are explained in detail in Chapter 12).

- *Nominal scale:* It is lowest and least precise scale of measurement. The nominal scale only provides number to the variables that does not give any quantitative meaning to variables. The number does not carry any quality of greater than or less than or make any inference about intervals between data points. In other words, nominal scales are used for labeling categories of variables, without any quantitative value. All these scales are mutually exclusive.

> **Box 10.1: Example of Nominal-Level Measurement.**
> - Blood group
>   - A
>   - B
>   - AB
>   - O
> - Gender
>   - Female
>   - Male

- *Ordinal scale:* Ordinal level data are next level of data set to nominal data. Ordinal data arrange the data in an inherent order. Data values such as strongly satisfied, satisfied, neither satisfied nor dissatisfied, dissatisfied and strongly dissatisfied have order. However, ordinal scale does not provide information about the differences between two data points.

> **Box 10.2: Example of Ordinal-Level Measurement.**
> - Socioeconomic status
>   - Low income
>   - Middle income
>   - High income
> - Level of knowledge
>   - Inadequate
>   - Adequate
>   - Good

- *Interval scale:* Interval scale is the next level of measurement after ordinal scale. It consists of all the qualities of a nominal and ordinal scale plus it adds the quality of equal distance between data point or intervals. This characteristic makes the researcher to draw conclusion regarding actual differences between two measures.

> **Box 10.3: Example of Interval-Level Measurement.**
> - Temperature (in degree centigrade)
>   - 20–70°
>   - 30–90°

- *Ratio scale:* Ratio scale is the highest level of measurement scale. Ratio scale consists all the qualities of previous measurement scale plus it adds the quality of an absolute zero. This absolute zero features enables to draw conclusion for presence or absence of a variable.

> **Box 10.4:** Example of Ratio-Level Measurement.
> - Height
> - Weight
> - Blood pressure
> - Pulse rate
> - Heart rate

A researcher should organize and process the data in their respective scale or level of measurement. The data should not be merged or collapsed to lower level of scale of measurement. However, a researcher may do so as per the mandate of the objectives. For example, the age (in years) of the participant is measured in ratio scale. The same data can be converted to category (<30 years and >30 years), which is ordinal scale, but the researcher loses the precision or accuracy of the data being analyzed. The statistical methods to be used to analyze the data depends on the scale in which the data is measured.

FREQUENCY DISTRIBUTION

A frequency distribution is a mathematical function showing the number of instances in which a variable takes each of its possible values. A frequency distribution of data can be shown in a table or graph. Some common methods of showing frequency distributions includes frequency tables, histograms or bar charts.

Visual depictions of frequency information is a quick and easy way to get an idea of the demographics of the whole sample. Frequency distribution can be plotted with the help of histogram, which is defined as the way that the variable of interest is clustered or spread across its continuum. It is shape of data when data are graphed so that the levels of the variable are on the *x-axis* and the number of cases found at each data point is on the *y-axis*. Most statistical software program such as SPSS (Statistical Package for the Social Sciences) can easily produce frequency data in the form of histogram.

NORMAL DISTRIBUTION CURVE

It is a bell-shaped curve. In symmetrical data distribution, the curve will divide in two halves and each half could be folded over one another and fit almost exactly. Skewed distribution have off center peaks with longer tail in one direction; if the longer tail is on the longer left, it is called *negatively skewed*; if the longer tail is on right, it is called *positively skewed*. An example of data that would be appear as a skewed distribution would be the age group of a group of stroke patients, since the majority would be older, thus pulling the hump to the right with long tail towards the left and making it a negatively skewed distribution (Fig. 10.1).

MEASURES OF CENTRAL TENDENCY

Measure of central tendency includes mean, median, and mode. The *mean* or '*averages*' is the most commonly used measure of central tendency. The *mean* (or average) is the most popular and best measure of central tendency. The mean is calculated by summing up all observations and dividing the total by number of observations. *The median* by definition refers middle value in a distribution. *Median* is the center value of a data set which divide whole data set in two

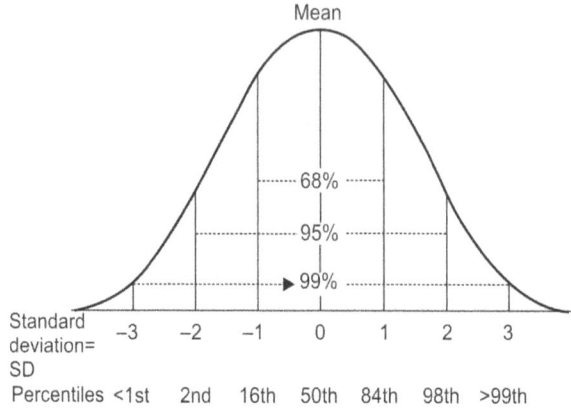

Fig. 10.1: Normal distribution curve.

halves at which half of the subjects lie above the value (median) and another half falls below it. *The Mode* is the most frequent possible value occurs in a given observation. It may be regarded as the '*most typical*' value of a series of values. The mode is the only useful measure of central tendency when a variable is measured on a nominal scale.

Box 10.5: Top 10 List of Common Statistical Methods.	
1. Mean	6. T-test (independent and dependent)
2. Frequency distribution	7. ANOVA, all kinds
3. Standard deviation (SD)	8. Correlation of coefficient (r)
4. Range	9. Cronback's alpha (α)
5. Percentages, percentile and quartile	10. Chi-square (X^2)

MEASURES OF DISPERSION/VARIABILITY

A researcher collects a set of data in which some of the observations are vary from the central value of data. In some observation, the difference may be less whereas in some other observation, it may be more. This property of deviation of the values from the average is called *dispersion or variation* and the measures used to measure this variation called *measures of dispersion/variation*. Measures of dispersion help us to study the important characteristics and distribution of an observation. The various measures of dispersion are as follows:

1. Range
2. Interquartile range or quartile deviation
3. Mean deviation
4. Standard deviation
5. Coefficient of variation (CV)

Range is the difference between highest and lowest values in an observation. The interquartile *range* represent the difference between first and third quartile. It describes the middle 50% of the observation of a data set. *Mean deviation* indicates the difference between the values of the observation from the arithmetic mean ignoring the sign of their deviation. *Standard deviation* is the square root of the squared deviation of the observation from the arithmetic mean. *Coefficient of variation* is the expression of standard deviation as a percentage of the arithmetic mean.

DATA PROCESSING

Data processing is the process of editing, organizing and coding of data to make the data amenable for analysis and interpretation. Data may proceed manually or with the help of computer software. However, a combine method is another good choice for a researcher to process the data.

Data Preparation, Input, Verification and Cleaning

Data need to transferred from the data collection tool (e.g. checklist, rating scale and questionnaire) into format that is suitable for analysis. This often takes the form of a grid, with respondents or cases in rows and variables in columns. Before analysis take place, a researcher should check the accuracy of the data to deal constructively with any missing values.

Data Editing

This is scrutinizing process of data and occur almost every phase of data collection or analysis. It ranges from the almost routine activities of correcting typographical errors to out of range entries done by a researcher. Further, data editing allow a researcher to claims the empirical findings on the variable under study.

Data Coding

It is almost impossible for a researcher to work with original data. It could be thousand of filled questionnaires, figures, checklist and observation of nursing staff in hospital. To make this job simplified, data are often coded. Data coding process follow following steps:

- *Developing a coding frame or coding sheet:* This is a process to prepare and assign code number to each information collected through research instrument. Researcher prepare a outline to assign the code for each information. It should be ensured that each information obtained from the sample should get a unique code and entered in the column mean for it. However, it is always good to pre-test the coding frame by taking few questionnaires to anticipate any problems in advance.
- *Coding the data:* Once the coding frame is finalized, it is time to code whole bunch of information into a separate sheet called transcription sheet or master data sheet. Master sheet is large and concise summary contains cods for all information collected in a research project. A sample master data sheet is given in Table 10.1.

Example,
Marital status (Please Tick)

Married	1	
Unmarried	2	
Widow	3	code numbers
Divorced	4	
Separated	5	

Note: Each category of marital status is coded with numbers but the numbers does not have any numerical meaning. The numbers are assigned for each category (e.g. Married = 1) for identification purpose and for the convenience of analysis with computer programs. The numbers will be decoded with respective category by computer or manually after analysis is done.

Table 10.1: Sample master data sheet.

Code No.	Gender	Age	Religion	SES	Weight	SBP	DBP
1	1	25	1	1	45	120	80
2	2	23	1	3	48	110	70
3	2	27	2	3	53	130	90
4	2	32	2	2	57	140	100
5	1	26	1	2	50	110	70
6	1	19	1	1	62	120	80
7	1	20	3	3	59	130	90

(SBP: systolic blood pressure; DBP: diastolic blood pressure; SES: socioeconomic status)
Note: The Dark columns indicate categorical (nominal variables)

Data Input

Data input is a process to enter data code into a data sheet. A researcher can directly enter the data code into a data analysis package (such as SPSS) or into a spreadsheet (such as MS excel). Direct imputation of data in SPSS or excel spreadsheet allow speedy preparation of frequency tables, figures and charts. However, online questionnaire provide an option to import data directly into a software package, thus saving data input time.

Data Verification

Once the data have been entered into computer package, they need to be checked carefully for accuracy. Verification is an attempt to ensure that error should not occur when transferring data from one source to another, for example, from rating scale to data base or software package. Strategies to achieve this include proofreading, checking 100% of data entry and double entry, when data are entered twice and compared for agreement. A random examination and re-examination of the coded data also make sure to find out any discrepancies.

Data Cleaning

Data cleaning aims to identify and correct the error or at least to minimize their impact on study results. Data cleaning deal with data problem once they have occurred. However, error prevention strategies during data imputation and transformation can reduce the problem but cannot eliminate them. Data cleaning involves two types of checks. The first check is for *outlier* and *wild codes*. Outliers are value that lie outside the normal range. Outliers can be found by inspecting frequency distribution, paying special attention to the lowest and highest values. Another problem is a *wild code*, a code that is not possible. For example, a researcher assign code for gender; (1) Male and (2) Female. If some of gender found with code 3, is the wild code.

Consistency check is another cleaning procedure focus on internal data consistency. In consistency check, researcher aims to check errors by testing compatibility of data within a case. For example, one question in survey asks current employment status of subjects and another might ask types of employment. If the data are internally consistent, respondent who answered 'not employed' for first question should have 'zero' for second question.

Steps of Data Processing

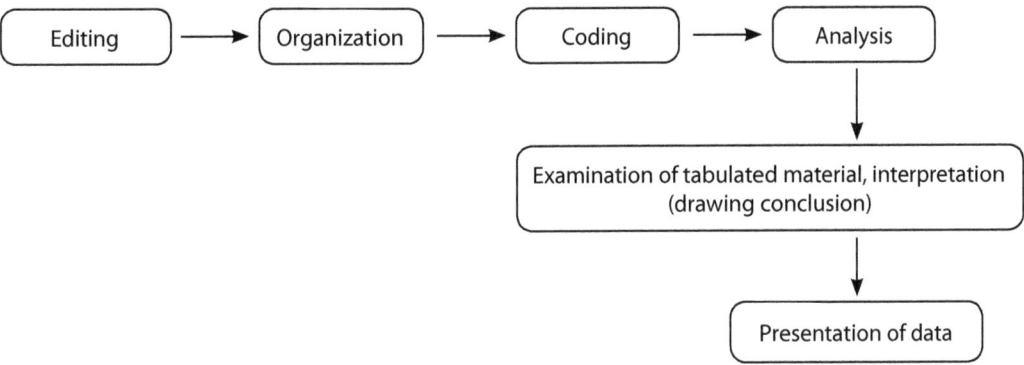

DATA PRESENTATION

Data presentation is an important step of data analysis in research. Information are usually gathered in raw format and thus inherent information is difficult to understand. Therefore, raw information need to be processed, summarized and analyzed to present in effective format. Data may be presented by using following methods:
- Table presentation
- Graph presentation

Table Presentation

Tabulation is a simple and attractive method of data presentation. It is orderly arrangement of data in column and rows. The arrangement of assembled data has to be done in concise and logical manner. Table is best suited for representing individual information and represent both qualitative and quantitative information. The tabulation technique applied for summarization and condensation of data. It helps in analysis of relationship, trends, drifts, inclination, leaning, tendency and other related summarization of the given data.

The tabulation may be simple or complex. Simple tabulation present result in one direction tables, which can be used to answer research question related to one characteristic of data. The complex tabulation generally results in two directional tables, which provides information about two interconnected characteristics of the data. Any researcher having knowledge of statistics can tabulate the data according to physical attribute or psychological approach. Structure of the table also depends on the character of the variables. An example of simple and complex table is given in Tables 10.2 and 10.3.

Example of Simple Table:

Table 10.2: Frequency and percentage distribution of sociodemographic characteristics of the study participants (N = 35).

	Demographic variables	(f)	(%)
Age (years)	20–24	11	31.4
	25–29	9	25.7
	30–34	7	20.0
	35–39	8	22.9
Gender	Male	21	60.0
	Female	14	40.0
Educational status	Illiterate	5	14.3
	Primary school	11	31.4
	Secondary school	13	37.1
	College	3	08.6
	Professional	3	08.6
Marital status	Unmarried	2	05.7
	Married	12	34.3
	Widow	21	60.0
Religion	Hindu	32	91.4
	Muslim	8	08.6

Example of Complex Table

Table 10.3: Frequency distribution of blood group among male and female students of a primary school (N = 148).

		Blood group				Total
		A	B	AB	O	
Gender	Male	15	20	13	25	73
	Female	18	17	18	22	75
Total		33	37	31	47	148

Principles of Tabulation

There is no definitive principle for making the tables. Tables are prepared according to the types of data and the purpose for which a table is essential. However, following guidelines may act as principle of tabulation:

- *The title of the table:* Each table should be labeled with an appropriate title. The title of the table should evidently fetch out the character of the data presented in the table.
- *Comparative and relative figures:* One of the main functions of tabulation is to present data in a comparative manner with a clear distinction between relation and proposition.

Therefore, it is advised that table is prepared in manner as would present quick and simple assessment. Generally comparative columns should be kept adjoining each others.
- *Emphasis:* The main items of information in the table should be properly emphasized by underlying the items or by using bold or italic letter or so on.
- *Source of information (reference):* Footnotes and source of information must be added whenever necessary and mandatory.
- *Unit of measurement:* Unit of measurement for data must be depicted accurately. Such as 'length in meters' and 'weight in kilograms'.

Discrete Frequency Distribution Table

The process of preparing a frequency distribution is very simple. In the case of discrete data, place all possible values of the variable in ascending order in one column, and then prepare another column of 'Tally' mark to count the numbers of times a particular value of the variable present. For example, number of children in a family is given here:

3	5	1	5	3
2	4	2	4	2
3	3	2	3	1
1	2	1	2	2

To condense this data into a discrete frequency distribution, we shall take the help of 'Tally' marks as shown in Table 10.4.

Table 10.4: Frequency distribution table.

No. of children	No. of families (Tally marks)	Frequency
1	////	4
2	//// //	7
3	////	4
4	//	2
5	//	2

Continuous Frequency Distribution Table

A researcher should keep following important points in mind while preparing a continuous frequency distribution table.

Class Limit or Interval

Class limit denote the lowest and highest value that can be included in the class. The two boundaries should be specifically defined before constructing a table. Class limit can be inclusive or exclusive type.

a. *Inclusive Class Interval:* When the lower and upper class limit is included, it is referred as inclusive class interval. This type is useful for the discrete type of variables (Table 10.5).

Table 10.5: Inclusive class intervals.

Age of participants	Frequency
25–30	5
31–35	6
36–40	4
41–45	3
46–50	2

b. *Exclusive Class Interval:* When the lower limit is included, but the upper limit is excluded, then it is an **exclusive class interval**. For example, 25–30, 30–35, etc. are exclusive type of class intervals. In the class interval of 25–30, 25 is included but 30 is excluded (Table 10.6).

Table 10.6: Exclusive class intervals.

Weight of the participants (in kg)	Frequency
44.5–49.5	5
49.5–54.5	6
54.5–59.5	4
59.5–64.5	3
64.5–69.5	2

In the above example, where will you place (or count) a participant whose weight is 49.5 kg? Note that 49.5 kg is mentioned in both first (44.5–49.5) and second (49.5–54.5) category.

In exclusive class interval, a participant with weight of 49.5 kg has to be counted under category 49.5–54.5 because the upper limit of 44.5–49.5 is 49.5 and it has to be excluded.

c. *Open End:* In open end distribution, the lower unit of the very first class and upper limit of the last class is not given. In distribution where there is a big gap between minimum and maximum values (Table 10.7).

Table 10.7: Open end table.

Income (₹)	Frequency
<1000	10
1000–2000	15
2000–5000	10
5000–15000	2
15000–25000	18
>25,000	10

d. *Cumulative frequencies:* As it name indicates, it cumulates the frequencies, starting at either the lowest or highest vale. The cumulative frequency of a given data interval, thus, represent the total of all previous class frequencies including the class against which it is written (Table 10.8).

Table 10.8: Cumulative frequency table.

Monthly salary (₹)	No. of employees	Cumulative frequencies
1000–2000	5	5
2000–4000	10	15
4000–6000	15	30
6000–8000	4	34

Significance of Tabulation

Tabulation play an important role to condense and summarize a bunch of information. It is easy and convenient way to present the information in attractive manner. Tabulation have following importance in data presentation.

- *To simplify complex information:* Tabulation helps in summarization and condensation of data. It avoid unnecessary details and duplication of information and save lot of time to study and understand information.
- *To facilitate comparison:* Table helps in comparison of information between two or more than two groups. Since, each part there is total and sub-total and this will help to study comparison and relationships between different groups.
- *To help references:* Each table presented with clear and concise title along with table name and number. This made a table a quick source of reference for others.
- *To save space:* Table helps to condense and summarize large group of information into rows and columns without consuming much space.
- *To depict pattern and trends:* Tabulation helps to provide information about the trends and pattern of study variables.
- *To facilitate statistical processing:* Tabulation helps application of statistical analysis. It is only possible after tabulation and classification that will make data used for statistical application.

Graph Presentation

Graph is another easy and simple way to represent the information. Graphs simplify the information by using images and figures and emphasizing data pattern of trends. Graphs are useful for summarizing, explaining, or exploring quantitative information. Graphs are effective way to represent a large bunch of information and hence, can be used in place of table. A right format of the graph helps to best represent the data to the readers and reviewers. There are various form of graphical presentation is possible to represent the data. Some the important methods of graphical presentation are given here:

- Bar graphs and histograms
- Pie or sector graphs
- Frequency curves
- Pictograms/pictographs
- Frequency polygons
- Cumulative frequency curve (Ogive)
- Scatter/dot diagrams
- Line diagrams
- Charts
- Maps
- Flowcharts.

Principles of Graphic Presentation

Graphical presentation is an easy and effective means of communicating finding to others. Therefore, it is important to understand about use of graphs, figures, audience and context in which you are communicating your findings. Though, there are no formal guidelines for graphical presentation but use of following points can help a researcher to communicate his data effectively to others.
- The figure/graph should be neatly and attractively drawn for voluntary attention of readers
- The figure should be concise and appropriate in terms of title, number and key words used in figure for clear understanding to readers
- Use of appropriate size of figure will helps to provide complete and clear information to others
- In case of multiple bars/graphs, it is recommended to use different colors for each bar or graph for easy identification
- A researcher should have knowledge about the audience before selection of a graph/figure.

Bar Graphs and Histograms

Bar graphs presents the data in the form of bars that can be drawn vertically or horizontally. The only difference between a histogram and bar chart is that there is no space between the bars in a histogram. The height of bars indicates the amount of information in a category. A bar chart used to indicate and compare value in a discrete category or group and the frequency or other measurement (i.e. mean).

There are three types of bar graphs:
1. Simple bar graph
2. Multiple bar graph
3. Proportional bar graph.

Simple Bar Graph (Table 10.9 and Fig. 10.2)

Table 10.9: Rice production per year (in tonnes).

Year	Production (in tonnes)
1991	45
1992	40
1993	42
1994	55
1995	50

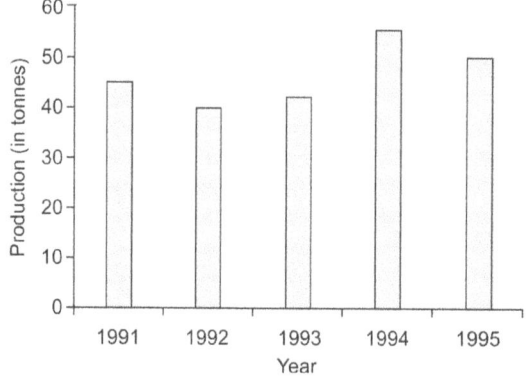

Fig. 10.2: Simple bar graph.

Multiple Bar Graphs (Table 10.10 and Fig. 10.3)

Table 10.10: Tax difference per year (in ₹).

Year	Profit before tax (in lakhs)	Profit after tax (in lakhs)
1998	195	80
1999	200	87
2000	165	45
2001	140	32

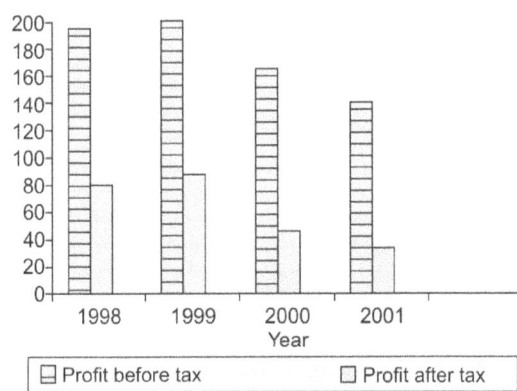

Fig. 10.3: Multiple bar graph.

Proportional Bar Graphs (Table 10.11 and Fig 10.4)

Table 10.11: Monthly expenditure on different items (in ₹).

Expenditure items	Monthly expenditure (in ₹)	
	Family A	Family B
Food	75	95
Clothing	20	25
Education	15	10
Housing rent	40	65
Miscellaneous	25	35

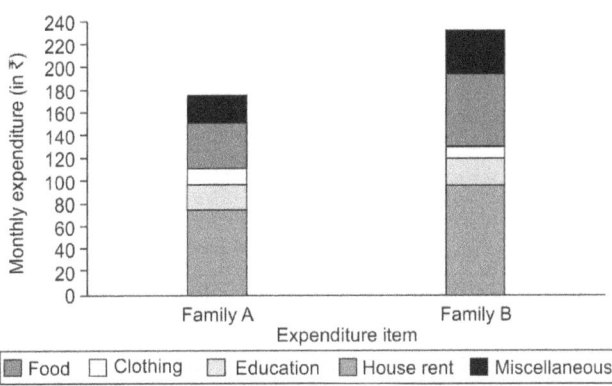

Fig. 10.4: Proportional bar graph.

Histogram (Table 10.12 and Fig. 10.5)

Table 10.12: Heights of 30 people.

Height	Frequency
139.5–149.5	6
149.5–159.5	9
159.5–169.5	7
169.5–179.5	5
179.5–189.5	2
189.5–199.5	1

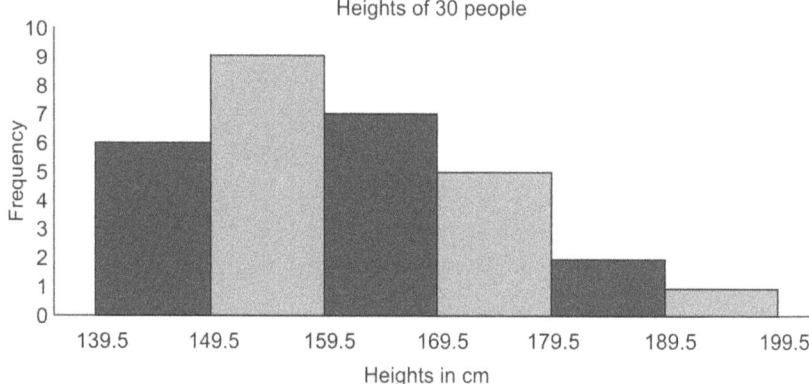

Fig. 10.5: Histogram.

Pie or Sector Graphs

Pie chart is the another most appropriate method to represent the data grouped into small number of categories. It is commonly used to depict nominal data, visually represent a distribution of categories. However, it also can be used to depict data which cannot be presented apart from a table (i.e. frequency distribution). It is most commonly used method to represent number of votes each candidates won in a election. It gives comparative difference at a glance. Size of each angle is calculated by multiple class percentages with 360° angle or use the given formula for calculating sector percentage, for example, distribution of seat won by different parties in parliament election (Table 10.13 and Fig. 10.6).

$$\text{Size of pie sector} = \frac{\text{Class frequency}}{\text{Total observation}} \times 360°$$

Table 10.13: Number of seats won a party in parliament election in India.

Party	BJP	Congress	AAP	BSP	Shivsena	Others
Seats	200	35	6	10	50	110
Degree	175	31	5	9	44	96

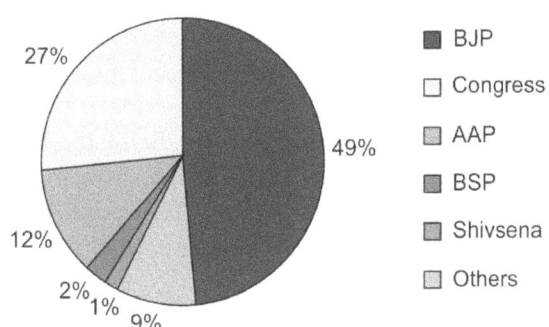

Fig. 10.6: Pie diagram: Number of seats won by parties at election.

Frequency Curves

Frequency polygon is a line diagram to present the frequency distribution. It looks similar to histogram except that midpoints are identified for each class and joined to each others. The diagram made is called frequency polygon. The frequency curve begins and ends at the base line. For example, hemoglobin level of patients attended health services at a tertiary care hospital at North India (Fig. 10.7).

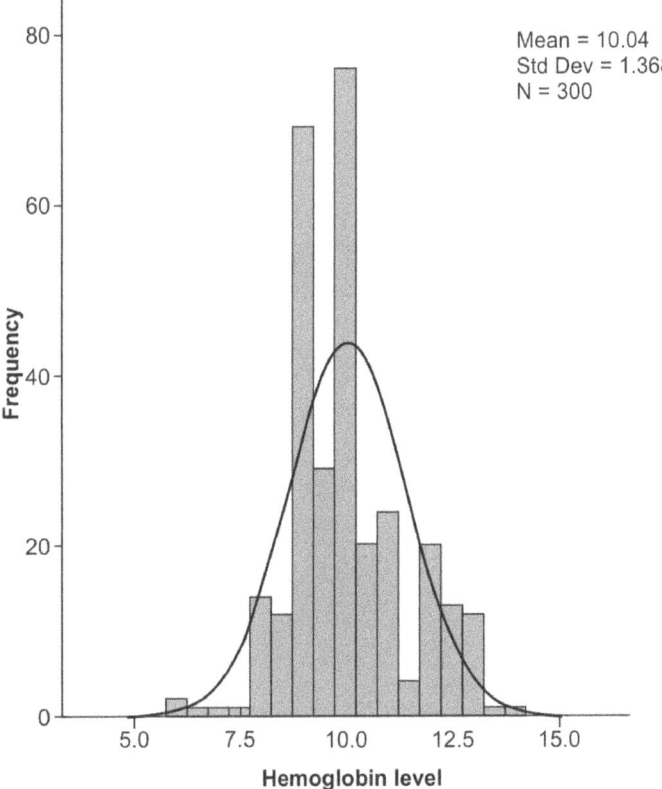

Fig. 10.7: Frequency curve.

Pictograms/Pictographs

Pictogram or pictograph is a popular method of data presentation. It is a line or bar graph uses symbols or pictures to depict its data.

Pictures are attractive and easy to comprehend and therefore, this method is particularly useful in presenting findings to the layman. In pictograph, data are presented through a pictorial symbol that is carefully selected. Pictorial symbols selected should be self-explanatory in nature. For example, production of apple and orange around the globe in a particular year (Fig. 10.8).

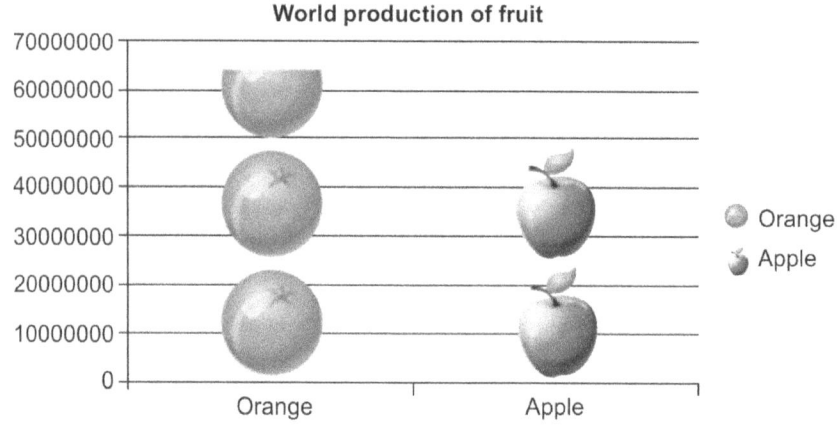

Fig. 10.8: Pictogram.

Frequency Polygons

A frequency polygon is a graph of frequency distribution. Frequency polygon constructed by joining the midpoint of the upper horizontal side of each rectangle of a histogram. It can also constructed by taking the midpoint of various class intervals. Frequency polygon is simpler than the histogram and it gives outline of data pattern more easily (Table 10.14 and Fig. 10.9).

Table 10.14: Weights of 245 people.

Weight in kg	Frequency
90–95	10
95–100	35
100–105	75
105–110	80
110–115	40
115–120	15

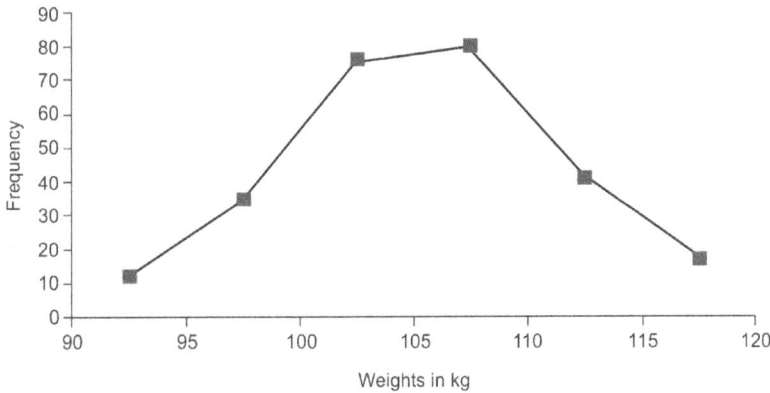

Fig. 10.9: Frequency polygon.

Cumulative Frequency Curve (Ogive)

Ogive is a graph of the cumulative frequency distribution. To draw this, an ordinary frequency table has to be converted to cumulative frequency table. It is obtained by cumulating the frequency of previous classes including the class in question. The cumulative frequencies are then plotted on graph to draw cumulative frequency graph. The Ogive can be drawn by taking lower or upper value of class interval. On joining the points by smooth free hand curve, the diagram appear is Ogive.

Ogive use to calculate median, quartiles and percentiles. It is also used to find out the number of observations, which are expected to lie below the two given value. For example, school going children test scores in mathematic paper at North India (Table 10.15 and Fig. 10.10).

Table 10.15: Psychology test scores of 642 students.

Marks	Frequency	Cumulative frequency
29.5–39.5	0	0
39.5–49.5	3	3
49.5–59.5	10	13
59.5–69.5	53	66
69.5–79.5	107	173
79.5–89.5	147	320
89.5–99.5	130	450
99.5–109.5	78	528
109.5–119.5	59	587
119.5–129.5	36	623
129.5–139.5	11	634
139.5–149.5	6	640
149.5–159.5	1	641
159.5–169.5	1	642
169.5–179.5	0	642

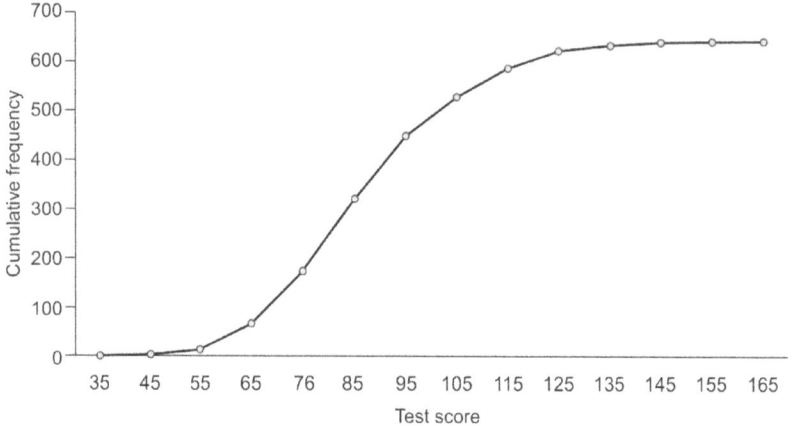

Fig. 10.10: Frequency polygon (Ogive).

Scatter/Dot Diagrams

It is graphic presentation made to shows the nature of correlation between two variables. For example, one variable is presented along the horizontal axis and other along the vertical axis. For each pair of observation of two variables, we put a dot in the plane. The direction of dots shows the scatter or concentration of various points along a plane. For example, relationship between height and weight of the school age children (Fig. 10.11).

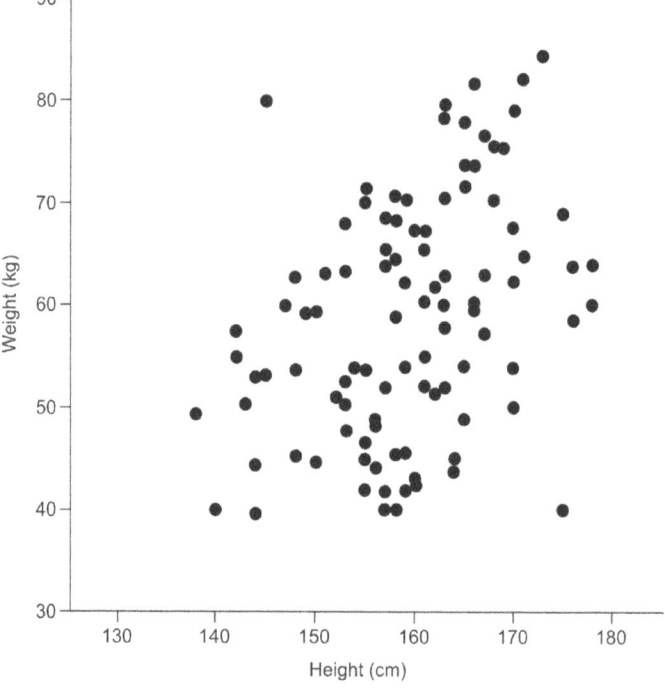

Fig. 10.11: Scatter plot.

Line Diagrams

This is frequency polygon presenting variation in observation over a period of time. It shows the trend of an event occurring over a period of time. In line diagram, vertical axis may not start from zero but at some point above when frequencies start at high level. To draw line chart, the data are plotted on x-axis or y-axis and points are joined by straight line.

For example, changes in suicide death rate over a period of years (Table 10.16 and Fig. 10.12).

Table 10.16: Number of suicidal death in a town between 2008 and 2012.

Year	Suicidal death in a town
2008	200
2009	220
2010	210
2011	270
2012	290

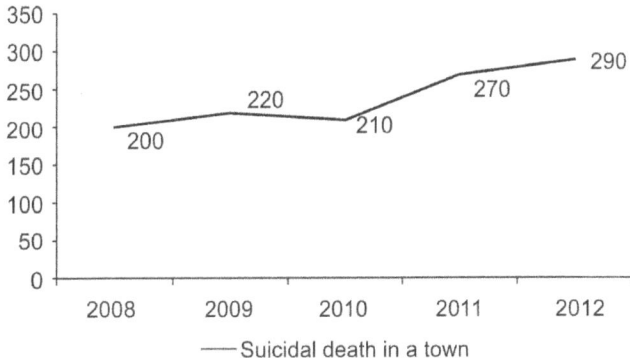

Fig. 10.12: Line diagram.

Charts

A chart is a visual representation of statistical data. Charts represents the data with the help of symbols such as bars or lines. It is a very effective tool as it displays data easily and quickly. It also helps to facilitate comparison and develop insight about trends and relationship within data.

Box 10.6: A Good Chart.

- Attract the reader's attention
- Display the information clearly, simply and accurately
- Does not mislead
- Display the information I condensed form
- Gives a overview of trends and pattern of an event
- Facilitate comparison and difference present the themes or messages in the accompanying text

Maps

Maps are very simple, and efficient means of communication and representation of data. Maps are especially useful tool for describing geographical variations, such as population distribution, voting pattern, crime rate, or labor force, etc.

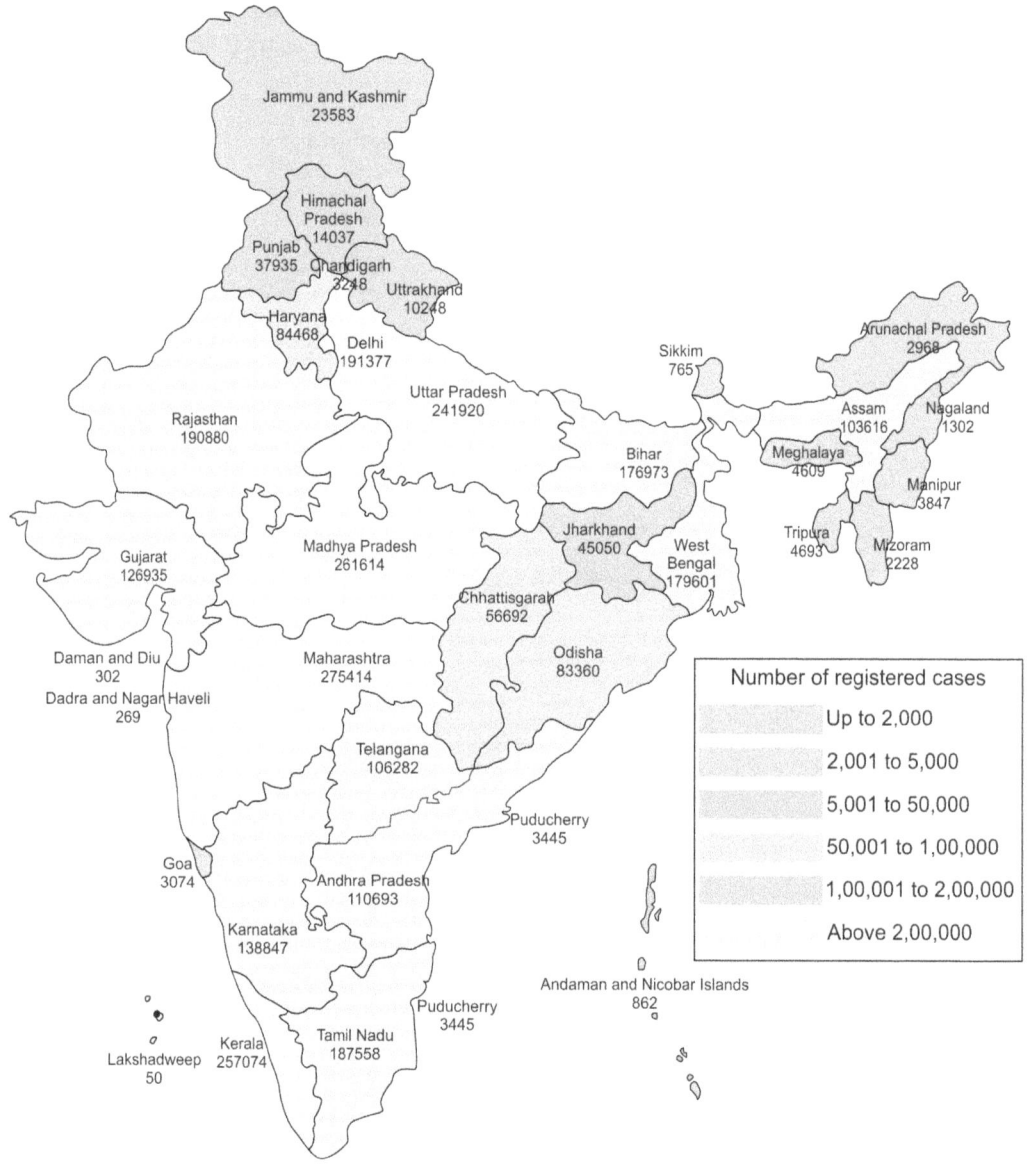

Cases registered under IPC crimes during 2015 (all India 29,49,400)
Source: NCRB

Flowcharts

Flowchart is a combination of map and graph. It is used to depict the flow of people from one place to another (usually origin to destination). It is also known as Dynamic Map. Transport map is the best example of flowchart.

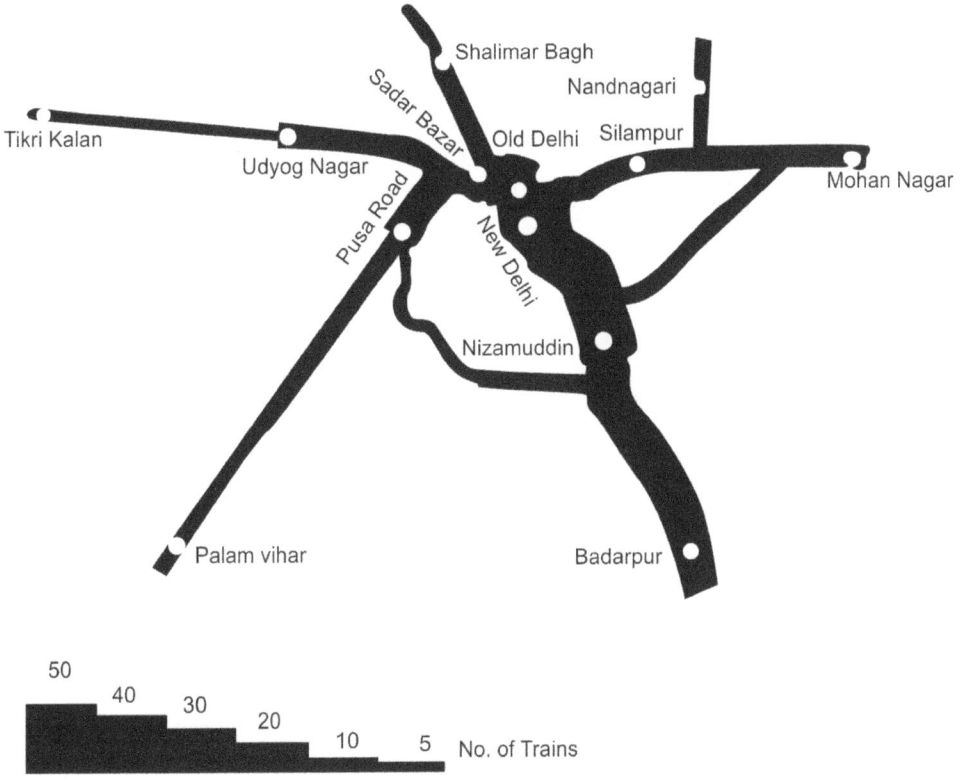

Fig. 10.13: Metro map of Delhi.

INFERENTIAL STATISTICS

Inferential statistics allow a researcher to make predictions about a specific study population based on information obtained from a representative sample. Nurse researcher ask many research questions and form hypotheses, which allow a researcher to determine whether the variance between two or more study groups can be explained ether by chance or by intervention. A researcher should also set a level of significance before conduct of study or statistics analysis in the form of probability or p value.

The significance value allow a researcher to reject or accept null hypotheses. Although, a significance level can be set at any value 0.1 and 0.5 are most preferred level of significance in nursing research. The level of significance means that there is 1 or 5% chance of rejecting null hypotheses, when, in fact, it is true.

Rejecting null hypotheses when actually it is true is called as *type I error* (false-positive results). Type I error also known as alpha error and denoted by Greek letter α. The lower the *p* value or significance level, the less chance it is that researcher will make type I error. *Type II errors* (false-negative results) occur when a researcher fail to reject null hypotheses when the research hypotheses is actually true. Type II errors also known as β errors (Table 10.17).

Table 10.17: Type I and type II errors.

Actual situation	Statistical decision	
	H_0 is not rejected (M1 = M2) No difference	H_0 is rejected (M1 ≠ M2) Significant difference
H_0 is true (M1 = M2) No difference	√	α Type I error
H_0 is false (M1 ≠ M2) Significant difference	β Type II error	√

Types of Inferential Statistics

Inferential statistics broadly deals with two types of test parametric test and non-parametric test.

1. *Parametric test* based on the assumptions that data are normally distributed, or on continuous scale (ration or interval level), and have equal variance. Parametric tests can be used to estimate population parameter. Example of parametric tests includes the one-way ANOVA, repeated measure ANOVA, Karl Pearson correlation, *t* test, simple and non-linear regressions, etc.
2. *Non-parametric* test are used when data are not normally distributed and on ordinal or nominal scale. Non-parametric tests rely on distribution free statistics methods and make fewer assumptions than parametric test. Example of non-parametric test includes Mann-Whitney U test, Median test, Wilcoxon rank sum test, chi-square test, Fisher exact test, etc. Inferential statistics are used to test exploratory and predictive middle range theories. Tests of explanatory theories require a statistic that measures the relationship between two or more concepts.

> **Box 10.7:** Application of Parametric and Non-parametric Statistics.
> - Kumar R (2018) used parametric measure of the Pearson product moment correlation coefficient to test personality dimensions, stress and adjustment styles among nursing students
> - Kumar R, et al. (2018) used a non-parametric test (Chi-square test) to test the significant association of types of family with stress level among nursing students

Hypothesis Testing

Hypothesis testing is an essential component of research process. Hypothesis is an empirically testable statement about a relationship between two or more than two variables or groups. Hypothesis testing allow a researcher to infer whether the difference between two or more than two groups is by chance or real intervention effect.

The null hypothesis: Null hypotheses postulate that there is no relationship between two or more than two variables or groups.

$$H_0 = \mu_1 = \mu_2$$

The research hypothesis: It postulate a predictive relationship between the variables under study. It is a positive statement of the null hypothesis. Acceptance or rejection of hypothesis is based on statistical significance, power, effect size, and sample size under study.

$$H_0 = \mu_1 = \mu_2$$

Interpretations of the Results

In quantitative research, results are either presented in the form of statistical value or *p*-value. A researcher must interpret the results to make it meaningful to others. Although, interpretation of results in descriptive study is easy job. For example, a research report present moderate self-esteem in 59.4% nursing students. Here, the results are easy and everyone can understand it. However, interpretations of results in experimental study is a challenging task for a researcher. For example, impact of structured training program on assertiveness skills in nursing officers. Here, a researcher need to interpret the results whether the test results is furious or by chance or caused by intervention. In-fact, if the results deemed to be true, that is, statistically significant, interpretations involves coming to the conclusion about internal validity when a casual inference is sought.

QUALITATIVE DATA ANALYSIS

The analysis and interpretation of qualitative data is distinct than quantitative data. Analysis is the investigator attempts to discover meaning of abstract or concept. It is both creative and interactive process, requires much time, critical thinking, and emotional and conceptual energy.

Qualitative findings contribute great deal of knowledge to nursing science, which has a primary purpose, excellence in theory development. As a part of healthcare reform and managed care, outcome of care that can be documented are receiving increased attention. Thus, the findings from qualitative research need to be evaluated for their potential to improve practice as well as for validity and credibility of their findings.

Purpose of Qualitative Data Analysis

Description and Exploration
Qualitative data analysis enable a researcher to gain understanding and insight about a particular phenomena or group of individuals.

Discovery and Explanation
- It helps to search the data to discover underlying themes, core pattern, and concepts that become the basis for inferences, interpretation and generating hypothetical statements about the meaning of the phenomena
- Analysis can be furthered to construct an explanatory scheme, model, or substantive grounded theory.

Qualitative Data Analysis Approach

- There are numerous approaches to analyzing qualitative data. Approximately 26 approaches to qualitative research analysis were identified, each one having a somewhat different approach to analysis. For example, analytical induction, thematic analysis, content analysis, phenomenological analysis, discourse analysis, narrative analysis, matrix analysis and constant comparison, etc.
- Within one approach, there may be various methods of analysis (e.g. phenomenology: Van Manen, Giorgi and Van Kaam)
- Analytic scheme or concept can be developed directly from the data; built upon the researcher's previous experience, or borrowed from the existing literature to organize or classify the data
- There are guidelines available for qualitative data analysis. However, each researcher has its distinct pattern of inquiry; the analytical method used will be distinct and unique, depending on knowledge, experience, skills, analytic abilities and style of the investigator.

Qualitative Data Analysis Overview

The analysis of qualitative material begins with a search for broad categories or themes. A *theme* is an abstract entity that brings meaning and identity to a current experience and its variant manifestations. As such, a theme captures and unifies the nature or basis of the experience to do a meaningful whole. Themes emerge from the data. They often develop with in categories of data. The search for themes involves not only discovering similarities across participants, but also seeking natural variation.

Some qualitative researcher use *metaphors* as an analytic approach. A metaphor is a symbolic comparison, using figurative language to evoke a visual analogy. Metaphor can be powerfully creative and expressive tool for qualitative analysis. As a literacy device, metaphors can permit greater insight and understanding in qualitative analysis and can help link together parts of the whole.

Element of Qualitative Data Analysis

Data analysis and collection occurs simultaneously in qualitative research. The researcher analysis data that have been collected and in light of that analysis, collects additional data until saturation or redundancy is reached, that is until no new information is forthcoming from additional participants or sources. It is a cyclical, integrative, and interactive process, while the researcher examines the themes and develops preliminary hypotheses throughout the progression of the study.

- *Emersion in the data:* The investigator becomes immersed in and dwells with the data.
- *Fraction of data:* The researcher divides the data into smaller unit for analysis (e.g. coding and categorization), reflects on what theses clusters mean, and when reintegrate them into a conceptualized whole, the result being a higher order synthesis.
- *Interpretation of data:* Interpretation is required, making inferences, assigning meanings, speculating, abstracting understandings, offering explication, and dealing with disconfirming evidence, difference in data, rival hypotheses, and alternatives explanation-all to test the feasibility of an interpretation.
- *Conclusion of findings:* There is a balance between the interpretation made and the data/evidence that serve as the support for the interpretation. Conclusions are directly grounded in description, quotation, or documentary evidences.

Processes of Qualitative Analysis

Qualitative data analysis process need reflection of data on personal and data-oriented level.
- *Personal reflection:* Feelings, assumptions, preconceived ideas, reactions, values explored and dealing with as necessary so that analysis is not merely a projection of what the researcher believes, thinks, or feels.
- *Data-oriented reflection:* The researcher interrogates contemplation, dialogues with, and critically appraise the data to develop clarity of meaning and to advance the descriptive evidence to a more abstract and conceptual level.
- *Comparison:* Comparison is used in describing conceptual similarities and differences, generating themes, and pattern, contrasting themes and pattern across individual cases/sites.
- *Creativity:* Use of metaphor, analogy, imagery and insight enable to make the data senseful.
- *Theoretical sensitivity:* Theoretical sensitivity provides meaning and understating by continual verification of interpretation, hunches, and hypotheses with the coded data.

Description of Data Analysis Process

A researcher should describe exactly what will be done in the study. It includes method of analysis, type of coding, category making, use of matrices, constant comparison, memoing, sorting and use of literature, etc. A researcher should also state that how the framework will inform the analysis of the study. Use of computer software package for data management should also be described.

Computer Software Application in Data Analysis

There is a wide variety of software tools to support different approaches to qualitative data analysis. Use of software depends on type of analysis, structure of data, ease of use and cost of the software. Qualitative software does not do the analysis—the researcher does. Use of qualitative data analysis (QDA) software provides techniques and tools that assist the researcher in the analysis and making sense of the data.

Use of QDA software will facilitate followings in the qualitative data analysis:
- Writing field notes and memos
- Editing
- Coding
- Storage
- Search and retrieval of texts and codes
- Data 'linking'
- Content analysis using frequencies, sequences, or location of words/phrases
- Data display
- Graphic making
- Repot writing.

Other QDA software are; hyper SEARCH, Ethnogrph V6, Frame WORK, MAXQDA 10 and Weft QDA, etc.

Data Quality and Rigor in Qualitative Research

A qualitative researcher should use certain measures for assessing quality and rigor of data including followings:

Credibility (Internal Validity)

The extent to which readers and participants can recognize the meaning that they give to the situation or context or the 'truth value' of the report. Credibility may be sought by using following measures:
- Prolonged engagement in the field of setting
- Triangulation
    - Investigator triangulation: A type of triangulation in which more than one investigator used to collect, analysis or interpret a set of data.
    - Theory triangulation: A type of triangulation in which multiple perspective are obtained and used from other researcher or published literature.
    - Method triangulation: A use of multiple data collection method (e.g. interviews, observation and document review) results in method triangulation.
- Ongoing peer review
- Negative case analysis (e.g. search and account disconfirming data)
- Member checking: A method of ensuring validity by having participants review and comment on the accuracy of transcripts, interpretation, or conclusions.

Dependability (Reliability)

Findings of the study need to be consistent and correct to be dependable, so that anyone reading the study will be able to evaluate the self-sufficiency of the analysis and results from the research process. For dependability, an auditor can inspect the inquiry process (audit trail) and the records relating to the inquiry in order to judge its authenticity. An audit trail is a through, conscientious reflection on and documentation of the decision that were made, the procedure that were designed, and the questions that were raised during analysis of data.

Transferability (Generalizability)

How the result in one context could be transferred to comparable situation or participants. In the cases, due to small-scale sample utilized, theoretical transferability could be achieved. Transferability can be achieved by going follow through:
- Provision of detailed data base and 'thick description'
- The concept of applicability (applying result of a study to another population when the sample is very similar)
- Fittingness—when findings fit into contexts different from the research situation and other find the findings meaningful and applicable to their own experiences.

Confirmability (Objectivity)

This method requires an audit or decision trail for readers who can judge the study for the intellectual honesty, researcher's bias and openness to sensitivity to the methods.

Qualitative Data Analysis Procedure

Qualitative data analysis is a process of examining and interpreting data in order to elicit meaning, gain understanding, and to develop empirical knowledge. Qualitative data analysis is a creative, challenging, time consuming and expensive task. Less experienced researcher may feel uncertain about how to proceed because the process feels ambiguous. The process of interpretation occurs in the mind of the researcher. Corbin and Strauss (2008) describe interpretation as translating the words and actions of participants into meanings that reader and consumers can utilized.

With most qualitative research traditions, analysis occurs simultaneously with data collection. This method of analysis is called *constant comparison*. It is a method of analysis in qualitative research that involves a review of data as they are gathered and comparison to data that have been interrelated to support or reject earlier conclusions.

In qualitative research, data may be collected through a variety of methods. Data are usually collected through a combination of methods, including observation, interactions, or documentation review. These data are often recorded on audiotape and transcribed for analysis. Qualitative data analysis may not be standard, but it does have some steps that are common to all approaches. All qualitative researchers must:
- Prepare the data for analysis
- Conduct the analysis by developing an in-depth understanding of the data
- Represent the data in reduced form
- Make an interpretation of the large meaning of the data.

Observation of body language, surroundings, and the other factors also important part of the data collection procedure in qualitative research. These are often referred to as field notes, and they enrich the data interpretation process with detailed description of the context, environment, and non-verbal communication.

Transcribing recorded data: Transcription of verbal data into written data is almost an assumption in qualitative research. Transcripts present the data in a form that allows the researcher to share the data with team members for analysis and validation. Data collected during qualitative study may be narrative descriptions of observation, transcript from audio recording of interview, entries in the researcher's diary reflecting on the dynamics of the setting.

Developing a Category Scheme

This phase of data analysis is essentially reductionist–data must be converted to smaller, more manageable units that can be retrieved and reviewed. Qualitative data analysis begins with classification and indexing of the data. The most widely used procedure is to develop a category scheme and then code data according to categories. Scrutinizing the data is a preliminary step in developing category system in qualitative study. There is no standard guideline for this task. Developing a high quality category scheme involves a careful reading of the data, with an eye to identifying underlying concepts and cluster of concepts. In creating category, researcher must break the data into segments, closely examine them and compare them to other segment for similarities and dissimilarities to determine the meaning of those segments.

Coding qualitative data: Coding is a means of naming and labeling. A code is a symbol or abbreviation used to label words or phrases in the data. Once a category scheme has been developed, that are read in their entirety and coded for correspondence to categories. Research may face many problems while finding a most appropriate code for developed theme. Through coding, the researcher explores the phenomena of a study. Sometimes researcher found initial categories incomplete, and a concept might not be well defined. In such a case, it would be necessary to reread all previously coded material to have a truly complete understanding of that category. The type and level of coding vary somewhat according to the qualitative approach being used. Table 10.18 display types of codes described in social sciences literature.

It is sometimes recommended that a single person code the entire data set to ensure the highest possible coding consistency across interviews or observations. Nevertheless, at least a portion of the interviews should be coded by two or more people early in the coding process, if possible, to evaluate and enhance reliability. It is wise to develop a code book to describe and define the exact definition of the various categories used to code the data.

Table 10.18: Types of coding in qualitative data analysis.

Type of code	Description
Axial coding	Findings and labeling connection between concepts; assigning codes to categories; also may be called level II coding in grounded theory approach
Open coding	Breaking data apart and delineating to stand for blocks of raw data; also called types I coding in grounded theory approach
Selecting coding	Building a story that comments the categories; the research may generate proposition or statements that bridge the categories
Substantive coding	Includes vivo coding (using words of participants) and implicit coding, in which the unspoken codes are constructed by researchers
Process coding	Incorporating previously assigned codes into an overall basic social process that is the core of the phenomena of interest; used in grounded theory studies.
Interpretative coding	Labeling coded data into more abstract term that represent merged codes
Explanatory coding	Connecting coded data to an emerging theory; describing coded data as pattern, themes, and links

Memoing (Reflective Remarks)

Memos are crucial aspect of grounded theory. In the grounded theory method, the coding process involves more than simply categorizing chunks of text. As you code data, you should also be using the technique of *memoing-writing memos or notes to yourself and other involved in the research project*. Strauss and Corbin (1998) highlighted three kinds of memos; code notes, theoretical noted and operational notes.

- *Code notes* identify the code labels and their meaning. It is particularly important because, as in all social sciences research, most of them we use with technical meaning also have meaning in everyday language. Therefore, it is essential to write down a clear account of what you mean by the codes used in your analysis.
- *Theoretical notes* cover a variety of topic: Reflection of the dimension and deeper meaning of concepts, relationship among concepts, theoretical proposition and so on. In qualitative data analysis it is vital to write down these thoughts, even those you will later discarded as useless.
- *Operational notes* deals primarily with methodological issues. Some will draw attention to data collection circumstances that may be relevant to understanding the data later.

The memo may be written to someone else involved in a study or may be just a note to yourself. The important thing is to value your ideas and document then quickly. Initially you might feel that ideas are so clear in your mind that you can unite and record later. However, you may soon forget the thought and be unable to retrieve it. So, whenever an idea emerges, even if its vague and not well thought out, develop the habit of writing it down immediately or recording it on a hand-held device such as a cell phone.

Concept Mapping

The graphic display of concepts and their interrelations are useful in the formulation of theory. It is clear by now that qualitative data analysis spend a lot of time committing thought to paper (or to a computer file), but this process is not limited to text only, often we think out relationship among concepts more clearly by putting the concept in a graphic format, a process is called *concept mapping*. Some researchers put all their major concepts on a single sheet of paper, whereas other spread their thoughts across several sheet of paper, blackboard, magnetic board, computer pages, or the other media.

Qualitative Content Analysis

Content analysis is technically not a specific qualitative research design; it is more accurately described as a data analysis method. The term, however, is commonly used to describe designs that rely on data collected via interviews or document analysis and that use interpretative coding to arrive at themes and patterns. In reality, content analysis is often used when no other classification 'fits'.

The purpose of content analysis is to describe and interpret the meaning in the words of respondents or in historical or written documents. Content analysis is an analytic method may be used in any of the other tradition, but when a qualitative study does not neatly fit into one of the more formal classification, study is often referred to simply as a content analysis study.

Strengths of Content Analysis

Content analysis is a common method applied to answer qualitative research question. It has some definitive advantages as an approach to qualitative study:
- Content analysis relatively uncomplicated to carry out
- Extended time period of observation are generally not needed; saturation may be achieved with relatively few interview or focus group
- Content analysis focus on general themes that enables a researcher to answer a question in a straight forward and concise way.

Limitations of Content Analysis

Content analysis not appropriate for all studies as it has certain limitations including followings:
- Content analysis relies on the informant's recall, ability to report, and willingness to take
- Selection bias may creeps as those who agree to respond to interviews may not be representative of all of those who are affected.

Semiotics

Semiotics is commonly defined as the '*science of signs*' and deals with symbols and meaning. It is commonly associated with content analysis. Although semiotics is based on language, and one of the many sign system of varying degree of unity, applicability, and complexity. Morse code, etiquettes, music, and even highway signs are examples of semiotics.

There is no meaning inherent in any sign, however, meaning reside in any particular sign means something to a particular person. However, the agreements we have about the meaning associated with particular sign make semiotics as a social science.

ETHNOGRAPHIC ANALYSIS

Ethnographer collects great quantities of material to discover what people believe and how they behave in everyday situation. This information primarily conveyed in written words compiled from transcribed interview of research participants, field notes of participants observation activities, and description of relevant documents. In an ethnographic approach, pattern of culture are observed and analyzed. Ethnographic approach describes and analysis pattern of people in their own environment. Thus, the central element in ethnography is culture. The purpose of ethnographic analysis is to organize the data and then make sense of what you have learned during the research experience. The written material is first categorized into meaningful pieces, when they are then examined for patterns that explain the phenomena of interest. In most ethnography reported in journal articles, however, explicit analysis strategies are not detailed.

Ethnographic analysis focuses on the cultural ideas that arise during the active data collection in ethnographic research. The cultural ideas then transformed, translated, or presented in a written document. Ethnographic analysis proceeds through many stages including followings:

- Shifting and sorting data to organize material
- Reading and thinking about the data
- Searching for inconsistencies and similarities
- Coding data to detect and interpret thematic categories.

Analysis of ethnographic data follows the tradition outlined in anthropology (Spradley, 1979). It follows four levels of data analysis; domain analysis, taxonomic analysis, componential analysis and themes analysis

- *Domain analysis:* This is the first level of data analysis. At this stage researcher find the unit of cultural knowledge that encompasses several smaller units in it.
- *Taxonomic analysis:* This is second step of data analysis, here researcher decides on number of domain under study. After making decision about number of domains, taxonomy (a system of classification and organization of domains) is developed. Taxonomy development will helps the researcher to illustrate internal organization of a domain and the relationship among the sub-categories of the domain.
- *Componential analysis:* Researcher examine the relationship among terms in the domains to identify similarities and differences among cultural term in a domain.
- *Theme analysis:* Finally, a cultural theme emerges. Domains are fitted in themes to provide a holistic view of the culture under study.

Narrative Analysis

Narrative analysis is a qualitative approach that uses stories as its data. Through a sense of life expectancies, people go through various stages and experience of life. Narrative analysis focuses on how participants give order to the sequence of experience in their lives, making sense of the element and actions in which they have participated.

Following models of narrative analysis are used in qualitative study:
- *Thematic analysis:* Emphasis on the content of the text, paying attention to the sequence of themes within the narrative description. In thematic analysis, researcher focuses on the

identification of behaviors, pattern and theme in the participant experiences from interview data. A researcher becomes familiar with the data through immersion by transcribing the data; reading, re-reading the data, noting down the initial ideas. A code may be developed for similar data to generate a potential theme from data. Defining and naming themes through ongoing analysis of each theme generate clear definition for each theme.
- *Structural analysis:* The way the story is told with a focus on form and content.
- *Interactional analysis:* The emphasis on the dialogic process between the teller (participant) and the listener (investigator).
- *Performative analysis:* Story telling seen as performance.

There are many other types of analysis possible for qualitative research; Table 10.19 provides a summary of additional types of qualitative data analysis.

Table 10.19: Qualitative data analysis.

Chronological analysis	Identifying and organizing major element in a time ordered description as events and epiphanies
Componential analysis	Identifying unit of meaning that are cultural attributes; process allow ethnographer to identify gaps in observation and selectively collect additional data
Direct interpretation	Identifying a single instance of the phenomena or topic and drawing out its meaning without comparing to other
Domain analysis	Focusing on a special aspect of a social situation such as people involved; used in ethnography
Taxonomic analysis	Identifying categories with a domain; used in ethnography research
Three-dimensional analysis	Thinking about and identifying continuum of interactions, and situation within a story

Source: Corbin and Strauss (1998), Creswell (2003).

GROUNDED THEORY ANALYSIS

Grounded theory analysis provides an overview of how qualitative researchers make sense of their data and extract them from insights into processes and behavior operating in natural settings. However, there are two common approaches used for grounded theory analysis.
1. Glaser and Strauss method (1967)
2. Strauss and Corbin method (1998)

Glaser and Strauss Method (1967)

This method based on the concept of constant comparative method of data analysis. *Constant comparative analysis* approach was given by Glaser and Strauss (1967) for grounded theory research. It involves taking one place of data such as one interview, one theme or one statement and comparing it with other that similar or different data to develop conceptualization of the possible relationship between various aspects of the data. The *concept of fit* is an important element of grounded theory analysis. Fit is the process of identifying characteristics of one piece of data and comparing them with other characteristics of another. Concept of fit enables a researcher to reduce the data and help the researcher to determine the placement of data in similar category. Coding in Glaser and Strauss (1967) method used to conceptualize data into pattern or concepts. This approach use substantive, theoretical and open coding. Table will provide an overview about different types of coding used in qualitative analysis.

Strauss and Corbin Method (1998)

The Strauss and Corbin approach is distinct from the Glaser and Strauss approach in term of method and outcomes. Table 10.20 summarizes major analytic differences between these two grounded theory approaches.

Table 10.20: Glaser and Strauss/Corbin's method.

Feature	Glaser	Strauss and Corbin
Initial data analysis	Breaking down and conceptualizing data involves comparison of incidents to incident so pattern emerge	Breaking down and conceptualizing data includes taking apart a single sentence, observation, and incident
Type of coding	Open, selective and theoretical	Open, axial and selective
Connection between categories	18 coding families	Paradigm model (conditions, contexts, action/interactional strategies, and consequences
Outcome	Emergent theory (discovery)	Conceptual description (verification)

Glaser (1978) stressed that to generate a grounded theory, the better problem must emerge from the data. Strauss and Corbin, however, state that research itself is only one of four possible sources of the research problem. This method involves following three types of coding:

1. *Open coding:* Data are broken down into part and compared to find out similarities and differences. In open coding, the researcher focuses on generating categories and their properties and dimensions.
2. *Axial coding:* The researcher systematically develop categories and links them with subcategories.
3. *Selective coding:* At this stage findings are integrated and refined.

PHENOMENOLOGICAL ANALYSIS

The fundamental principle of the phenomenological approach is that the researcher must remain true to the facts and how they reveal themselves (Husserl, 1960).

Nurse researchers find phenomenological analysis intuitively appealing because it focuses upon the individual's experience and the context of that experience. This is a central concern for nursing, thus frequently used in qualitative research. This section deals with the process of phenomenological analysis. Schools of phenomenology have developed different approaches for data analysis. The most common approaches used for phenomenology analysis are:

1. Vaan Kaam (1966) approach
2. Colaizzi method (1978)
3. Giorgi method (1985)

However, these methods are different to each other in analytic approach. For example, Colaizzi's method is the one that calls for validation of results by returning to study participants. Girogi's method relies solely on researcher and Van Kaam's method requires that intersubjective agreement be reached with other experts personals.

Vaan Kaam (1966) Approach

Vaan Kaam (1969) first described the six steps of analysis in his study 'really feeling understood'. These six steps are explained here:

Step I (The classification of data into categories): Researcher collect a large pool of cases randomly from the pool of protocols and prepare a list of statement of common response of participants for phenomenon under investigation. A group of expert used to judge the data in order to ensure the validity of response and procedure. A final list of concrete, intricate, vague, and overlapping response occur in the protocol.

Step II: (Reduction and linguistic transformation of statement): A researcher describe the list of experience of subjects in his own words. Transformation is a challenging job for a researcher and distinct to quantitative research. Linguistic expression carried out by means of the ordinary human capacity to understand the meaning of statement. In this case, experience is redescribed from prescriptive concerned in precise descriptions.

Step III (Element elimination): Statement that merely express aspects of the experience that relate to a specific situation and elements that are blending of several parts are removed from the statement list.

Step IV (The hypothetical identification): Once the classification reduction and elimination over, the resulting list considered as fist hypothetical identification and description of the experience of participants.

Step V (Application and testing): The hypothetical statement is testes on randomly selected protocols in order to ensure necessary and sufficient summary of the topic under investigation. At this stage, a researcher may add or delete the experience, which he find wild, and not relate to hypothetical statement.

Step VI (Validity of statement): Once the previous phases are over, the statement can be considered valid descriptions of statement and experience. However, these statement valid only for population represented by the sample. The validity continue until new cases of the experiences can be appear and correspond to necessary and sufficient to change in the valid statement.

Colaizzi Method (1978)

Phenomenology use semi-structured face to face interview to collect data from participants buy using interview guide. Researcher encourage the participants to talk freely and discuss the issue in their own language and words. Interview conducted by principal researcher and may extend for 45 minutes to one hour. The extent of data saturation is determined by principal researcher and other researcher who are parallel engaged in data collection.

The following steps (Fig. 10.14) represent Colaizzi process for phenomenological data analysis (cited in Sanders, 2003; Speziale and Carpenter, 2007).

1. Each transcript should be read and re-read in order to obtain a general sense about the whole content.
2. For each transcript, significant statements that pertainto the phenomenon under study should be extracted. These statements must be recorded on a separate sheet noting their pages and lines numbers.
3. Meanings should be formulated from these significant statements.

4. The formulated meanings should be sorted into categories, clusters of themes, and themes.
5. The findings of the study should be integrated into an exhaustive description of the phenomenon under study.
6. The fundamental structure of the phenomenon should be described.
7. Finally, validation of the findings should be sought from the research participants to compare the researcher's descriptive results with their experiences.

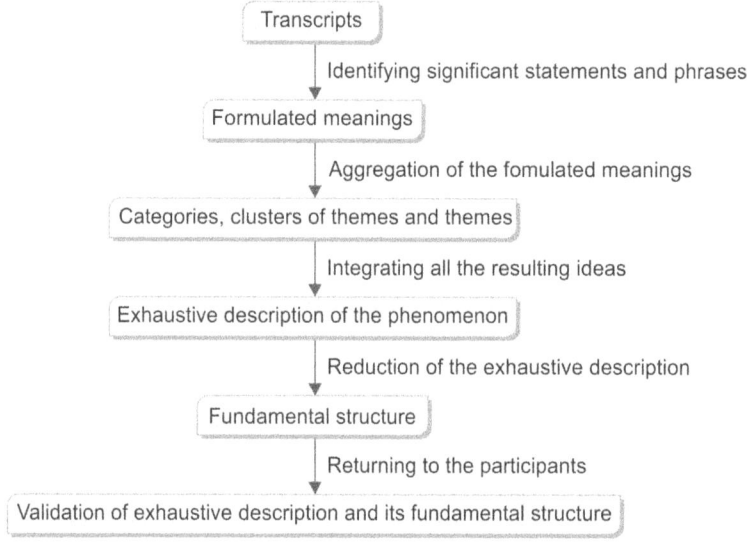

Fig. 10.14: Phenomenological data analysis: Colaizzi approach.

Giorgi Method (1985)

This is another analysis approach to phenomenological study proposed by Giorgi and colleagues at Duquesne University, USA. This approach based on the principle of Husserl's philosophy. This method helps an analyst to describe the essential features of any given phenomenon experienced by the research participants. This approach has following stages:

Stage I (Reading through the manuscript): A phenomenologist should read the whole manuscript in full before carrying out any further analytic steps. Throughout the subsequent process, each aspect of data must be analyzed in the context of awareness of the participants' whole account.

Stage II (Discrimination of meaning units): This is transformation stage in which data will be transformed and structured description is provided to data. It is pragmatic step to attach meaning to data. In this stage, transcript in divided in many small parts and researcher define every unit independently.

Stage III (Transformation): Once the meaning units are defined, they go through one or more stages of transformation. This stage sensitize the researcher about what each unit might suggest about the nature of the phenomenon under investigation. Here, each unit considered as independent, whole, and summarized separately.

Stage IV (Individual description of the unit): The final stage of analysis to write structural description of the phenomenon that has been studied. This is very concise and condensed description of 'typical essential' of the phenomenon. This step involves understanding, judgment of relevance, and coherent organizing. Sometimes, description of matter is not coherent and not related to the phenomenon that is investigated. Therefore, relevant and constituents are put together accordingly to their intertwining meaning so that they can express lived experiences.

Stage V (The general description of the phenomenon): It is the point of analysis where each individual structure is compared to others to establish similarities and differences in meaning constituents.

Utrecht School of Phenomenology

This is the second approach for phenomenological analysis. It is combination of descriptive and interpretative phenomenology. This school believes that thematic experience to be studied by using following three methods:
1. *Holistic approach:* Researcher read text as whole and extracts the meaning from it.
2. *Selective approach:* Researcher highlights statement or phrases that seem essential to study.
3. *Detailed approach:* Here, researcher analysis each sentence to get a common themes. Once themes have been identified, they become the objects of reflection and interpretation through follow-up interview with participants.

Heideggerian Hermeneutics School of Phenomenology

Diekelmaan, Allen and Tanner (1989) have described seven stages process of hermeneutics phenomenological data analysis. The steps are as follows:
1. All the interview or texts are read for an overall understanding.
2. Interpretative summaries of each interview written.
3. Analysis of transcribed data.
4. Resolution of any disagreement on interpretation.
5. Develop a common meaning by comparing and contrasting text.
6. Identify the relationship among themes.
7. Develop a final draft of themes along with explicit examples from text.

REVIEW QUESTIONS AND ANSWER

Long and Short Answer Questions

1. Explain about qualitative analysis. *(AIIMS, MSc N-2002)*
2. What are statistical procedures elaborate? *(KUHAS, MSc N-2004)*
3. What is data processing? *(RGUHS, MSc N-2007)*
4. Steps in testing hypothesis. *(PGI, MSc N-2001)*
5. Qualitative analysis. *(AIIMS, MSc N-2013)*
6. Explain the use of computer in nursing research. *(PGI, MSc N-20015)*
7. List the steps of analysis of data. *(TNMGRMU, MSc N-2000)*
8. Explain the guidelines for formulating a table. *(BFUHS, MSc N-2002)*

Multiple Choice Questions

1. Type of graphical presentation used to explain correlation between two variables is termed as:
   a. Scatter plot
   b. Bar diagram
   c. Histogram
   d. Pie chart

2. A process that renders data from into numbers that can be entered into a database is known as:
   a. Editing
   b. Coding
   c. Matrixing
   d. Transcribing

3. Which of the following is an example of interval level data?
   a. Age in years
   b. Height in meters
   c. Pain on a scale
   d. Temperature in Kelvin

4. In exclusive type of class interval, the value 20 will be put under:
   a. 10–20
   b. 20–30
   c. Either a or b
   d. Both a and b

5. Type II erros also known as:
   a. False positive
   b. False negative
   c. True positive
   d. True negative

6. Which of the following is true for a normal distribution curve?
   a. Man >Median >Mode
   b. Mode >Median >Mean
   c. Median <Mode >Mean
   d. Mean =Mode =Median

7. Which of the following component is not needed to calculate power (1-beta) of a study?
   a. The effect size
   b. Sample size
   c. Standard deviation
   d. Level of significance (alpha)

8. Which of the following is a measure of dispersion?
   a. Mean
   b. Median
   c. Mode
   d. Standard deviation

9. Which of the following measure of central tendency is very sensitive to extreme values?
   a. Mean
   b. Median
   c. Mode
   d. Standard deviation

10. The only difference between a histogram and bar chart is best understood by following explanation:
    a. No space between the bars in a histogram
    b. Bars in histogram are taller than bar chart
    c. Bars in histogram is smaller than bar chart
    d. Both are synonymously used

11. The method of statistics used to draw conclusion from a data collected from a sample of population instead of entire population is termed as:
    a. Descriptive statistics
    b. Inferential statistics
    c. Sample survey
    d. Population statistics

12. The indices calculated from a sample is termed as:
    a. Statistics
    b. Inference
    c. Conclusion
    d. Result

13. While testing the hypothesis, rejecting the null hypothesis when it is actually true is known as:
    a. Type I error
    b. Type II error
    c. Sampling error
    d. Standard error

14. Which of the following correlation coefficient value indicates strongest relationship between stress and anxiety among nursing students?
    a. r = 0.50
    b. r = −0.70
    c. r = 0.45
    d. r = −1.20

Answer Key

1.	2.	3.	4.	5.	6.	7.	8.	9.	10.	11.	12.	13.	14.
a.	b.	d.	b.	d.	d.	c.	d.	a.	a.	b.	a.	a.	b.

SUGGESTED READING

1. Aradilla–Herrero A, et al. Association between emotional intelligence, depression and suicide risk in nursing students. Nurse Education Today; 2013. pp. 1-6.
2. Balan R. Sandeep BB, Sandhay J. Can Indian classical instrumental music reduce pain felt during venepunture? Ind J Pediatr. 2009;76(5):469-73.
3. Burn N, Grove SK. Understanding nursing research—building an evidence-based practice, 4th edition. St Louis: Saunders Elsevier; 2007.
4. Colaizzi PF. Psychological research as the phenomenologist views it. In: Valle R, King M (Eds). Existential phenomenological alternatives for psychology, New York: Oxford University Press; 1978.
5. Creswell J. Research designs: Qualitative, quantitative and mixed method approaches. Thousand Oaks, CA: Sage Publication; 2003.
6. Dickelmann NL, Allen D, Tanner C. The NLN criteria for appraisal of baccalaureate program: A critical hermeneutic analysis. New York: NLN Press; 1989.
7. Fain E. Reading, understating and applying nursing research. Philadelphia: FA: Davis; 2008.
8. Garrett HE. Statistics in psychology and education. New Delhi: Paragon International Publishers; 2007.
9. Giorgi A. Phenomenology and psychological research. Pittsburg, PA: Duquesne University Press; 2008.
10. Giuliano KK, Polanowicz M. Interpretation and use of statistics in nursing research. AACN Advanced Critical Care. 2008;19(2):211-22.
11. Glaser B. Theoretical sensitivity. Mill Valley, CA: Sociology Press; 1978.
12. Glaser BG, Strauss A. The discovery of grounded theory: Strategies for qualitative research. New York: Aldine de Gruyter; 1967.
13. Gupta SK. Statistical methods. New Delhi; Sultan Chand and Sons; 2008.
14. Harting D, Touchette D. Overview of the clinical research design. American Journal of Health System Pharmacy. 2009;66(15):398-407.

15. Kerliner F. Foundation of behavioral research, 3rd edition. New York: Halt, Rinehart and Winston; 1986.
16. King N, Horrocks C. Interview in qualitative research. Sage; 2010. pp. 198-204.
17. Kumar R. Personality traits, academic stress and adjustment styles among nursing students. The Nursing Journal of India. 2018;ICX(4):184-8.
18. Makoe M. A phenomenological analysis of experiences of learning in the South African distance education context, in Enhancing Higher Education, Theory and Scholarship, Proceedings of the 30th HERDSA Annual Conference, Adelaide; 2007. pp. 341.
19. Munhall P. Nursing research: A qualitative perspective, 4th edition. Sudbury MA: Jones and Bartlett; 2006.
20. Nieswiadomy RM. Foundation of nursing research. India: Person Education; 2008.
21. Parahoo K. Nursing research: principle, process and issues. London: Macmillan; 1997.
22. Polit DF, Beck CT. Nursing research—principle and methods, 7th edition. Philadelphia: Lippincott William Wilkins; 2004.
23. Sanders C. Application of Colaizzi's method: Interpretation of an auditable decision trail by a novice researcher. Contemporary Nurse Journal. 2003;14(3):292-302.
24. Shosha GA. Employment of Colaizzi's strategy in descriptive phenomenology—a reflection of a researcher. European Scientific Journal. 2012;8(27):31-43.
25. Singh AK. Tests measurement and research methods in behavioral sciences: Bharti Bhawan (P and D); 2013.
26. Speziale HJ, Carpenter DR. Qualitative Research in Nursing: Advancing the Humanistic Imperative, 4th edition. Philadelphia. Lippincott, Williams and Wilkins; 2007.
27. Spradley J. The ethnographic interview. New York: Holt, Rinehart and Winston; 1979.
28. Stevens SS. On the theory of scales of measurement. Science. 1946;103:677-80.
29. Strauss A, Corbin J. Basics of qualitative research: Grounded theory procedure and techniques, 2nd edition. Thousand Oaks: Sage; 1998.
30. Talbot LA. Principles and practice of nursing research, 1st edition. St Louis: Mosby Year Book Inc; 1995.
31. Valle RS, Hailing S. Existential phenomenological perspective in psychology: exploring the breadth of human experiences. Springer Sciences and Business Media; 2013. pp. 51-3.
32. Van Kaam A. Existential foundation of psychology. Pittsburg, PA: Duquesne University Press; 1966.

Chapter 11
Communication and Dissemination of Research Findings

INTRODUCTION

Communication and dissemination of research findings is one of the essential step of research process. Research is not complete unless it is written up and the findings have been communicated to others. Patricia Grady, Director of National Institute of Nursing Research, referred to the old saying that 'research not published is research not done'. Winslow (1996) made a plea for nurses to publish the findings of their studies. She wrote that failure to publish study findings in her opinions; is a form of scientific misconduct. Usually, researcher communicates their research findings to other scientists by written or oral presentation or by publishing the findings in a peer reviewed scientific journal. The internet is revolutionizing the dissemination of research findings in a way never thought before. Furthermore, in a funded research, a researcher has an obligation to submit periodic report to the funding agencies before publishing findings.

Purposes of Dissemination of Research Findings
- Communication of research findings generate pool of data which make a strong base for sound clinical practice
- Communication of research findings promote personal and professional growth of an individual and organization
- A planned and systematic research findings improve the body of knowledge and therefore, fill the gap between theory and practice
- Use of empirical information and research evidence to clinical practice leads to better quality care and improve patient satisfaction
- Use of best evidence improve quality, safety, and promote effective care that can positively impact patient outcomes.

COMMUNICATION OF RESEARCH FINDINGS

Research communication defined as the process of interpreting or translating complex research findings into a language, format and context that nonexpert can understand. It goes way beyond mere dissemination of research result. Even if you are gifted in communication, there is no guarantee that you will be able to disseminate the result of your study. A researcher should keep in mind certain tips before communicating research findings including followings:
- As a researcher be always humanize for his remarks. It is always good to talk about your study findings but it is equally good to discuss your failure story
- It is point less to discuss all the findings at a time in one publication. You should limit your study findings

- Always present the findings with the help of figures, graphs and table to attract the audience/target group
- It is always good to make your remarks colorful and bring them to life with metaphor and analogies
- Be passionate while disseminating the findings to others.

Steps of Disseminating Research

Although, the communication of research findings is frequently considered to be last step in the research process, but it is only the beginning of the most important phase of research—the utilization of research findings. Disseminating research findings is a systematic process and a researcher should use appropriate method to transmit their research findings to target group effectively.

- *Select the audience:* It is necessary to know about audience before communicating research findings. A researcher should ask to self, 'who will read and listen my research and who will get benefited from research?' The answer of above question may be physician, staff nurses, nurse educators, administrator, nurse manager, community leaders or local public, etc. Knowledge about audience will helps in the selection of method of communicating research findings.
- *Select method of communication:* Selection of appropriate method to communicate research findings is also important. There are many methods for communication available like publishing in scientific journal, books, oral or poster presentation at conference and workshop, etc. In case of journal, there are more than 500 nursing journals are indexed in Cumulative Index to Nursing and Allied Health Literature (CINAHL). Journals are vary in prestige and it can be assessed in term of impact factors (IF). An impact factor is a measure of citation frequency for an average article in a journal. Researcher should also follow a standard reporting guideline for reporting findings of a specific study (Table 11.1).
- *Avoid technical jargon:* The presentation should be efficiently prepared by avoiding technical jargon and self-created abbreviations. It is not a good way to impress audience to use technical jargon and using ambiguous language in presentation. It may confuse and distract the audience from main theme.

Table 11.1: Reporting guidelines for research studies.

Research study	Guidelines
Randomized control trails (RCTs)	CONSORT (Consolidated Standards of Reporting Trails)
Nonrandomized designs	TREND (Transport Reporting of Evaluations with Nonrandomized Designs)
Journal article reporting guidelines	TREND + CONSORT (APA Publication guidelines) JARS (Journal Article Reporting Standards)
Observational epidemiological study	STROBE (Strengthening of Reporting Observational Studies in Epidemiology)
Systemic review	PRISMA (Preferred Reporting Items for Systematic Reviews and Meta-Analyses)
Meta-analysis of observational studies	MOOSE (Meta-analyses of Observational Studies in Epidemiology)
Genetic risk predisposition studies	GRIPS (Genetic Risk Prediction Studies)

- *Do not overload presentation:* The presentation should be well written and concise. Adding unnecessary information in presentation and report can make the audience/reader to loss their interest. Avoid duplication of the findings by putting the finding in text and tables and figures simultaneously.
- *Prepare systematically:* The presentation should prepare systematically by following steps as followed in scientific investigation with emphasis on conclusion and recommendation.
- *Effective writing:* A successful writing is the result of effective planning and organization of research report. A research presentation should be clear, accurate and concise. Use of technical and scientific language should be discouraged. The result of the study should be presented in an interesting and informational manner. The major part of research report should be written in past tense, hypothesis and conclusion in present tense and implications and recommendations are directed to future.

Methods of Communication Research

There are two major ways for researcher to communicate the research findings; either they can talk about their findings or write about them.

- *Written report:* A written report is a written summary of the study. Even when oral presentation is planned, a report should be written out in it's entirely. Publishing a research article in scientific journals involves preparation of manuscript (unpublished documents submitted to a journal for review) in a suggested format named '*journal guidelines*'. Once the manuscript prepared, it should be send to selected journal through appropriate manner (either online or offline mode). Written report could either be theses, dissertations or periodicals. A sample of conference abstract is given here for better understanding.

Box 11.1: Sample Format of Abstract for a Conference.

Personality Traits, Academic Stress and Adjustment Styles among Nursing Students
Rajesh Kumar, *Assistant Professor, College of Nursing, All India Institute of Medical Sciences (AIIMS), Rishikesh (Uttarakhand) -249203; Email: rajesh.nur@aiimsrishikesh.edu.in*

Introduction: Nursing students face an extremely high level of stress in their beginning years. Certain personality traits make the students more vulnerable for using adjustment styles and handle the stress in subsequent years of study. The aim of this study is to see the impact of academic stress on personality traits and adopted adjustment styles among nursing students.

Material and methods: Study was conducted on 114 randomly selected nursing students. They were administered a sociodemographic data sheet, The Short Form revised Eysenck Personality Questionnaire- A Hindi edition (EPQRS-H), Academic Stress Scale and the Brief COPE. The data was analyzed by using chi-square test, one-way ANOVA and Pearson's correlation.

Results: Students reported more use of active and healthy coping styles and reported more environmental stressors. Academic stress shows negative correlation to extroversion ($p < 0.05$), neuroticism ($p < 0.05$), lie $p < 0.05$) and psychoticism ($p < .05$) personality domains of nursing students. Students having extroversion had significantly use more of support seeking style ($p = 0.05$), avoiding ($p = 0.05$), venting negative feelings ($p = 0.05$) and less use of substance abuse ($p = 0.05$) styles. A significant group difference was observed higher in academic ($p = 0.015$), personal ($p = 0.015$) and environmental areas ($p = 0.004$) and was associated to psychoticism ($p = 0.029$) in students.

Conclusion: Academic stress shows negative correlation with different dimensions of personality of nursing students. Students had extroversion had significantly more use of positive and less use of negative coping styles in order to get adjust in environment.

Key words: Personality, academic stress, adjustment styles, coping

- *Presenting research at professional conferences:* Research findings can be presented at professional conferences and meeting before experts of fields. The following two methods can be used to present the research in scientific conference.
    - *Oral report:* Presentation of research findings at local, regional, national and international conferences and meetings also promotes communication of research findings. A nurse can present their research findings at nursing conferences as well as interdisciplinary conferences (i.e. medical conference, biostatistical conference, etc). Researcher should submit the abstract or complete research report to conference organizers in a given conference format (usually **IMRaD** format).

        Most conferences requires presenter to submit abstract (usually, 250-300 words) of research report. Abstract should contains purposes, research question(s), hypothesis(es), design, methodology, major findings and conclusion. During oral presentation, presenter is asked to present the report within stipulated time period (usually 10-15 minutes) followed by 5-10 minutes for discussion. The discussion (question-answer session) can be a good opportunity for presenter and audiences to improve the depth understanding regarding certain aspects of research report.
    - *Poster presentation:* Poster presentation is another way to present the research findings in a conference. Abstracts must be sent to conference organizers as according to suggested format or guidelines. Once the abstract approved, a researcher has to prepare poster as per given guidelines or instructions of conference. Usually, a poster presentation session continue for 1-2 hours and presenter has to stand near to his poster to clarify doubts or quarry of audience. A poster can be presented by a lead author or co-author. Usually, IMRaD format is used to prepare a poster to present in a conference.

RESEARCH REPORT

The research report is an end product of the research process. The research report should be presented in order of the research process, beginning with the problem and end with conclusion, implications and recommendations for future researchers.

Salient Features of a Good Research Report

Research report writing is not as simple as it sound. Writing a research report is an acquired skill through long standing experience of theoretical and practical aspects of a research process. A researcher has to immerse in practical research to learn the writing skill and continually polished. A successful research report is the collective efforts of team. It is always good to have a team of different field experts such as data collector, statistician, writer or editor to write a comprehensive research report. However, a well written research report should have following essential characteristics.
- A well written research report should be clear, easy to read and concise
- A research report should be based on the steps followed in the research process
- It is always good to present the findings with the help of figures and diagram. It will attract the audience and maintain the interest to read
- A research report should be complete in all aspects. It should reflect the balance in different part of a research process. Do not over emphasize a single part of research in report
- A researcher should control his personal biases, prejudices and avoid plagiarism and fabrication while writing a research report

- A research report should be free from use of technical jargons, personal pronouns, abbreviations or any ambiguity.

Preparation of a Research Report

The preparation of a good research report is an art and skill. Usually, the format of research report is varying from different universities and institutions. However, the format of a report may differ depending on the requirements of academic institution/university or journal. Usually, quantitative research report follows **IMRaD** format; I–Introduction, M–Methods, R–Results, and D–Discussion. Despite slight variation in styles, following steps can be followed to write a standard report:

- *The title:* A research report should have a clear, brief and concise title (not more than 15 words, preferably less). The title should be an accurate reflection of the research that has been performed. It must be both meaningful and brief. Usually, title should contain population, setting and variables under study.
- *Introduction to the study:* The body of the paper should be open with introduction that present specific problem under study and give an overview about research study. The introduction contains existing current literature, need of the study, conceptual framework, the problem, research question, hypothesis and objectives for the study. The introduction should be written in pyramid shape; beginning broadly and progressing to specific problems.
- *Methods:* This section describes in detail about material and methods used to complete the research study. This section helps the reader to evaluate credibility and worth of the study. This section includes design, population, setting, duration, sampling technique, sample size, variables in the study, and analytical and statistical procedures. For various studies, explicit guidelines available for reporting methodologic informations (Table 11.2).
- *Result:* This section considered heart of the research report. This section summarizes the result of the statistical or qualitative analysis performed on the data. This can includes tables and figures that depict the research findings. However, If statistical analysis is performed to analyze the result, it is mandatory to mention the level of significance.

Table 11.2: Sample outlines for a research report.

Introduction	Methods
- Background of the study → Introduction of the study - Need of the study - Review of literature - Research problem - Objectives - Hypotheses - Operational definitions - Conceptual framework	- Research design - Research setting - Population under study - Sample size - Sampling technique - Research instruments - Validity and reliability of research instruments - Tryout/pilot study - Ethical consideration - Plan for data analysis - References - Appendices

- *Discussion:* Discussion discusses the thoughtful analysis of the research findings. Here, researchers free to examine and interpret their result as well as draw inferences from them. The discussion should answer the following questions—what have study contribute to literature?; How has my study helped to resolve the original problem?; What conclusion and theoretical implications can be drawn?; What are the limitations of the study?; What are the implications for future research and practice?; etc. Typically, the discussion section begins with main findings. The summary of findings should be brief as the main focus of discussion is on inferring the findings.
- *Abstract:* This is brief concise and nonevaluative summary of research report (not more than 100-200 words) that describes the research problem, the research methods, and findings. The abstract must summaries the report in no more than a few short paragraphs. It must include all elements of a research report. An abstract should give an overview of the research process to audiences.
- *References:* A list of sources must appear in the reference list.

Other aspects of a research report:

- *Key words:* Key words help other researcher to locate or index your study. A list of key words can be added. The key words should be three to five in numbers.
- *Acknowledgment:* The people who helped in research process but does not fulfill the criteria of authorship should be recognized in acknowledgment list. These may be people like authority who gave permission for study, statistician and data collectors.
- *Checklist:* A few journals require the completion of an author checklist. The checklist may contain information regarding copyright form, key words, ethical permission, instruments permission letter, etc.

Table 11.3: Format of a research report.

Division	Sections	
Preliminary material	Title of report	
	Abstract	
	Copyright (plagiarism) report	
	Approval page	
	Acknowledgment page	
	Table of contents	
	List of tables	
	List of figures	
	List of appendices	
Body of report	Chapter I	Introduction
	Chapter II	Review of literature
	Chapter III	Methodology
	Chapter IV	Result
	Chapter V	Discussion, implications, recommendations and limitations
Supplementary material	References or bibliography	
	Appendices	
	Curriculum vitae (if needed)	

REFERENCES AND BIBLIOGRAPHY

An objective research report is based on many sources. Usually, a list of references and bibliography come at end of the report. There are many styles used for writing references and bibliography. However, some of the commonly used styles for reference and bibliography writing recommended by guidelines of publication journal are discussed here.
- *Vancouver style:* It is formulated by Council of Science Editors (CSE) and used in medical and allied sciences for writing references.
- *APA style:* It is given by American Psychological Association (APA). It is often used in social sciences, medical and scientific research for reference writing.
- *Other style:* Harvard style, Chicago style, IEEE (The Institute of Electrical and Electronic Engineers) and OSCOLA style, etc.

Vancouver Style References

Journal

Math SB, Chandrashekar CR, Bhugra D. Psychiatric epidemiology in India. Indian Journal of Med. Res. 2007; 126:183-92.

For more than 6 authors

In case of more than 6 authors, a list of first six authors should be written followed by 'et al' to give credit to remaining authors.
Vijayalakshmi P, Reddy D, Math SB, Thimmaiah R, Raman TR, Jamal K, et al. Attitudes of undergraduates towards mental illness: A comparison between nursing and business management students in India. S Afr J Psych. 2013; 19(3):66-73.

Book

For single author or editor
Scheff TJ. Being Mentally Ill: Sociological Theory. Chicago: IL: Aldine; 1986 : 55.

For more than one author
Burn N, Grove SK. Understanding Nursing Research–Building an Evidence-based Practice.4th ed. St Louis: Saunders Elsevier; 2005.

Conference Proceeding

Kimura J, Shibaski H, editors. Recent advances in clinical neurophysiology. Proceeding of the 10th International Congress of EMG and clinical neurophysiology; 1995 Oct 15-19; Tokyo, Japan, Amsterdam: Elsevier; 1996.

Thesis and Dissertation

Kumar R, Mehta S, and Kalra R. A study to identify the learning needs of staff nurses working in psychiatric nursing unit regarding legal and ethical responsibilities in the field of psychiatric nursing with a view to develop and evaluate the guidelines on legal and ethical responsibilities for nurses in a selected hospital of Jaipur, Rajasthan. An Unpublished Master Dissertation: Delhi University; 2010.

E-Thesis

Mary Kohler. Exploring the relationship among work related stress, QoL, job satisfaction and anticipated turnover on nursing unit with clinical nurse leaders, Graduate school thesis and Dissertations University of South Florida; 2010.
Available from: URL: http://scholarcommons.usf.edu/etd/3648

E-Journals

Virk KC. Occupational stress and work motivation in relation to age, job level and type behavior in nursing professionals, J Indian Academy Applied Psycho. 2001; 27 (1) 51-55.
Available from: URL: http://works.bepress.com.

Newspaper Article

Rana P. Fighting with cancer. A Motivational Approach for Western people. The Tribune 2009 July 15; Sect. A : 3 (Col. 5)

Internet and Other Electronic Sources

Morse SS. Factors in the emergence of infectious diseases. Emerg infect dis [Serial online] 1995 Jan-Mar [cited 1999 Dec 25]; 1(1).
Available from: URL: http://www.cdc/gov/ncidoc/EID/eid.htm

APA Style of References

Book

Parahoo, K. (2006). Nursing research, principles, process and issue. (2 ed). Palgrave, Houndmills.

For more than one author

Burn, N. and Grove, S. K. (2007). Understanding nursing research: Building an evidence-based practice. (4th ed). St Louis: Saunders Elsevier.

Journal

Younger, P. (2004). Using the internet to conduct literature review, Nurs Stand, 19 (6): 45-51.

Dissertation and Thesis

Rajesh, K. (2010). A study to identify the learning needs of staff nurses working in psychiatric nursing unit regarding legal and ethical responsibilities in the field of psychiatric nursing with a view to develop and evaluate the guidelines on legal and ethical responsibilities for nurses in a selected hospital of Jaipur, Rajasthan, Unpublished Thesis, University of Delhi.

CRITICAL APPRAISAL OF RESEARCH REPORT

A clinical nurse should be aware about the best evidence to use in patient care. The adage *'All that glitter is not gold'* is also true in research. Not all nursing research is of same quality and standard and therefore, a nurse should be careful while using research evidence in clinical setting.

Research critique should not confuse with criticism which only looks for limitations. It is an intellectual critique to evaluate limitations and strengths of a research work.

Definitions

'A critical estimate of a piece of research which has been carefully and systematically studied by a critic who has used favorable and other general features of the research study'.
(Leninger, 1968)

'Critiquing is a systematic method of appraising the strengths and limitations of a piece of research in order to determine its credibility and or its applicability to practice'.
(Valente, 2003)

Purposes of Research Critique

Research critique refers to planned, systematic and careful evaluation/appraisal of a research work. Research critique based on some prespecified standard criteria to judge the strengths and limitations of a research work. It involves a careful examination of all aspects of study to judge the merits, limitations, meaning and significance based on previous research experience and knowledge of topic.

Critical appraisal serve following purposes:
- A researcher read and review the entire report to identify flaws and limitations and therefore, expand his own body of knowledge about the topic, area and process of research
- Critical appraisal gives an idea about the level of research understanding of the student completed the work
- It point out the flaws in a research work and hence, develop insight into an investigator to improve upon the deficit areas of a research
- It also study methodological and analytical aspects of a research work and therefore, recommend appropriate suggestions in order to improve the research report.

Principles of Research Critique

The following principles should be kept in mind while appraising a research work:
- *Be objective:* A critique should be objective. The evaluator should make the comments specific to work irrespective of name, job and related information of author.
- *Be constructive:* The critical appraisal of research should be oriented to improve the research process rather than criticizing it negatively. The expert/evaluator should start commenting on strengths points of the report first than reflect on negative points in diplomatic manner for improvement in research study.
- *Be balanced:* The report should be considered in a balanced way, i.e. identify inadequacies as well as adequacies. The evaluator should not focus on a particular aspect of research report like taking about only adequacies or inadequacies on a particular part of a research report.
- *Be a good adviser:* An evaluator should advise the scope of improvement in weak areas and suggest alternatives to make things more trustworthy and rigor.
- *Be specific:* A researcher should be very specific to discussion and avoid passing vague comment for strong and weak areas. A specific comment will help the student or novice researcher to improve upon the weak areas.
- *Critique whole report:* It is important to read whole research report before passing any comment on any part. It is always better to read entire report and then discuss strengths and weakness one by one for better improvement. Comment on each dimension of the research report and suggest alternative to improve in each area.

- *Principle of uncertainty:* A reviewer should appraise a work on realm of probability where anything is possible and nothing is certain or permanent.

Dimensions of Research Critique

A research report is divided in many dimensions. Critical appraisal of a research report should look into each dimension to find out the strengths and weakness of research report in a whole. Critical appraisal cover following dimensions of a research report:
- *Substantive dimension and theoretical dimension:* This dimension refers to use of theoretical application in research and congruency between theory and research concepts. This dimension explain how research variables are fit into theoretical framework and linked together
- *Methodologic dimension:* It deals with methodology part like approach, design, population, sample size, sampling technique, research instruments, validity, reliability and pilot study of a research report
- *Ethical dimension:* It consider the various ethical issues, like obtaining ethical permission, consent, confidentiality, assessing risk benefit ratio and anonymity, etc.
- *Interpretive dimension:* It deals with the result and their interpretation section.
- *Presentation and stylistic dimension:* It consider issues related to font size, type, spacing, color, use of paper, grammatical mistakes and other guidelines of research report.
  The research report can be evaluated on given guidelines (Table 11.4).

RESEARCH PROPOSAL

A research proposal is a detailed outline of the research process prepared by the researcher for the certification and approval of the proposed program. The research proposal is formal description of research process. Research proposal helps in communicating research process steps to higher authority, funding agencies and ethical committee member for approval of project.

Significance of Research Proposal

A well written research proposal serves the following purposes:
- Research proposal describe What you will do?, How you will do?, Why you will do? and Where you will do? So, well clear proposal form a backbone of your thesis/dissertation
- Proposal helps to communicate your things to higher authority, funding agencies and institutional ethics committees for granting necessary support, fund, cooperation and resources to carry out research process
- It helps to complete the proposal in given time period
- It gives direction to researcher to carry out project
- A well written proposal helps department to make right decision about other aspects of the project, i.e. allotment of guide and co-guide
- Proposal helps to estimate the necessary resources for project, i.e. money material, man, machine and time, etc.

Research Proposal Development

Although, it is very difficult to explain the process of writing a research proposal as each and every researcher use their own strategy to write research proposal. Writing a research proposal

Table 11.4: Guidelines for critiquing a quantitative research.

Dimension	Question
Writing styles	Is the research work concise, written well, free from grammatical errors, jargon and personal pronouns? Is it well organized in form of research process.
Author	Do the researcher well qualified in the field or area of research topic? Does he have experience of working in this area? Does his position allow him to take such work?
Purpose and significance	Is the purpose of the study clear? Is the significance (importance) of the problem discussed? Does the study have the potential to solve a problem that is currently faced in clinical practice?
Problem statement and research question	Is the problem statement being clear and concise? Is the problem statement clearly articulated? Does the investigator identify key research questions and variables to be examined?
Aim/objectives/research question/hypotheses	Have aims and objectives, a research question or hypothesis been identified? If so, Are they clearly stated? Do they reflect the information presented in the literature review?
Literature review	Does the literature review follow a logical sequence leading to a critical review of supporting and conflicting prior work? Is the relationship of the study to previous study is clear? Does the investigator desirable gaps in the literature and support the necessity of the present study?
Conceptual framework	Is the framework identified and appropriate for the study? Are the variables explained and fit to the conceptual framework?
Sample	How the sample were selected? Was it non-probability or probability sampling technique? Is the sample size analyzed? Are the exclusion and inclusion criteria laid down?
Ethical consideration	Were informed consent obtained? Was the confidentiality/autonomy of the subjects assured? Were the measures taken to protect the participants from any harm? Was ethical permission sought for the study?
Methodology	Is the research design being appropriate? Has the research instrument been described and relevant to population? Whether it is self-developed or standardized? Were the validity and reliability tested for the study? Was a pilot study undertaken?
Data analysis and results	What types of statistical test was employed? Was it according to objective and hypotheses? Implications of the findings.
Discussion	Are the findings compared with the existing work? Was hypothesis was rejected or accepted? Were the strengths and limitations are laid down? Was a recommendation written for future researchers?
References	Were all the journals, books and other media used as resource for work are included in reference list?

can be challenging, frustrating, daunting and time consuming task. The process starts by identifying a general area or research and then developing a specific research question to be answered. The protocol need to be appropriate to the research question, but also feasible in term of time, resources and ethical consideration.

When you are ready to start writing research proposal, the first step is to carefully read over the guidelines of whatever agency you are submitting to it. These guidelines will give the deadlines for submission and certain instructions for author like length of proposal, structure, format of the proposal, etc. Therefore, it is well worth effort to obtain and carefully read the guidelines prior to writing research proposal.

> **Box 11.2:** Essentials of Research Proposal.
> - Research proposal should be concise, clear and succinct
> - Use of technical jargons, abbreviations and personal pronounces should be avoided
> - A proposal should be divided under separate heading for individual variable for better presentation
> - A researcher should encourage to use short and simple sentence. Use of lengthy sentence are confusing for the audiences
> - Use of small paragraph is attracting and arouse interest of audience to read the proposal
> - Use of image, figures and diagram may help to break monotony and draw the attention of experts quickly

Format of a Research Proposal

The format of proposal vary from one organization or university to another. However, if you are not given any guidelines for preparing research proposal, you could adopt the following given format:

- *The title:* Title of the research study should be clear and concise. The title should be smart enough to give information regarding who, where, what and how the study will be conducted.
- *Investigator(s):* The research title should be presented with the name of the investigators(s) with their complete official designation and address like name of the investigator, designation, official address, contact number, mail Id, name and details of data collector (if any). A proposal can also submitted with a detailed curriculum vitae of all investigators, data collector and trainees (if any).
- *Background of the study:* The background work provides details of magnitude of problem, its consequences and impact on health sector. Generally, it presents the current and existing work on the study topic.
- *Need of the study:* In this section, the importance of research should be justified by the researcher. Investigator should tell why your study should be done. The need of study should answer following questions:
    - Will this study generate new knowledge?
    - Will this study benefits to patient, nursing, staff and faculty?
    - Will study helps to refine or update the old practice?
- *Objectives:* The research proposal should be presented with general as well as specific objectives.
- *Hypotheses:* Research proposal should include hypotheses based on study objective(s). A hypothesis helps to direct the research process.
- *Methodology:*
    - *Research approach:* Quantitative or qualitative.
    - *Research design:* Details of design used in the study, i.e. experimental, non-experimental, etc.

- *Research setting:* The details of the place where collection will be conducted.
- *Study duration:* Tentative duration of the research study in days, months and years.
- *Population:* The group in which a researcher is interested in the study.
- *Sample size:* The group of individuals selected from the population.
- *Sampling technique:* The details about the types of sampling technique and process of randomization for samples in the study.
- *Research instruments:* The details of research tools that will be used in research study to collect information from subjects like knowledge questionnaire, attitude scale and opinionnaire, etc. The instruments reliability and validity should also mentioned.
- *Ethical consideration:* Need and type of ethical issues like consent, maintaining confidentiality, privacy and anonymity, etc.
- *Plan for data collection:* A detail about what information will be collected and who will collect the information should be given in proposal.
- *Plan for data analysis:* Detail of data analysis, and type of statistical tests should be mentioned in the proposal.
- *Budget estimation:* Detail of financial expenditure; whether it is self-financed or sponsored by some authority or agency.

- *References:* A list of search resources should be provided in list of references.

RESEARCH AND PUBLICATION MISCONDUCT

The pressure of publication is tremendously increasing day by day in medical field. There is increasing competition to publish the work in a high impact factor journal. However, the research and publication misconduct are also kept on rising. Commercialization into the scientific societies also drawing attention of researchers to publish their work quickly. The first research misconduct scandal exposed in United States (1980s) when a researcher republish the work of another researchers (Steneck, 2007).

Research misconduct can be broadly classified into two headings:

1. *Research integrity violations:* It refers to plagiarism, falsification and fabrication, etc.
2. *Publication ethics violations:* It includes authorship abuse, duplicate publication and self-plagiarism, etc.

The integrity of scientific writing intoday's world is essential for scientific community. The research and author should practice ethics in scientific writing to promote their credibility, honest and openness in data sharing. Ethics in writing is shared responsibility of authors, reviewers, editors and publishers. Research misconduct occurs when a researcher fabricate, falsifies and plagiarism information or ideas within a research report or article.

Usually, the research misconduct are intentional in nature. The definition of misconduct also extends to breach of confidentiality and authorship abuses.

'Research misconduct is fabrication, falsification, plagiarism in proposing, performing and reviewing research or reporting research result'. *(US Public Health Service Regulation, 2005)*

Violation of certain ethical principles in publication and writing research report and paper is considered scientific misconduct. The most common misconducts are:

- *Authorship abuses:* Authorship obliviously convey professional benefits. Students in many biomedical graduate research program cannot earn higher degree (PhD in nursing at INC consortium) without publishing one or more first authored paper. Authorship should be defined on the basis of contribution in the research study. Sometimes, authorship defined

on inappropriate criteria known as abuse of authorship like (as given by ICMJE, www.icmje.org.)
- *Promiscuous author:* It is awarding authorship to someone who has not contributed in an intellectually significantly way to paper.
- *Coercive authorship:* Authorship conferred to an individual in response to their exertion of seniority or supervisory status over subordinated and junior investigators. For example, using coercion when a department head requires authorship on all paper published from his/her department, but has little or no intellectual inputs into them.
- *Ghost author:* Author who made a significant contribution in research project (in any section; planning, doing or analyzing or writing) and do not get name in publication paper is called as ghost author. There can be many deceitful reasons for ghost authorship. For example, pharmaceutical companies hires some professional author to write their paper and then a bonafide author is asked to sign their name to the paper to improve legitimacy.
- *Guest, honorary, gift author:* Granting authorship out of appreciation, respect or friend for an individual in an attempts to increase the credibility of publication or to give the paper a great sense of legitimacy.
- *Authorship order:* There is no formal guidelines for defining authorship order. However, the lead author and contributed authors may mutually decide the authorship order based on their contribution in research project. Further, it is always better to decide the authorship in the beginning to avoid any conflict of interest in future.

- *Plagiarism:* It refers to use of others' opinion, scientific work, expression and ideas without appropriate citation; that is revealing sources. It is theft of intellectual property. Plagiarism can be intentional and unintentional in nature. United Grant Commission (UGC) approved new draft to prevent plagiarism (Promotion of Academic Integrity and Prevention of Plagiarism in Higher Education Institutions) in April, 2018. This draft made provision of stringent penalty for students and teacher found involved in plagiarism act.
- *Self-plagiarism:* It refers to use of one's own scientific and published work in future publication without appropriate citations. However, there is no formal guidelines indicates what the *'appropriate mean'* is.

Term 'recycling fraud' is also used to denote self-plagiarism. Self-plagiarism may be further classified in following ways:
- *Duplicate or redundant publication:* It is publishing or sending manuscript for publication in two or more than two journals. It can be in the form of:
  - *Shot gunning:* Submission of a manuscript for review in two or more journals at a time
  - *Salami slicing:* It refers to publication of a single set of findings into different journals or in articles. It can leads to distortion of the literature by leading unsuspecting readers to believe that presented in each segment or paper is derived from different subject sample.
  - *Duplicate publication:* It refers to publishing one's own work by copying of the entire published manuscript or scientific work.
  - *Text recycling:* It refers to use of same text published in earlier publication into recent publications.
- *Copyright issue:* The authors should submit a copyright form to journal along with manuscript. Copyright form should be dully signed by all the authors in the order of authorship.

Copyright form submission gives legal protection to author and prevents others from copying the content.
- *Protecting the right of individual in publication:* Author should keep in mind privacy, confidentiality and anonymity of subjects and organization while writing manuscript and sending it for publication.
- *Fabrication:* It involves making or cooking up the data or study results and recording and reporting them. In fabrication, researcher or author never visit field or setting and interact with subject to collect data or sometimes prepare the study results by sitting at one place, at home or office.
- *Falsification:* It involves deliberate manipulation of research materials, equipment or processes to get the choice of finding. It may also involve changing the data or result intentionally. For example, making the non-significant findings to significant for early acceptance of manuscript in a high impact journal.
- *Register clinical trials:* An experimental research conducted on human being should get register before starting data collection. The clinical trials can be registered on Clinical Trials Registry India (CTRI) or online at www.ctrl.nic.in.

RESEARCH UTILIZATION (RU)

One of the important goals of research is to generate new knowledge and establish an evidence base within the profession. Research may not solve problem or make decision, but can provide empirical information that can be used in clinical decision-making process. The need for quality patient outcomes and cost effective care has made it essential that nurses base their practice on research evidence. Ever since, Florence Nightingale also used research evidence to bring about significant changes in the delivery of health care. However, despite an increase in research output, utilizing research evidence by nurses in clinical setting remains a challenge.

Definitions

'Research utilization is the process by which scientifically produced knowledge is transferred to practice'. *(Bransteiner and Prevost, 2002)*

'Research utilization refers to the review and critique of scientific research and then the application of the findings to the clinical practice'. *(Estabrooks, 1998)*

'The process of synthesizing, disseminating and using research generated knowledge to make an impact on or a change in the existing practices in the society'. *(Burns and Grove, 2005)*

The concept of research utilization should not confuse and mix with evidence-based practice. However, a few of the principles of evidence-based practice and research utilization are similar, but evidence-based practice goes beyond just the rigorous scientific research step.

EVIDENCE-BASED PRACTICE

Evidence-based practice (EBP) is a problem-solving approach that incorporate the conscientious use of current best clinical practice from high quality research, a clinician's expertise, and patient value and preferences. Evidence-based practice result to improve patient's satisfaction and safety, improve clinical outcomes, reduced healthcare expenditures and decreased variation in patient outcomes. The importance of evidence-base practice is visible and significant in healthcare sector.

Definitions

'Evidence-based practice is an integration of the best available, nursing experience, and the values and preferences of the individuals, families and communities who are served.'

(Sigma Theta Tau, 2005)

'Evidence-based practice is the conscientious, explicit and judicious use of theory derived, research based information in making decision about care delivery to individual or group of patients and in consideration of individual needs and preferences.' *(Ingersoll, 2000)*

For example, despite the new evidence about pain assessment, wound care, pain-free injections, preoperative fasting and preoperative shaving, many nurses do not apply this knowledge to their practice. A comparison of research utilization and evidence-based practice is given in Table 11.5. [Refer chapter 1 for detail description for evidence-based practice (EBP)].

Barriers to Research Utilization

The concept of research utilization is at the forefront of evidence-based practice. This involves taking the best available evidences from research to the bedside. However, the literature and clinical experience in clinical settings reveals that it is difficult for staff nurses to apply at the bedside. Some of the main constraints to the research utilization are given below: Funk et al. (1991) categorized these barriers in following four categories:

1. *Barriers related to nurses:* These are individual barriers related to nurses includes lack of knowledge about the scientific research process, lack of interest of higher authority to change and adopt new practices, lack of supportive colleagues, lack of knowledge of technical language of research process published in scientific work, overwhelming patient load, and lack of time to do quality research, etc.
2. *Barriers related to organization:* Organizational qualities that may negatively influence evidence-based practice includes lack of recognition in organization in terms of salary, incentive and promotion, lack of resources, apathy of nurse administrator towards novel ideas and lack of decentralization and formalization in an organization.

Table 11.5: Research utilization and evidence-based practice: A comparison.

Research utilization (RU)	Evidence-based practice (EBP)
In RU, findings of one conveniently selected study are utilized	In EBP, findings of multiple studies are used in integration of clinical expertise, patient preferences and values
Findings are usually applied at individual and organization level	Findings are applied in the bedside and are tailored to individual patient care
It is easy and economic process	It is time consuming and effortful process as researcher has to select rigorous evidences from multiple studies and integrate them with clinical expertise, patient values and preferences
RU has narrow scope in health care setting	EBP has broader scope in health care setting in prevention, promotion and treatment areas of a health problem
RU, as such do not have any formal process or protocol	EBP has a pretested specified protocol and process; selection of a clinical research question, review relevant literature, compare and integrate findings with clinical expertise, patient value and preference and determine the result

3. *Barriers related to research:* These are another very common issues faced by a nurse researcher. These includes lack of knowledge about scientific research process, knowledge of statistical analysts and tests, writing research report, inability to organize voluminous amount of information, and lack of resources related to publication and literature, etc.
4. *Barriers related to communication:* These are another common reported barriers includes lack of communication skills to higher authorities like administrator, research committee, funding agencies, and long standing time for acceptance of manuscript, and inadequate knowledge about method of research communication, etc.

FACILITATING RESEARCH UTILIZATION

The application of evidence-based practice can be challenging and requires collaboration and team work among nurses working in clinical and academic setting. A consistent educational programs may help to build up positive attitude and knowledge to use EBP. A successful leadership behavior also encourages nurses to use evidence-based practice. However, use of following measures may anticipate use of EBP in nursing profession.

- *Development of specialized research department or wing:* The organization should have a separate research block devoted to the promotion, and education of staff nurses in research conduction, evaluation, utilization and implementation. Improving knowledge of staff nurses about research process will help to carry-out research project independently.
- *Design educational program before implementing research utilization concept:* It has been proved that nurses feel ill-prepared to institute changes because of lack of training and adequate knowledge of research. So, it is better to prepare an educational event aimed to improve knowledge of research and utilization of research findings in practice. By participating in educational events specifically developed to further the knowledge and comfort level of nurses, research utilization can be increased.
- *Develop reward system for nurses:* Positive reinforcement (i.e. promotional, salary hikes and other benefits plans, etc.) can also designed for staff nurses to improve the utilization of research findings.
- *Organize continuing education events:* The organization can organize continuing education period time to time to refine or update the old knowledge and practice of staff nurses. Even, organization can make continuing education hours mandatory to take the advantage of promotion, hikes in salary and other organizational welfare benefits, etc.
- *Administrative support:* Administration support is a mandatory prerequisite to conduct and implement research in practice. Administration can provide necessary resources like money, staff, equipment and other resources to carry-out good quality research.
- *Open communication channels:* An effective communication line between higher authority and subordinates will help to resolve many barriers related to conducting and using research findings in practice. Administrators and managers should held periodic meeting with subordinates to discuss and resolve the related barriers and can plan line of attack to deal them effectively.
- *Change the attitude to welcome research in practice:* Developing a favorable attitude towards learning, conducting and implementing research can bring lot of changes in practice. Organizational higher authority as well as subordinates should change their perception towards research findings based care and can become a role model for others.

REVIEW QUESTIONS AND ANSWER

Long and Short Answer Questions

1. What are the characteristics of a well written scientific paper? (BFUHS, MSc N-2004)
2. What is research report? (KUHAS, MSc N-2006)
3. Report witting and communication of research. (AIIMS, MSc N-2008)
4. Discuss in detail what are the various steps involved in writing research protocol? (AIIMS, MSc N-2009)
5. Steps in research critique. (TNMGRMU, MSc N-2009)
6. What are the research and publication misconduct? (BFUHS, MSc N-2011)
7. What are the barriers of research utilization? (PGI, MSc N-2013)
8. Steps in evidence-based practice. (RGUHS, MSc N-2016)

Multiple Choice Questions

1. This section of a research report includes interpretation and evaluation of the results of a research study.
   a. Abstract
   b. Method and material
   c. Results
   d. Discussion

2. Ideally, the abstract of the research article should be limited to:
   a. 100 words
   b. 100–200 words
   c. 150–250 words
   d. 250–500 words

3. In Vancouver styles reference styles, et al is used if the authors number exceeds:
   a. 3
   b. 4
   c. 5
   d. 6

4. Which of the following part of a journal article is read most by research users?
   a. Introduction
   b. Material and methods
   c. Discussion
   d. Abstract

5. It is a research misconduct in which a researcher publish one set of data in two or more journals?
   a. Shot gunning
   b. Plagiarism
   c. Salami slicing
   d. Authorship abuse

6. A following number of key words is appropriate for a research report:
   a. 1–2
   b. 2–3
   c. 3–5
   d. >6<10

7. Author who made a significant contribution in research project (in any section; planning, doing or analyzing or writing) and do not get name in publication is termed as:
   a. Guest author
   b. Ghost author
   c. Coercive author
   d. Honorary author

8. It is a common publication misconduct refers to use of others' opinion, scientific work, expression and ideas without appropriate citation; that is revealing sources is termed as:
   a. Plagiarism
   b. Fabrication
   c. Falsification
   d. Self-plagiarism

9. Which of the following is/are common method of dissemination of research findings?
   a. Oral presentation
   b. Publication in journal
   c. Poster presentation
   d. All of the above

10. A careful and intellectual appraisal of the strengths and weakness of the study is termed as:
    a. Research critique
    b. Research action
    c. Research rigors
    d. Evidence-based practice

Answer Key

1.	2.	3.	4.	5.	6.	7.	8.	9.	10.
d.	c.	d.	d.	c.	c.	b.	a.	d.	a.

SUGGESTED READING

1. Arumugam A, Aldhafiri FR. A researcher's ethical dilemma: Is self-plagiarism a condemnable practice or not? Physiotherapy Theory and Practice. 2016;32(6):427-9
2. Brnsteiner J, Prevost S. How to implement evidence based practice. Reflection on nursing leadership/Sigma Theta Tau International, Honor Society of Nursing. 2002; 28(2): 18-21, 45.
3. Burn N, Grove SK. Understanding nursing research—building an evidence based practice, 4th edition. St Louis: Saunders Elsevier; 2005.
4. Burn N, Grove SK. Understanding nursing research—building an evidence based practice, 4th edition. St Louis: Saunders Elsevier; 2007.
5. Bush CT. Nursing research 1st edition. Virginia: Reston Publishing company: Inc. 1985.
6. Callaham ML. Journal policy on ethics in scientific publication. Ann Emerg Med. 2003; 41: 82-9.
7. Claxton LD. Scientific Authorship Part-2. History, recurring issues, practice, and guidelines. Mutat Res. 2005;589; 31-45.
8. Considine J, McGillivray B. An evidence-based practice approach to improving nursing care of acute stroke in an Australian emergency department. J Clin Nurs. 2010;19(1-2):138-44.
9. Coughlan M, Cronin P, Ryan F. Step by step guide to critiquing research part-I: Quantitative research. British Journal of Nursing. 2007;16(11):658-61.
10. de Pedro-Gomez J, Morales-Asencio JM, Bennasar-Veny M, et al. Determining factors in evidence-based clinical practice among hospital and primary care nursing staff. J Adv Nurs. 2012;68(2):452-9.
11. Estabrooks CA. Will evidence based nursing practice make practice perfect. Canadain Journal of Nursing Research. 1998; 30(1): 15-36.
12. Eysenbach G. Medical students see that academic misconduct is common. Br MedBMJ. 2001; 322-7.
13. Fineout-Overholt E, Melnyk B, Schultz A. Transforming health care from the inside out: advancing evidence-based practice in the 21st century. J Prof Nurs. 2005;21:335-44.
14. Flanagin A, Carey LA, Fontanarosa PB, Philip SG, Pace BP, Lundberg GD, et al. Prevalence of articles with honorary authors and ghost authors in peer reviewed journals. JAMA. 280; 222-4.
15. Funk SG, Champagne MT, Wiese RA, Tornquist E M. Barriers: The barriers to research utilization scale. Applied Nursing Research. 1991 a; 4: 39-45.
16. Funk SG, Champagne MT, Wiese RA, Tornquist EM. Barriers to use research findings in practice: The clinician's perspective. Applied Nursing Research. 1991b; 4: 90-5.

17. Funk SG, Champagne MT. Administrator's view on barriers to research utilization. Applied Nursing Research. 1995; 8: 44-9.
18. Grady PA. News from NINR. Nursing Outlook. 2000; 48: 54.
19. Harvard University (2000). Authorship guidelines. Faculty of Medicine, Harvard University [online]. President and fellows of Harvard College, Boston, MA. http://www.hms.harvard.edu/fa/guide_doc.html. [14 Nov 2014].
20. Hicks CM. Research Methods for clinical therapies—applied project design and analysis, 3rd edition. London: Churchill Livingstone; 1999.
21. Horsley JA, Crane J, Crabtree M, Wood D. Using research to improve nursing practice: A guide. New York: Grune and Stratton; 1983.
22. Hutchinson AM, Johnston L. Bridging the divide: A survey of nurses' opinions regarding barriers to, and facilitators of, research utilization in the practice setting. Journal of Clinical Nursing. 2004; 13: 304-15.
23. Ingersoll GL. Evidence based nursing: What it is and what it isn't. Nursing Outlook. 2000; 48(4):151-2.
24. Kajermo KN, Nordstrom G, Krusebrant A, Bjorvell H. Barriers to and facilitators of research utilization, as evidenced by a group of registered nurses in Sweden. Journal of Advanced Nursing. 1998;27: 798-807.
25. Kim HS. Interdisciplinary relation to establish research ethics. In: The Theme and Prospect of Research Ethics. The 1st 2010 Research Ethics Forum, 2010; pp. 13-30, (The Korean Association of Academic Societies, Seoul).
26. Kwok LS. The White-Bull Effect: Abusive coauthorship and publication parasitism. J Med Ethics. 2005; 31: 554-6.
27. Leninger MM. The research critique: Nature, function and art. Nursing Research. 1968.
28. Mc-Gratch JP, Polit DF, Beck C T. Canadian essential of nursing, Lippincott William and Wilkins; 2010.
29. Peterson ED, Bynum DZ, Roe MT. Association of evidence based care processes and outcomes among patients with acute coronary syndromes: performance matters. J Cardiovasc Nurs. 2008;23(1):50-5.
30. Polit DF, Beck CT. Nursing research: Principle and methods, 7th edition. Philadelphia: Lippincott William Wilkins; 2004.
31. Polit D, Beck C. Essential of nursing research: Methods, appraisal and utilization. 6th edition. Philadelphia: Lippincott William Wilkins; 2006.
32. Rohwer A, Young T, Wager E, Garner P. Authorship, plagiarism and conflict of interest: views and practices from low/middle-income country health researchers. BMJ Open. 2017;7:1-10.
33. Sigma Theta Tau international. (2005). Position statement of evidence based practice. Available at http://www.nursingsociety.org/aboutus/positionpapers/pages/EBN_positionpaper.aspx [Accessed Nov. 2014].
34. Spielmans GI, Biehn TL, Sawrey DL. A case study of salami slicing: Pooled analyses of duloxetine for depression. Psychother Psychosom. 2010;79:97-106.
35. Steneck NH. ORI (The Offi ce of Research Integrity) Introduction to the Responsible Conduct of Research. Revised edition. (Department of Health & Human Services, Bethesda). 2007.
36. Talbot LA. Principles and practice of nursing research, 1st edition. St Louis: Mosby Year Book Inc. 1995.
37. Valente S. Research dissemination and utilization: Improving care at the bedside. J Nurs Care Quality. 2003;18(2):114-2.
38. Winslow E. Failure to publish: A form of scientific misconduct? Heart and Lung. 1996; 25,:169-74.

Chapter 12

Introduction to Statistics

INTRODUCTION

In the modern world of computer and information technology, the importance of statistics is very well-recognized by all disciplines. Statistics has originated as science of statehood and found application slowly and steadily in agriculture, economics, commerce, biology, medicine and nursing. Statistics is a set of tools used to organize and analyze data. Analyzing 'real' data helps investigator to understand both the mechanical of statistical testing and the meaning of the outcomes. Research is structural and there are basic steps depending on the subjects matter and researcher. Moreover, statistics is one step in research process that enables researcher to organize, interpret and communicating numeric information.

Meaning and Definition

It may be interesting to point out that statistics is not a new discipline but as old as human life existing. The word 'statistics' comes from the Italian word *'statista'* (meaning 'statesman') or the German word *'statistik'* which means a 'political state.' It was first used by Professor Gottfried Achenwall (1719-1772), a professor in Marlborough in 1749 to refer the subject matter as a whole. Statistics is defined differently by different authors over a period of time. In the olden days statistics was confined to only state affairs but in olden days it embraces almost every sphere of human activity. Therefore, a number of old definitions were replaced by new statistical definitions.
Achenwall defined statistics as 'the political science of the several countries.'
'Statistics is the science and practice of developing human knowledge through the use of empirical data expressed in quantitative form. It is based on statistical theory which is branch of applied mathematics. Within statistical theory, randomness and uncertainty are modeled by probability theory.' *(Wikipedia Encyclopedia)*
'Statistic is defined as collection, presentation, analysis and interpretation of numerical data.' *(Croxton and Cowden)*
'Statistics are numerical statement of facts in any department of inquiry placed in relation to each other.' *(AL Bowley)*
'Statistics is a science which deals with collection, classification and tabulation of numerical facts as the basis for the explanation, description and comparison of phenomena.' *(Lovitt)*
'Statistics is the science which deals with the methods of collecting, classifying, presenting, comparing and interpreting numerical data collected to throw some light on any sphere of inquiry.' *(Seligman)*
Biostatistics is the science and art of collection, compilation, presentation, analysis and interpretation of numerical data concerned with biological events.

Therefore, statistics is a branch of mathematics used to summarize, analysis and interpret a group of numbers or observation.

CHARACTERISTICS OF STATISTICS

The followings are the main characteristics of statistics:
- *Statistics must be numerically expressed:* All statistics are expressed in numbers. Qualitative expressed statements do not come under statistics. For example, evaluation of students expressed in percentage and percentile over a period of time are statistics but expressed as 'good', 'fair' and 'poor' are not statistics.
- *Statistics are aggregates of facts and figures:* A single event or incident is not statistics but figures relating to event or incident are statistics. For example, number of road accidents, birth over a period of time.
- *Statistics should be collected to serve a purpose:* The purpose of statistic should be clear and definite. Stray collections of facts are not statistics. For example, we may collect information about the number of road traffic accidents in a coming year to compare it with previous years to reach on some conclusion, whether it is increased or decreased.
- *Statistics should be estimated according to reasonable standards of accuracy:* The data collection for statistical purposes should be collected either by counting or measuring a particular event or attribute. The reasonable standard of accuracy is a relative term depends upon the purpose for which statistics are collected. For example, in measuring height of the college student one-tenth of a centimeter is material importance, but in measuring distance between two or more city even a few meters can be left out to record reasonably a correct distance.
- *Statistics are affected to a marked extent by a number of causes:* There are many factors responsible to bring change in figures and facts. For example, statistics of price are affected by a number of factors like condition of supply, demand, imports, exports and value of currency, etc.

FUNCTIONS OF STATISTICS

Almost all organization take help of statistics in planning, formulation and revision of existing quality of work. Statistic play a essential role in collecting, summarizing and interpreting data assigned to empirically evaluate a principle. Statistics facilitate drawing general conclusion based on specific data. In this way, statistics serve following important functions.
- Statistics enable a researcher to condense large pool of data into concise figures and number to reach on a specific conclusion
- Statistics summarize the observation or data in such a manner that they provide answer to the research question or hypothesis
- Statistic answers how closely or distinctly certain features or relationship exist between two or more variables in a observation
- Statistics expand body of knowledge and experience by collection, compilation and presentation of data
- Statistics helps to differentiate normal to abnormal in an observation and therefore, help in planning and policy revision. For example, acceptable limit of infection in an ICU
- It helps in testing hypotheses to reveal results, therefore, It helps to develop and test evidence-based intervention for practice
- It helps to control and maintain quality level.

COMMON STATISTICAL TERMS

- *Data:* Piece of information obtained in the course of a study.
- *Data set:* A collection of related items.
- *Database:* A collection of data organized for rapid research and retrieval, usually by a computer; often a consolidation of many records stored separately.
- *Data collection:* The gathering of information needed to address research question.
- *Observation:* An event and its measurement such as blood pressure (event) and 120/80 mm Hg (measurement).
- *Parameter:* It is summary of characteristic that describe a sample such as mean, median, standard deviation and correlation coefficient, etc.
- *Raw data:* Data recorded in an arbitrary manner from the field of inquiry. For example, collection of information about level of self-esteem through Rosenberg self-esteem scale from a group of nursing students. The information will be called 'raw data' unless it will not analyze and presented through appropriate method of presentation.
- *Continuous data:* The data which can assume any value from zero to infinity. Therefore, measurement in fraction and decimal is possible. For example, height and weight and distance, etc.
- *Discrete data:* A data which cannot be measured in fraction or decimal. Discrete data present a specific value of a variable. For example, RBC count, male and female, etc.

LEVELS OF MEASUREMENT

Level of measurement refers to the amount and extent of the degree of detail of information present in a data set. Stevens (1946) categorized data elements in four categories—*nominal (categorical), ordinal, interval* and *ratio (continuous)* level.

Nominal Measurement

The term nominal (or categorical) refers to data that can only categorize into groups. For example, the demographic data of marital status are measured at nominal level which only group the variable into categories such as married, unmarried, divorced, separate and so on. Here, no category is better or worse than one another and there is no quantitative difference between one another. They are just unique category in thyself. The only possible interpretation is that both subjects are not same on said variable. It just gives information about name or categorization of variables. Nominal measurement must have category that are mutually exclusive and exhaustive in nature.

> **Box 12.1:** Example of Nominal-Level Measurement.
>
> - Blood group
>   - A
>   - B
>   - AB
>   - O
> - Gender
>   - Female
>   - Male

Ordinal Measurement

Ordinal level data are next level of data set to nominal data. Ordinal data arrange the data in an inherent order. Data values such as strongly satisfied, satisfied, neither satisfied nor dissatisfied, dissatisfied and strongly dissatisfied have order. An individual would interpret strongly dissatisfied as being highest level of dissatisfaction than strongly satisfied. However, it cannot be interpreted that strongly dissatisfied is double or triple in dissatisfaction to satisfied or strongly satisfied. The possible interpretation is that one's greater in dissatisfaction to other or vice versa. Ordinal data rank objects based on their relative standing on a specific scale without difference in magnitude. Visual analogue scale (VAS) is the most common example or ordinal data used in clinical setting.

Box 12.2: Example of Ordinal-Level Measurement.

- Socioeconomic status
  - Low income
  - Middle income
  - High income
- Level of knowledge
  - Inadequate
  - Adequate
  - Good

Interval Measurement

The interval level of measurement determine the distance between data element.

An interval scale consists of all of the qualities of a nominal and ordinal scale plus it add the quality of equal distance between data points or intervals. This characteristic allows the researcher to make conclusions regarding actual differences between measures rather than just saying one measure is greater than another. Most standardized psychological and educational tests used in nursing research. However, interval data level do not have true zero, hence multiplication is not possible. Consequently, you cannot say that 30° is twice hot as 15°. Lack of true zero and reference point does not allow to say that 30° is twice hot as 15°.

An interval scale consists of all of the qualities of a nominal and ordinal scale plus it add the quality of equal distance between data points or intervals. This characteristic allows the researcher to make conclusions regarding actual differences between measures rather than just saying one measure is greater than another. Most standardized psychological and educational tests used in nursing research are on interval scale.

Box 12.3: Example of Interval-Level Measurement.

- Temperature
  - 20–70°
  - 30–90°

Ratio Measurement

Ratio level measurement are highest level of measurement among all and contain all features of lower level of measurement (nominal, ordinal and interval). Ratio level data have the key feature of a true zero and a reference value. Ratio level data may undergo by addition, subtraction, multiplication and division. These level of data required use of most powerful statistical (parametric) test. Weight, height, heart rate, and money quantities are examples of ratio level measurement. Many ratio scales are found in biologic measures rather than psychological measures.

Box 12.4: Example of Ratio-Level Measurement.

- Height
- Weight
- Blood pressure
- Pulse rate
- Heart rate

DESCRIPTIVE STATISTICS

Descriptive statistics helps to organize and present the large volume of information in meaningful way.

Descriptive statistics present and summarize the data with the help of table, graph and summary of data in the form of mean, median and mode.

Descriptive statistics helpful when it is not possible to examine each members of an entire population. So, it deals with presentation of numerical findings, or observation, in either graphs or tables form and make the data meaningful to others.

METHODS OF DATA PRESENTATION

Once the data will be collected, it should be analyzed purposively in order to bring out the important points clearly. These data will not serve any purpose until we classify and organize them in some fashion. Therefore, it is important to choose a method which can facilitate the presentation of data in a meaningful manner. Broadly, there are two main methods of presenting data:
1. Table presentation
2. Graph presentation.

Table Presentation

Tabulation is the most common and preferred method of data presentation. Tabulation helps in presenting data from a mass of statistical information. Tabulation is a systematic presentation of information contained in the data in the rows and columns in accordance with their respective features.

Construction of a Good Table

Construction of a table is an art and skill as researcher should learn. A table contains all the information within a smallest possible space without losing data. A researcher should keep in mind purpose and presentation in mind while preparing a table. An ideal table should have following parts in it.
- *Table number:* A table should be numbered for reference and identification purpose. Table number should be placed at center of the top of table. Sometimes, it is also written just before title of table.
- *Title:* A good table should have a clearly worded but unambiguous title explaining the nature of the data. It should be placed at the center and top of the table.
- *Caption or column heading:* Caption in table are brief and self-explanatory heading of vertical columns.
- *Stub or row heading:* It is brief self-explanatory heading for horizontal rows.
- *Body:* The body of table contains main information about the observation in frequency and percentage style.

Title of table (Demo table)

Subheading	Caption heading	Total
	Caption subheading	
Stub subheadings	Body	
Total		

- *Footnotes:* Footnotes are given at the end of the table for explanation of any facts or abbreviation used in table.
- *Source of data:* Lastly, the table should be given name of source from where table and information sought by investigator.

Essentials of a Good Table

Table are prepared according to the purpose and presentation of data. However, following points can be considered principles of tabulation.
- A table should be precise and self-explanatory in nature
- The arrangement of rows and columns should be in logical and systematic order
- The rows and columns should be separated by using double dark line
- In case of large table, it is good to either split the table in two or more small tables or prepare two or three small tables
- Use of symbols and code in a table should be explained in footnote for quick reference.
- Unit of measurement for data must be depicted accurately. Such as 'length in meters' and 'weight in kilograms'.
- A good table should maintain consistency throughout chapter or protocol in terms of format, decimal level and footnotes, etc.
- Table should be prepared in accordance to given format or guidelines of university or board.

Graph Presentation

Graph is another easy and simple way to represent the information. Graphs simplify the information by using images and figures and emphasizing data pattern of trends. Graphs are useful for summarizing, explaining, or exploring quantitative information. Diagrammatic presentation is one of the most convincing and appealing way in which result may be presented through diagram, graph and charts, etc. It is easy to present a bunch of information through diagram.

Moreover, even a layman who has nothing to do with numbers can also understand diagram. Evidence of this can be found in newspaper, magazines, journals and advertisement, etc.

Significance of Graphical Presentation
- Graphs and figures are economic and convenient method of presenting bunch of information to others
- Graphs facilitates understanding as it present the phenomenon as a unit
- Figures are attractive way of data presentation and enable others to memorize the information easily
- Graphical presentation is an easy and inexpensive method of data presentation
- Graph and figures are self-explanatory in nature and can easily comprehend by others.

Principles of Graphic Presentation
- The figure/graph should be neatly and attractively drawn for voluntary attention of readers
- The figure should be concise and appropriate in terms of title, number and keywords used in figure for clear understanding to readers
- Use of appropriate size of figure will helps to provide complete and clear information to others

- In case of multiple bars/graphs, it is recomended to use different colors for each bar or graph for easy identification
- A researcher should have knowledge about the audience before selection of a graph/figure.

Methods of Graphical Presentation

Graphs are effective way to represent a large bunch of information and hence, can be used in place of table. A right format of the graph helps to best represent the data to the readers and reviewers. There are various form of graphical presentation to represent the data. Some of the important methods of graphical presentation are given here:
- Bar diagrams and histograms
- Pie or sector graphs
- Frequency curves
- Pictographs/pictograms
- Frequency polygons
- Cumulative frequency curve (Ogive)
- Scatter or dot diagrams
- Line diagrams.

Bar Diagrams and Histograms

Bar graphs presents the data in the form of bars that can be drawn vertically or horizontally. The only difference between a histogram and bar chart is that there is no space between the bars in a histogram. The height of bars indicates the amount of information in a category. A bar chart used to indicate and compare value in a discrete category or group, and the frequency or other measurement (i.e. mean).

There are three types of bar graphs:
1. Simple bar graph
2. Multiple bar graph
3. Proportional bar graph.

Example 1: Construction of a simple bar graph using production of rice in particular year (Fig. 12.1 and Table 12.1).

Table 12.1: Production of rice in a year (in tonnes).

Year	Production (in tonnes)
1991	45
1992	40
1993	42
1994	55
1995	50

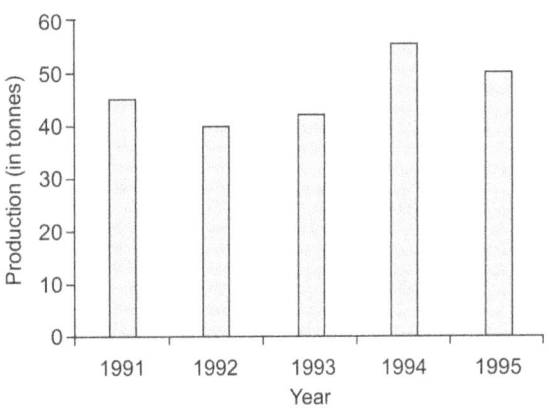

Fig. 12.1: Simple bar diagram.

Example 2: Construct a multiple bar diagram using profit before and after tax in a particular financial year (Table 12.2 and Fig. 12.2).

Table 12.2: Profit amount (in lakhs) before and after tax in a particular year.

Year	Profit before tax (in lakhs)	Profit after tax (in lakhs)
1998	195	80
1999	200	87
2000	165	45
2001	140	32

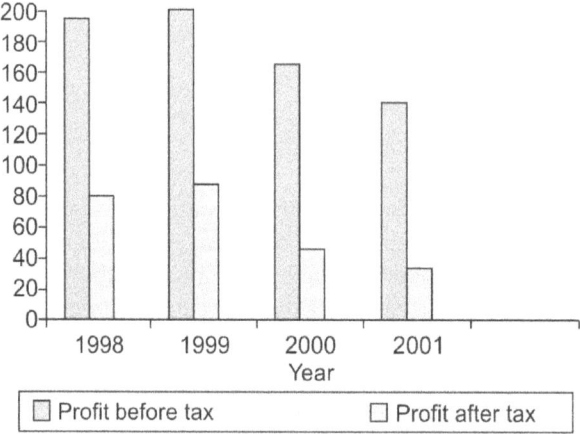

Fig. 12.2: Multiple bar diagram.

Example 3: Construct the subdivided bar diagram using different expenditure items in families (Table 12.3 and Fig. 12.3).

Table 12.3: Monthly expenditures (in rupees) in a particular year.

Expenditure items	Monthly expenditure (in ₹)	
	Family A	Family B
Food	75	95
Clothing	20	25
Education	15	10
Housing rent	40	65
Miscellaneous	25	35

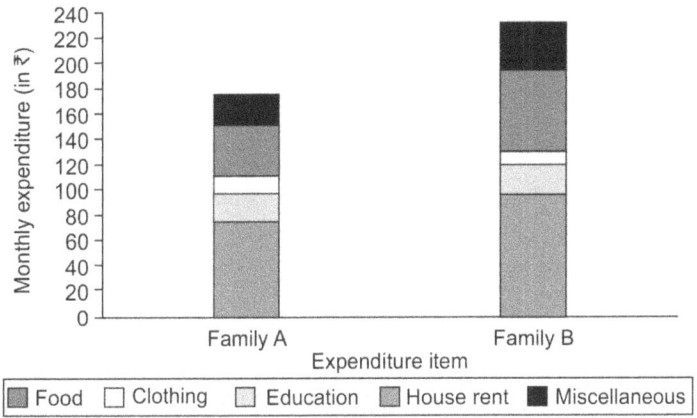

Fig. 12.3: Subdivided bar diagram.

Example 4: Construct the histogram using number of worker and their daily wages (Table 12.4 and Fig. 12.4).

Table 12.4: Number of worker and their daily wages.

Daily wages	Number of workers
0–50	8
50–100	16
100–150	27
150–200	19
200–250	10
250–300	6

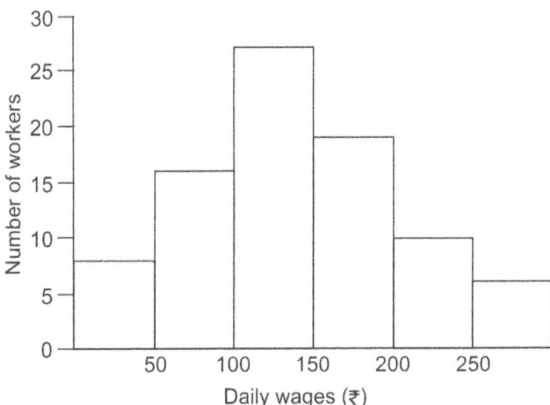

Fig. 12.4: Histogram.

Pie or Sector Graphs

Pie chart is the another most appropriate method to represent the data grouped into small number of categories. It is commonly used to depict nominal data, visually represent a distribution of categories. However, it also can be used to depict data which cannot be presented apart from a table (i.e. frequency distribution). It is most commonly used method to represent number of votes each candidates won in an election. It gives comparative difference at a glance. Size of each angle is calculated by multiple class percentages with 360° angle or use the given formula for calculating sector percentage.

$$\text{Size of pie sector} = \frac{\text{Class frequency}}{\text{Total observation}} \times 360°$$

Example 5: Construct a pie chart using number of seats won a party in Parliament Election in India (Table 12.5 and Fig. 12.5).

Table 12.5: Number of seat won by different parties at parliament election.

Party	BJP	Congress	AAP	BSP	Shivsena	Others
Seats	200	35	6	10	50	110
Degree	175	31	5	9	44	96

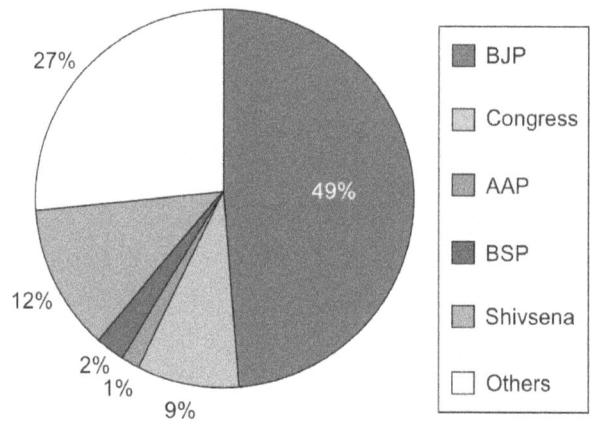

Fig. 12.5: Pie diagram showing number of seats won by different party at parliament election.

Frequency Curves

Frequency curve is a line diagram to present the frequency distribution. It looks similar to histogram except that midpoints are identified for each class and joined to each others. The diagram made is called frequency polygon/curve. The frequency curve begins and ends at the baseline.

Example 6: Construct a frequency curve using number of family and their monthly wages (₹) (Table 12.6 and Fig 12.6).

Introduction to Statistics

Table 12.6: Monthly wages of families in India.

Monthly wages (₹)	Number of family
0–1000	21
1000–2000	35
2000–3000	56
3000–4000	71
4000–5000	63
5000–6000	40
6000–7000	29
7000–8000	14

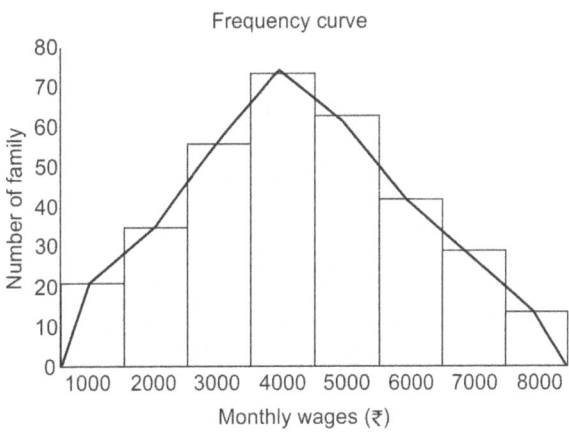

Fig. 12.6: Frequency curve.

Pictograms/Pictographs

Pictogram or pictograph is a popular method of data presentation. It is a line or bar graph uses symbols or pictures to depict its data.

Pictures are attractive and easy to comprehend and therefore, this method is particularly useful in presenting findings to the layman. In pictograph, data are presented through a pictorial symbol that is carefully selected. Pictorial symbols selected should be self-explanatory in nature.

Example 7: Production of apple and orange around the globe in a particular year (Fig. 12.7).

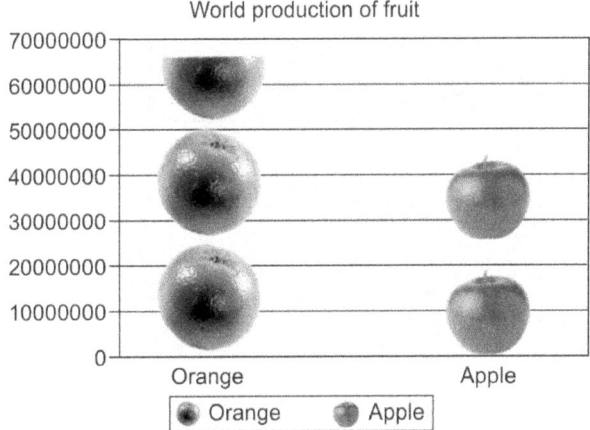

Fig. 12.7: World production of fruit in 2012.

Frequency Polygon

A frequency polygon is a graph of frequency distribution. Frequency polygon constructed by joining the midpoint of the upper horizontal side of each rectangle of a histogram. It can also constructed by taking the midpoint of various class intervals. Frequency polygon is simpler than the histogram and it gives outline of data pattern more easily.

Example 8: Construct a frequency polygon using scores of nursing students (Fig. 12.8 and Table 12.7).

Table 12.7: Score of nursing students.

Score	Frequency
44.5	0
54.5	5
64.5	10
74.5	30
84.5	40
94.5	15
104.5	0

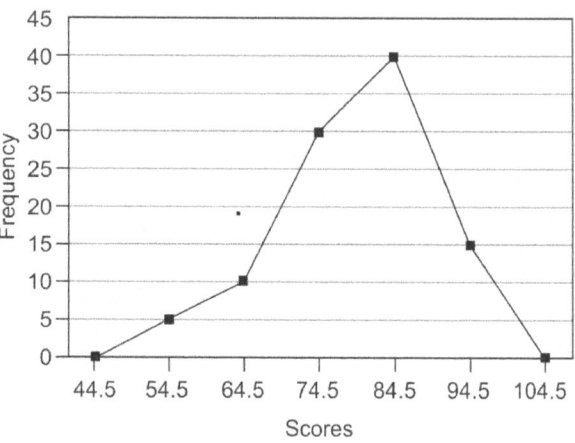

Fig. 12.8: Frequency polygon.

Cumulative Frequency Curve (Ogive)

Ogive is a graph of the cumulative frequency distribution. To draw this, an ordinary frequency table has to be converted to cumulative frequency table. It is obtained by cumulating the frequency of previous classes including the class in question.

Example 9: Construct an Ogive for the frequency distribution given in Table 12.8.

Table 12.8: Marks of nursing students.

Marks	Number of students
30	4
40	6
50	15
60	24
70	35
80	43
90	48
100	50

The cumulative frequencies are then plotted on graph to draw cumulative frequency graph. The Ogive can be drawn by taking lower or upper value of class interval. On joining the points by smooth free hand curve, the diagram appear is Ogive.

Ogive use to calculate median, quartiles and percentiles. It is also used to find out the number of observations which are expected to lie below the two given values (Fig. 12.9).

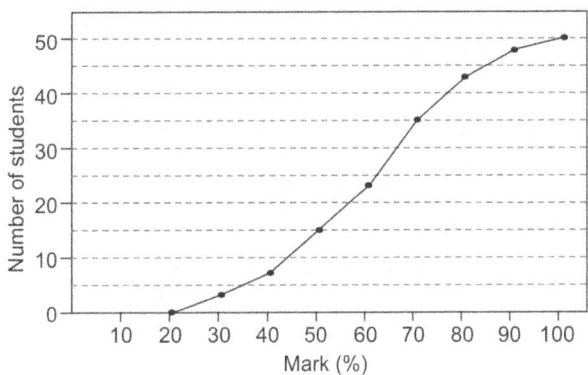

Fig. 12.9: Ogive.

Scatter or Dot Diagrams

It is graphic presentation made to shows the nature of correlation between two variables. For example, one variable is presented along the horizontal axis and second variable along the vertical axis. For each pair of observation of two variables, we put a dot in the plane. The direction of dots shows the scatter or concentration of various points along a plane (Table 12.9).

Table 12.9: Height and weight of adolescent.

Height (cm)	140	150	160	170	176
Weight (kg)	45	55	60	75	85

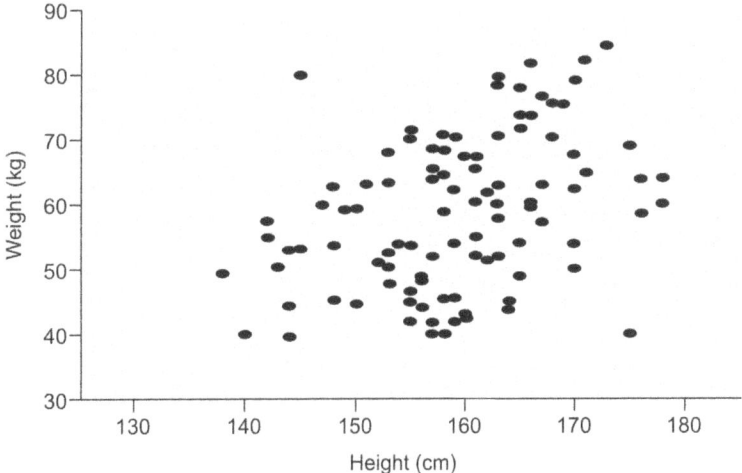

Fig. 12.10: Scatter plot.

Line Diagrams

This is frequency polygon presenting variation in observation over a period of time. It shows the trend of an event occurring over a period of time. For example, changes in infant mortality rate over a period of years. Vertical axis may not start from zero but at some point above when frequencies start at high level. To draw line chart, the data are plotted on X-axis or Y-axis and points are joined by straight line.

Example 10: Construct a line diagram using given data (Table 12.10 and Fig 12.11).

Table 12.10: Number of children in Indian families

Number of children	0	1	2	3	4	5
Frequency	10	14	9	6	4	2

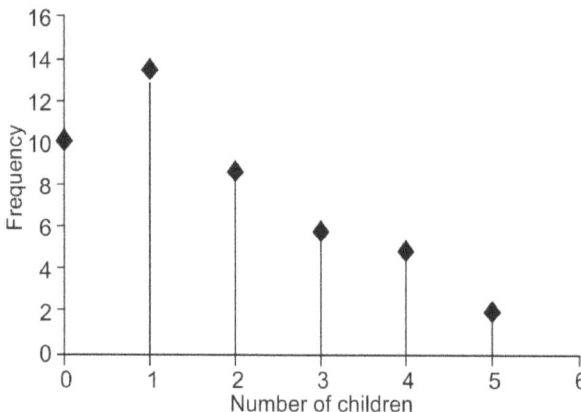

Fig. 12.11: Line diagram.

MEASURES OF CENTRAL TENDENCY

The extent to which the observation cluster around a central location is explained by the measures of central tendency. Measures of central tendency pick up the middle or central value of an observation. Measure of central tendency provide information about where majority of the value lie in an observation. Mean, median and mode are measures of central tendency.

The mean and median are used to describe continuous level data, while the mode is used to describe both continuous and nominal data.

The three common measure of central tendency are:
1. Mean
2. Median
3. Mode

MEAN

The mean (or average) is the most popular and best measure of central tendency. The mean is calculated by summing up all observations and dividing the total by number of observations. It is also known as arithmetic mean. It is denoted by $\bar{X}$ (read x bar).

Mean is more sensitive to outliers and more affect by the pattern of distribution of an observation (or data). The use of mean is limited for interval and ratio level data set. However, use of means for nominal or ordinal data is not possible.

Properties of Arithmetic Mean

Arithmetic mean have following important properties.
- The sum of deviation of items from the arithmetic mean is always zero.
  For example:

X	(X - X̄)
5	-10
20	5
15	0
20	5
ΣX = 60	Σ(X - X̄) = 0

- The sum of squared deviation of the items from mean is minimum, that is less than sum of the squared deviation of the items from any others value.
  For example:

X	(X - X̄)	(X - X̄)²
4	0	0
3	-1	1
4	0	0
5	1	1
ΣX = 16	Σ(X - X̄) = 0	Σ(X - X̄)² = 2

- The sum of the deviation is equal to two in above case. If the deviations are taken from any other value then sum of the square deviation would be greater than zero. Follow the example:

X	(X - 3)	(X - 3)²
4	1	1
3	0	0
4	1	1
5	2	4
ΣX = 16	Σ(X - X̄) = 0	Σ(X - X̄)² = 6

Mean for Ungrouped Data

$$\bar{X} = \frac{X_1 + X_2 + X_3 + X_4 + \ldots\ldots X_N}{N}$$

$$\bar{X} = \frac{\Sigma X}{N}$$

Where,
$\bar{X}$ = Arithmetic mean
ΣX = Sum of all the observations
N = Number of observation

Example: Calculate mean for monthly income of 5 nursing employees at nursing college.

Employees	1	2	3	4	5
Monthly income	20000	30000	35000	45000	15000

$$\overline{X} = \frac{20000 + 30000 + 35000 + 45000 + 15000}{5} = \frac{145000}{5} = 29{,}000$$

So, mean income of nursing employees is 29,000

Calculation of Mean by Assumed Mean Method

The arithmetic mean can be calculated by following method also

$$\overline{X} = A + \frac{\Sigma d}{N}$$

Where,

$\overline{X}$ = Arithmetic mean
A = Assumed mean
Σd = Sum of deviation of all the observations
N = Number of observation

For example, calculate arithmetic mean of IQ test result of 10 students

Students	1	2	3	4	5	6	7	8	9	10
IQ test	110	90	80	105	115	120	90	80	90	80

Students	X	d = (X − X̄)
1	110	10
2	90	−30
3	80	−40
4	105	−15
5	115	−5
6	120	0
7	90	−30
8	80	−40
9	90	−30
10	80	−40
		Σd = −230

Suppose assumed mean is 120 for given data.
Apply all figures in assumed mean formula to calculate arithmetic mean

$$\overline{X} = 120 + \frac{(-230)}{10} = 97$$

So, mean IQ level of students is 97.

Calculation of Mean for Grouped Data

$$\overline{X} = \frac{\Sigma fm}{N}$$

Where,

$\bar{X}$ = Arithmetic mean
$\overline{X}$ = Arithmetic mean
f = Frequency of each class
m = Mid value of class interval $\left(\dfrac{\text{Lower limit + Upper limit}}{2}\right)$
Σfm = Sum of fm
N = Number of observation

For example, score of 50 nursing students in psychology examination is as below. Calculate mean for given data.

Marks	Frequency (f)	Midpoint (m)	fm
0–10	5	5	25
10–20	12	15	180
20–30	25	25	625
30–40	8	35	280
	X = 50		Σfm = 1110

Substitute the given value in formula

$$\bar{X} = \dfrac{\Sigma fm}{N}$$

$$\bar{X} = \dfrac{1110}{50} = 22.2$$

So, mean score in psychology examination is 22.2.

Merits of Mean

- Mean is the most useful method in practice as it is most easy to calculate and understand
- Mean is the calculated value and its not affect by position change such as median
- Mean is the only measure of central tendency used to compare two or more than two sets of data.

Demerits of Mean

- Mean cannot be calculated for nominal or nonnominal ordinal data. Even though if you calculate mean for ordinal data, it does not provide meaning, e.g. grading of cancer
- In case of very small sample, mean is sensitive to extreme value or outliers. Therefore not a appropriate measure of central tendency for skewed distribution.

MEDIAN

The median by definition refers middle value in a distribution. Median is the center value of a data set which divide whole data set in two halves at which half of the subjects lie above the value (median) and another half falls below it.

In this case, one half of observation (50%) in distribution have a value smaller than median and rest one half have a value higher than median. Hence, median is 50% of the observation.

It is denoted by Mdn and also called 'positional average'. Median calculated by arranging the data in ascending or descending order, then (n + 1)/2th observation is the median. Median is not influenced by an accidental grouping or extreme case values away from the true center of data. However, median can only use for ordinal.

Calculation of Median for Ungrouped Data

a. *Median for odd observations (Grouped data)*

9, 4, 6, 8, 7, 5, 3

Arrange the observation in a order (Ascending or descending order)
3, 4, 5, 6, 7, 8, 9
Select the middle value, it is 6 here
So, median is 6 for given observation.

b. *Median for even observations*
In case of even number of observation, use following formula to compute median

$$Md = \left(\frac{n+1}{2}\right)^{th}$$

Example, 8 students score in English is given below, compute median for the score
80, 85, 70, 75, 90, 95, 80, 85

Arrange the observations in order
70, 75, 80, 80, 85, 85, 90, 95

$$Md = \left(\frac{n+1}{2}\right) = \frac{8+1}{2} = 4.5$$

$$4\text{th item} + \left(\frac{1}{2}\right)(5\text{th} - 4\text{th item})$$

$$80 + \frac{1}{2}(85-80) = 82.5$$

So, median is 82.5.

Calculation of Median for Grouped Data

The given steps can be followed to calculate median from grouped data.
- Arrange the data in ascending or descending order
- Compute cumulative frequency
- Determine the particular class internal in which median is lie by dividing total observations by two, i.e. $\frac{N}{2}$
- Select lower limit of median class interval
- Choose cumulative frequency of the median class interval
- Select frequency of the median class interval
- Choose the class interval of the observation

Use following formula:

$$Mdn = L + \frac{\frac{N}{2} - cf}{f} \times i$$

Where,

L = Lower limit of median class interval
cf = Cumulative frequency of a class just before the median class
f = Simple frequency of median class
i = Class interval of the data

For example, score of nine nursing students on biophysics is given in table, compute median for the score.

Marks	f	cf
5–10	7	7
10–15	15	22
15–20	24	46
20–25	31	77
25–30	42	119
30–35	30	149
35–40	26	175
40–45	15	190
45–50	10	200
	N = 200	

Here, $\frac{N}{2} = 100$

So, median class is 20–25

$$L = 20, cf = 46, f = 31, i = 5$$

Substitute the value in given above formula and get the median

$$20 + \left(\frac{100 - 46}{31}\right) \times 5$$

$$Mdn = 31.25$$

So, student median score is 31.25.

Merits of Median
- It is easy to comprehend and compute
- It is not affected by outliers/skewed data
- It can also be calculated for ratio, interval, and ordinal scale.

Demerits of Median
- Median does not take into consideration the precise value of single observation and therefore does not use all information available in a observation
- Unlike mean, median is not used for advance mathematical calculation and hence its scope in use of statistics is limited
- Unlike mean, median cannot be expressed in a single value for two or more than two observations.

MODE

Mode is the easiest measure of central tendency to determine. Mode is the most frequent possible value occurs in a given observation. It may be regarded as the *'most typical'* of a series of values. Sometimes, data set do not have a mode (amodal) because each value occurs only once. On the other hand, some data set have more than one mode called *bimodal*. Modality refers to number of modes found in a data set.

Table 12.11: Types of mode.

Data points	Type of mode	Location of mode
0, 1, 2, 3	Amodal	N/A
0, 1, 1, 2, 3	Unimodal	1
0, 1, 1, 2, 2, 3	Bimodal	1, 2

Calculation of Mode for Ungrouped Data

For example, the score obtained by 10 GNM nursing students in pediatric nursing is given below. Compute mode for this score:

15, 10, 10, 15, 18, 19, 20, 21, 10, 23, 25, 10, 9

Since 10 is most frequent score in given score. So, mode for above given score is 10. In some ill-defined case mode may be absent or more than two modes called bimodal.

Calculation of Mode for Grouped Data

Mode is calculated using following formula:

$$\text{Mode} = L + \frac{f_m - f_1}{2f_m - f_1 - f_2} \times i$$

Where,

L = Lower limit of modal class
f_m = The frequency of modal class
f_1 = The frequency of the class interval preceding modal class
f_2 = The frequency of the class interval succeeding modal class
i = The class interval of observation

For example, the wages of 60 white people is given in dollar. Compute the median for wages.

Wages	30–35	35–40	40–45	45–50	50–55	55–60
White people (f)	3	8	12	20	15	2

Since, the class interval 45–50 has highest frequency, so, 45–50 will be modal class interval for above data

Here, L = 45, f_m = 20, f_1 = 12, f_2 = 15, i = 5

Substitute the value in given formula to compute mode

$$\text{Mode} = 45 + \frac{20 - 12}{2 \times 20 - 12 - 15} \times 5$$

$$= 48.08$$

So, mode of wage is 48.08 for white people.

Merits of Mode

- Value of mode is not affected by extreme events
- It is easy to calculate and in some case mere observation is sufficient for selecting mode
- Mode can be computed for open ended classes without ascertaining class interval
- Mode can be used for qualitative phenomena.

Demerits of Mode
- In some cases, mode is ill-defined and more than one mode possible called bimodal. So, calculation of mode is difficult
- Mode is most unstable measure of central tendency and its value is difficult to determine.

MEASURE OF DISPERSION REPLACE OR WITH/OR VARIABILITY

A researcher collects a set of data in which some of the observations are vary from the central value of data. In some observation, the difference may be less whereas in some other observation, it may be more. This property of deviation of the values from the average is called *dispersion or variation* and the measures used to measure this variation called *measures of dispersion/variation*. Measures of dispersion help us to study the important characteristics and distribution of an observation. The various measures of dispersion are as follows:
1. Range
2. Interquartile Range or Quartile Deviation
3. Mean Deviation
4. Standard Deviation
5. Coefficient of Variation (CV).

Characteristics of Good Measure of Dispersion
- It should be easy to calculate and understand
- It should take in consideration each and every items of the distribution
- It should not affect with extreme value.

RANGE

The range is the easiest and simplest method of studying dispersion. It is defined as the difference between the highest and lowest value in an observation. Range has advantage of easy calculation and has lot of disadvantages that it affect with outliers (extreme values) and does not count all observation in a data set. It is good to provide minimum and maximum value rather than range. It can be represented as follow:

$$\text{Range (R)} = H - L$$
$$H = \text{Highest value}$$
$$L = \text{Lowest value}$$

For example, the score of 10th class students on general aptitude test is given below, calculate range for score

$$5, 7, 9, 11, 13, 18, 15, 17, 24, 25, 35$$
$$\text{Range (R)} = 35 - 5 = 30$$

Therefore, the range of score is 30 for above data.

INTERQUARTILE RANGE OR QUARTILE DEVIATION

The interquartile range represent the difference between first and third quartile. It describes the middle 50% of the observation of a data set. A larger interquartile range indicates that the middle 50% of observation are wide spaced out.

Interquartile range is not affected by extreme values and can be used as a measure of variability for missing extreme values. However, it has limitation that it is not amenable to mathematical manipulation.

$$\text{Interquartile range} = Q_3 - Q_1$$

When the average of interquartile range is calculates it is known as Quartile Deviation (QD)

$$\text{Quartile Deviation (QD)} = \frac{Q_3 - Q_1}{2} \text{ (for ungrouped data)}$$

Quartile deviation is the absolute measures of dispersion. The relative measures corresponding to this measure called the coefficient of quartile deviation.

$$\text{Coefficient of Quartile Deviation (QD)} = \frac{\frac{(Q_3 - Q_1)}{2}}{\frac{Q_3 + Q_1}{2}} = \frac{Q_3 - Q_1}{Q_3 + Q_1}$$

Calculation of Quartile Deviation for Ungrouped Data

For example, the score of 7 MBBS students in anatomy subject is given below. Compute the quartile deviation for given score.

Students	1	2	3	4	5	6	7
Score	20	28	40	12	30	15	50
Ascending order	12	15	20	28	30	40	50

$$Q_1 = \text{Size of } \frac{N+1}{4} = \frac{7+1}{4} = \text{2nd value}$$

So, Q_1 is 15 for given score

$$Q_3 = \text{Size of } 3\left(\frac{N+1}{4}\right) = 3\left(\frac{7+1}{4}\right) = \text{6th value}$$

So, Q_3 is 40 for score

$$QD = \frac{Q_3 - Q_1}{2} = 12.5$$

Calculation of Quartile Deviation for Grouped Data

$$Q_1 = L + \frac{\frac{N}{4} - cf}{f} \times i$$

$$Q_3 = L + \frac{\left(3\frac{N}{4} - cf\right)}{f} \times i$$

Where,

L = Lower limit of class interval on which quartile is found
cf = Cumulative frequency of previous class interval
f = Frequency of quartile deviation class interval
i = Class interval

$$\frac{N}{4} = \text{Size of quartile for } Q_1$$

$$\frac{3N}{4} = \text{Size of quartile for } Q_3$$

Example, Calculation of quartile deviation for grouped data.

Class	Frequency (f)	Cumulative frequency (cf)
5–9	2	2
10–14	4	6
15–19	9	15
20–24	12	27
25–29	6	33
30–34	3	36
	N = 36	

$$Q = \frac{Q_3 - Q_1}{2}$$

$$Q_1 = \frac{L + \frac{N}{4} - cf}{f} \times i$$

Where, L = Lower limit of quartile class interval
cf = Cumulative frequency of previous class interval
f = Frequency of quartile class interval
i = Class interval

$$\frac{N}{4} = \frac{36}{4} = 9$$

Here, L = 15, cf = 6, i = 5, f = 9

$$Q_1 = 15 + \frac{9-6}{9} \times 5 = 16.66$$

Similarly, for

$$Q_3 = \frac{3N}{4} = \frac{3 \times 36}{4} = 27, \text{ here } L = 20, cf = 15, f = 12, i = 5$$

$$= 20 \frac{27-15}{12} \times 5 = 25$$

Now, Q is $\frac{Q_3 - Q_1}{2} = \frac{25 - 16.66}{2} = 4.17$

MEAN DEVIATION

The mean deviation is also known as average deviation. It is average difference of the items in the distribution and the median or mean of that total score. Theoretically, the deviation of item from median is minimum when sign is ignored. However, in practice mean is mostly used for calculating the value of average deviation. So, it is known as *mean deviation*. It is denoted by MD.

Steps:
- Calculate average mean of the observation
- Calculate deviation—by ignoring sign of + and − and present these deviation |D|
- Compute total of these deviation, i.e. Σ |D|
- Divide the deviation from number of observation Σ |D|/N

Where,
$$MD = \frac{\Sigma |D|}{N}$$

$$|D| = X - A$$
X − A = Average value of deviation irrespective of sign (absolute value)

For example, Calculate mean deviation for following data.

X	4000	4200	4400	4600	4800	
X − A	−400	−200	0	200	400	Σ|D| = 1200

Mean for above data is:
A

So,
$$\bar{X} = \frac{\Sigma X}{N} = \frac{22000}{5} = 4400$$

$$= \frac{1200}{5} = 240$$

Substitute the value in given formula to get mean deviation. The mean deviation is 240.

Merits of Mean Deviation
- It is not much affected by fluctuation of sampling.
- It is rigidly defined.
- It is better utilized for comparison
- It is flexible to calculate from any measure of central tendency.

Demerits of Mean Deviation
- It is not very accurate measure of dispersion
- Mean deviation is not suitable for further mathematical application
- It is rarely used measure of dispersion

STANDARD DEVIATION

The concept of standard deviation (SD) is given by Karl Pearson in 1893. It is most widely used and important measure of dispersion. It has strength over weakness of all previous discussed measures of dispersion. It is also called *Root Mean Square Deviation* and denoted by a small Greek letter σ (read as *sigma*).

The standard deviation measure the absolute dispersion (variability) of distribution. The greater the amount of variability in distribution in data; greater the standard deviation.

Calculation of Standard Deviation for Ungrouped Data
For individual

$$\sigma = \sqrt{\frac{\Sigma x^2}{N}} = \sqrt{\frac{\Sigma (X - \bar{X})^2}{N}}$$

Where,

$(X - \bar{X})$ = Deviation of each item
$(X - \bar{X})^2$ = Square of deviation
$\Sigma(X - \bar{X})^2$ = Sum of square of deviation

For discrete data,

$$\sigma = \sqrt{\frac{\Sigma fx^2}{N}}$$

Where,

$x = (X - \bar{X})$ deviation of each item
N = Total number of observation
f = Number of observation

For example, a score of 10 engineering students in final examination is given below. Calculate the standard deviation for score.

X	x = X - X̄	x²
240	−24.1	580.81
260	−4.1	16.81
290	25.9	670.81
245	−19.1	364.81
255	−9.1	82.81
288	23.9	571.21
272	7.9	62.41
263	−1.1	1.21
277	12.9	166.41
251	−13.1	171.61
		Σx² = 2688.9

Substitute the value in above given formula to get standard value

$$SD = \sqrt{\frac{2688.9}{10}} = 16.39$$

So, standard deviation for score is 16.39.

Calculation of Standard Deviation by Assumed Mean Method

Apply following formula to calculate standard deviation

$$\sigma = \sqrt{\frac{\Sigma d^2}{N} - \left[\frac{\Sigma d}{N}\right]^2} = \frac{1}{n}\sqrt{n\Sigma d^2 - (\Sigma d)^2}$$

Where,

d = Deviation from assumed mean
N = Total number of observation
Σd = Sum of deviation from assumed mean
Σd^2 = Square of sum of deviation from assumed mean

Steps

- Assume any one of the value in the series as a mean
- Find out deviation from assumed mean (X - A)
- Square the deviation and sum up the square of deviation, i.e. Σd^2
- Substitute the value in given formula to get value of standard deviation

In case of frequency distribution also given, then use the following formula:

$$s = \sqrt{\frac{\Sigma fd^2}{N} - \left[\frac{\Sigma fd}{N}\right]^2} = \frac{1}{n}\sqrt{n\Sigma fd^2 - (\Sigma fd)^2}$$

For example, calculate the standard deviation of distance covered by 8 runners in Olympic race competition: (Where Assumed mean = 31)

X	f	d (X – A)	fd	fd²
20	5	–11	–55	605
22	12	–9	–108	972
25	15	–6	–90	540
31	20	0	0	0
35	25	4	100	400
40	14	9	126	1134
42	10	11	110	1210
45	6	14	84	1176
	N = 107		$\Sigma fd = 167$	$\Sigma fd^2 = 6037$

Substitute the values in given formula

$$= \sqrt{\frac{6037}{107} - \left(\frac{167}{107}\right)^2} = \sqrt{53.98} = 7.35$$

So, standard deviation of distance is 7.35.

Calculation of Standard Deviation for Group Data

Marks of 88 students on mental health nursing are given here:

Marks	f	Mid interval x	fx	fx²
0–10	6	5	30	150
10–20	16	15	240	3600
20–30	24	25	600	15000
30–40	25	35	875	30625
40–50	17	45	765	34425
	n = 88		$\Sigma fx = 2510$	$\Sigma fx^2 = 83,800$

$$\text{Mean } \bar{x} = \frac{\Sigma fx}{n} = \frac{2510}{88}$$

$$SD = \sqrt{\frac{\Sigma fx^2}{n} - \bar{x}^2} = \sqrt{\frac{83800}{88} - \left(\frac{2510}{8}\right)^2} = \sqrt{138.73}$$

$$SD = 11.78$$

Example, calculate standard deviation from the following data:

Class (X)	f	m	$d = \frac{(X - A)}{C}$	fd	fd²
0–10	8	5	–3	–24	72
10–20	12	15	–2	–24	48
20–30	17	25	–1	–17	17
30–40	14	A = 35	0	0	0
40–50	9	45	1	9	9
50–60	7	55	2	14	28
60–70	4	65	3	12	36
	N = 71			Σfd = –30	Σfd² = 210

Use of following formula will give standard deviation for the above data

$$SD = \sqrt{\frac{\Sigma fd^2}{N} - \left(\frac{\Sigma fd}{N}\right)^2} \times i$$

$$SD = \sqrt{\frac{210}{71} - \left(\frac{30}{71}\right)^2} \times 10$$

$$SD = 16.67$$

Calculation of Standard Deviation for Combined Observation

Sometimes, investigator has two or more than series of observation to compute combined standard deviation. We can compute combined mean and combined standard deviation by using the following formula:

Example, For a group of 50 male industry workers, the mean and standard deviation of their salary are ₹ 62 and ₹ 9 respectively. For another female group, salary is ₹ 54 and ₹ 6 respectively. Standard deviation for 90 industry workers is:

Characteristics	Group		Combined group
	Male	Female	
Size	$N_1 = 50$	$N_2 = 40$	$N_1 + N_2$
Mean	$\bar{X}_1 = 63$	$\bar{X}_2 = 54$	$\bar{X}_{12} = ?$
Standard deviation	$\sigma_1 = 9$	$\sigma_2 = 6$	$\sigma_{12} = 7$

$$\text{Combined Mean} = \bar{X}_{12} = \frac{N_1 \bar{X}_1 + N_2 \bar{X}_2}{N_1 N_2}$$

$$\bar{X}_{12} = \frac{50 \times 63 + 40 \times 54}{50 + 40}$$

$$d_1 = \overline{X}_{12} - \overline{X}_1 = 59 - 63 = -4$$
$$d_2 = \overline{X}_{12} - \overline{X}_2 = 59 - 54 = 5$$

$$\sigma_{12} = \sqrt{\frac{N_1\sigma_1^2 + N_2\sigma_2^2 + N_1 d_1 + N_2 d_2}{N_1 + N_2}}$$

σ_{12} = Combined standard deviation
σ_1 = σ of first set
σ_2 = σ of second set
$d_1 = \overline{X}_1$ - Combined mean
$d_2 = \overline{X}_2$ - Combined mean

$$= \sqrt{\frac{50 \times 9^2 + 40 \times 6^2 + 50(-4)^2 + 40 \times 5^2}{50 + 40}} = \sqrt{\frac{7290}{90}} = \sqrt{81} = 9$$

A comparison between standard and mean deviation is discussed in Table 12.11.

Table 12.11: Mean deviation and standard deviation: A comparison.

Standard deviation	Mean deviation
It is calculated from mean only	It can be calculated from any measure of central tendency, mean, median or mode
Mathematically, it is bit difficulty to analyze	It is comparatively easy to calculate
It takes algebraic signs into consideration therefore, considered mathematically sound	It does not take algebraic sign into consideration and therefore considered weak

COEFFICIENT OF VARIATION

The standard deviation is not a useful measure to compare the variability of two or more series of data with different unit of measurement and mean value. For example, consider a series with 5 as standard deviation and 30 as mean value. On the other hand, another series is with 10 as standard deviation and 100 as mean value. Here, standard deviation is not a useful measure to compare the variability between two groups.

The coefficient of variation (CV) developed by Karl Pearson as a relative measure of dispersion. The coefficient of variation can be used to measure the variability of two or more set of data with different unit of measurement and mean valves.

Coefficient of variation is obtained by dividing the standard deviation by the mean value and multiplying it by 100.

$$CV = \frac{SD}{\overline{X}} \times 100$$

In case of less value of CV, the group is less variable, more stable, more uniform and more consistent or homogenous in nature.

Example 1: In two factories X and Y, the average weekly wages (in rupees) and SD as follows:

Factory	Average	SD	No. of employees
X	40	5	500
Y	45	4.5	300

Calculate which factory pay large pay scale for employees?
Given values, $N_x = 500$, $N_y = 300$, $\overline{X}_x = 40$, $\overline{X}_y = 28.5$, $SD_x = 5$, $SD_y = 45.5$
Substitute the values in above given formula

$$CV_x = 625, CV_y = 300$$

So, factory X pays more salary to employees.

Example 2: In two factories X and Y, working in same industrial area the average weekly salary (in Indian Rupees) and standard deviation is given below. Calculate which factory has greater variation in salary?

Factory	Average	Standard Deviation	No. of workers
X	34.5	5	476
Y	28.5	4.5	524

Coefficient variation (CV) of weekly distribution of salary in factory X

$$CV(X) = \frac{\sigma}{\overline{X}} \times 100 = \frac{5}{34.5} \times 100 = 14.49\%$$

Coefficient variation (CV) of weekly salary distribution of factory Y

$$CV(Y) = \frac{4.5}{28.5} \times 100 = 15.79\%$$

So, faculty of factory Y has greater variability in individual salary.

COEFFICIENT OF CORRELATION

The correlation is a statistical measure for finding out the degree (or strength) of the relationship between two variables. It is also called as *Pearson's product Moment coefficient correlation* or Pearson's coefficient correlation. There are many types of correlation coefficient but this section is limited to Pearson correlation coefficient. The Pearson r measures of linear relationships between two variables. Pearson's coefficient correlation is use when both observation are on interval or ratio level.

A *positive correlation* between two variables indicates that as the measures on one variable increase. So do the measures of another.

A negative relationships means that the observation for two variables are moving in different directions. As the measures of one variable increases, they tend to decreases on second variable. It can be also understood in the form of inverse relationship between two variables.

Pearson's coefficient correlation only work on assumption of linear relationships between two variables. Since relationship between two variables are not linear, one should prepare a scatter plot. A scatter diagram can be constructed by plotting one variable (x) (abscissa) on the horizontal axis and another variable (y) on vertical (ordinate) axis. A linear relationship between two variables come as straight line in scatter plot.

The value of correlation coefficient index range from –1.00 for *'perfect negative'* correlation, through zero for *'no relationship'*, to +1.00 for *'perfect positive relationship'*. The higher the value (absolute) of correlation coefficient indicates strength of relationship. For example, a value of –0.35 is stronger than a value of +0.25. Correlation coefficient ranging from 0 to 0.19 are considered *very weak*; correlation coefficient ranging from 0.2 to 0.39 are considered *weak*, correlation coefficient ranging from 0.4 to 0.59 are considered *moderately weak*; correlation coefficient ranging from 0.6 to 0.79 are considered *strong*; and correlation coefficient ranging from 0.8 to 1.00 are considered *very strong*.

Types of Correlation Coefficient (Fig. 12.11)

Pearson's product moment coefficient correlation represent linear relationship between two variables. Linear relationship range from –1.00 (perfect negative) to +1.00 (perfect positive). Following types of relationship can be possible between two variables.
1. *Perfect positive relationship:* Both variables increase or decrease in same direction.
2. *Perfect negative relationship:* Both variables increase or decrease in opposite direction.
3. *Absolute no correlation:* No impact of change in one variable on other variable.
4. *Moderate +ve correlation:* Slight impact of change in one variable on other in same direction.
5. *Moderate –ve correlation:* Slight impact of change in one variable on other variable in opposite direction.

Significance of Coefficient Correlation

- Coefficient correlation is used to assess strength and direction of linear relationships between two variables
- Correlation coefficient used to assess reliability of a research instrument or intervention going to be used in a research
- It helps to test null hypotheses and thus able to make conclusion for acceptance or rejection about a intervention.
- Correlation matrices (generally Pearson) are among the most widely used techniques for studying the construct validity of data in factor analysis, whether exploratory or confirmatory.

Calculation of Coefficient Correlation (r)-Direct Method (Ungrouped Data)

The coefficient correlation can be calculated by using the following formula:

$$r = \frac{N\Sigma XY}{\sqrt{[N(\Sigma X)^2][N(\Sigma Y)^2]}}$$

$$r = \frac{\Sigma(X-\bar{X})\Sigma(Y-\bar{Y})}{\sqrt{[\Sigma d(X-\bar{X})^2][\Sigma d(Y-\bar{Y})^2]}} = \frac{\Sigma dx\, dy}{\sqrt{\Sigma dx^2\, \Sigma dy^2}}$$

Where,
$$dx = X - \bar{X} \text{ and } dy = Y - \bar{Y}$$

Box 12.5: Interpretation of Coefficient Correlations.

a. 0.90 to 1.00 (–0.90 to –1.00): Very high positive (negative) correlation
b. 0.70 to 0.90 (–0.70 to –0.90): High positive (negative) correlation
c. 0.50 to 0.70 (–0.50 to –0.70): Moderate positive (negative) correlation
d. 0.30 to 0.50 (–.030 to –0.50): Low positive (negative) correlation
e. 0.00 to 0.30 (0.00 to –0.30): Negligible correlation

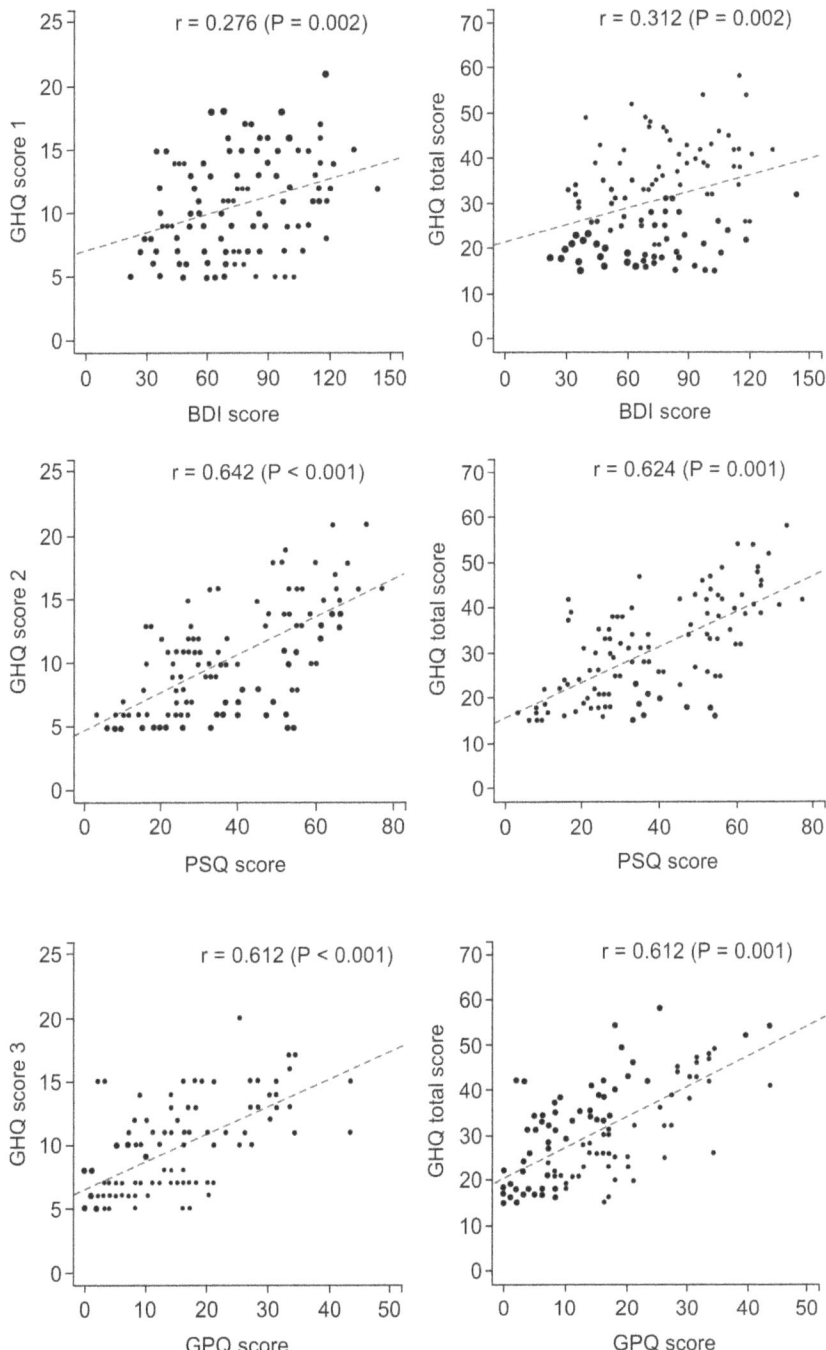

Fig. 12.11: Types of correlation coefficient.

A data on X and Y variables are given in table. Calculate correlation coefficient by direct method.

X	X²	Y	Y²	XY
9	81	15	225	135
8	64	16	256	128
7	49	14	196	98
6	36	13	169	78
5	25	12	144	60
4	16	11	121	44
3	9	10	100	30
2	4	8	64	16
1	1	9	81	9
ΣX = 45	ΣX² = 285	ΣY = 108	ΣY² = 1356	ΣXY = 597

$$r = \frac{N\Sigma XY}{\sqrt{\left[N(\Sigma X)^2\right]\left[N(\Sigma Y)^2\right]}}$$

$$r = \frac{\Sigma(X-\bar{X})\,\Sigma(Y-\bar{Y})}{\sqrt{\left[\Sigma d(X-\bar{X})^2\right]\left[\Sigma d(Y-\bar{Y})^2\right]}} = \frac{\Sigma dx\,dy}{\sqrt{\Sigma dx^2\,\Sigma dy^2}}$$

N = 9, ΣXY = 597, ΣX = 45, ΣY = 108, ΣX² = 285, ΣY² = 1356.
Substitute the values in given formula to calculate correlation coefficient. For this data r is 0.95.

Calculation of Coefficient Correlation (For Group Data)

$$r = \frac{N\Sigma xy - \Sigma x \Sigma y}{\sqrt{N\Sigma x^2 - (\Sigma x)^2}\sqrt{N\Sigma y^2 - \Sigma y^2}}$$

Where,
x = Deviation of x series from mean, i.e. (X - $\bar{X}$)
y = Deviation of y series from mean, i.e. (Y - $\bar{Y}$)

When deviation are taken from assumed mean method, use following formula:

$$r = \frac{N\Sigma dxdy - \Sigma dx \Sigma dy}{\sqrt{N\Sigma dx^2 - (\Sigma dx)^2}\sqrt{N\Sigma dy^2 - \Sigma dy^2}}$$

Where,
dx = Deviation of x series from an assumed mean, i.e. (X - $\bar{X}$)
dy = Deviation of y series from an assumed mean, i.e. (Y - $\bar{Y}$)
Σdxdy = Sum of the product of deviation of x and y series from their assumed mean.
Σdx² = Sum of the square of the deviation of x series from an assumed mean.
Σdy² = Sum of the square of the deviation of y series from an assumed mean.

SPEARMAN'S RANK CORRELATION COEFFICIENT

Spearman's rank correlation is a non-parametric test which describe a linear relationship between two variables. Spearman coefficient is abbreviated by symbol (ρ) rho. It is an appropriate index for nominal and ordinal level data. Pearson correlation is calculated by the rank of value of each of the variable rather than instead of their actual value.

$$\rho = 1 - \frac{6\Sigma D^2}{N(N^2 - 1)}$$

Where,

D = Difference between ranks of two series
N = Number of pair of observation

Marks of 5 students on subjects X and Y are given here:

X	Y	Rank Rx	Rank Ry	D = Rx − Ry	D²
78	84	7.5	10	−2.5	6.25
45	55	2	4	−2	4
36	50	1	3	−2	4
78	60	7.5	5	2.5	6.25
62	82	6	9	−3	9
					ΣD² = 29.50

Substitute the value in above formula

$$\rho = 1 - \frac{6 \times 29.5}{5(25 - 1)} = -0.45$$

So, rank correlation coefficient is −0.45.

NORMAL DISTRIBUTION CURVE

The normal distribution has another place in statistics. Although, normal distribution is remain mysterious concept to many. When a large pool of information is called we call the pattern of value obtained distribution. A large set of biological/experimental observation may follow symmetrical or asymmetrical distribution. If the data are normally distributed on both sides of mean and form a bell-shaped curve in frequency distribution curve, the distribution of data is called normal or Gaussian distribution. Majority of biological parameters usually lie around a central point, with symmetrical negative and positive distribution about this central point. The standard normal distribution curve is *'bell shaped'*. The distribution of normal score is presented as follows:

50% score lies within ± 0.68 SD
68% score lies within ± 1 SD
95% score lies within ± 1.96 SD
95.45% score lies within ± 2 SD
99% score lies within ± 2.58 SD
99.73% score lies within ± 3 SD

The modal probably originated in 1733 by Abraham Demoivre. Karl Pearson Gauss found a new deviation of the formula curve in 1809s and thereafter normal curve also known as the *'Gaussian Curve'*.

Salient Features of Normal Distribution

- The normal distribution is bell or breast shaped and symmetric about mean
- In a normal distribution, total area under the curve is equal to one

- It is universal applicable to biological phenomena occurring to nature
- All measures of central tendency are coincide or equal to each other at highest level of normal distribution curve, i.e. Mean = Median = Mode
- It is symmetrical and asymptotic, i.e. the distribution graph approached towards end but never touch the horizontal line
- In a normal distribution curve, the greatest proportions of scores lie close to the mean
- Almost all the scores (0.9997 of them) lie within the 3SD of the mean (Mean ± 3SD = 99.73). Example is shown in Figure 12.12.
- The area under the curve to left of equals to the area under the curve to right of both of these area are equal to ½
- Both parts are mirror image of each other and can cover each one.

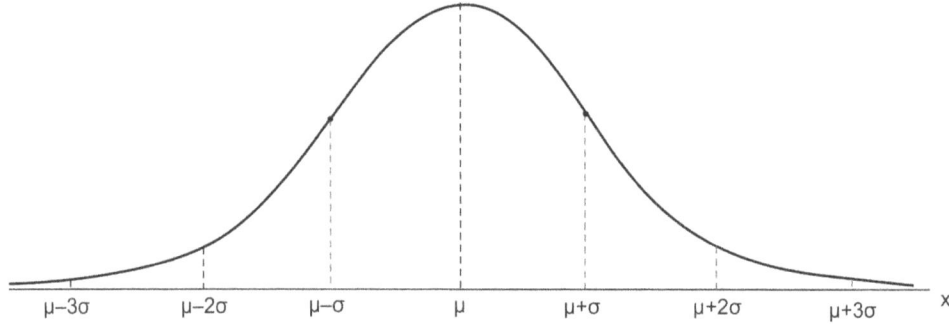

Fig. 12.12: Normal distribution curve.

The value of standard deviation determines the spread. The bigger the σ; the more spread out or flat the curve. The value of mean fixes the location of normal curve, where it is centered. In all of the normal curves half of the scores lies to left of the mean and half to the right.

Significance of Normal Distribution Curve
- The probability of any observation or number of observation lying below or above at any distance from the mean can be estimated
- It used to compute confidence limit of the population parameter
- It form the basis for testing hypotheses
- It helps to study sample mean and standards deviation in large defined sample
- It helps to define normal and abnormal limit of biological parameters, i.e. blood pressure, weight, height, etc.

Shape of Normal Curve
Normal distribution curve is bell shaped and thus often called bell curve. It is symmetrical representation of observation; that is, the left and right halves of the curve are mirror image of each other and can cover each one. However, in few observations, the distribution curve change from symmetrical to asymmetrical. This is called *skewness*. For example, income level of Indian population. Here, a small group of population has a tail of extreme very low or high earning side and therefore, shift the curve towards left or right side.

In order to use the normal distribution, it is necessary to be able to determine areas under the curve of the normal distribution. These are given in the figure here. As given in the diagram, this is the area under the normal distribution between the center, Z = 0 and the value of Z indicated.

Example, distribution of area under normal probability curve (Fig. 12.13).

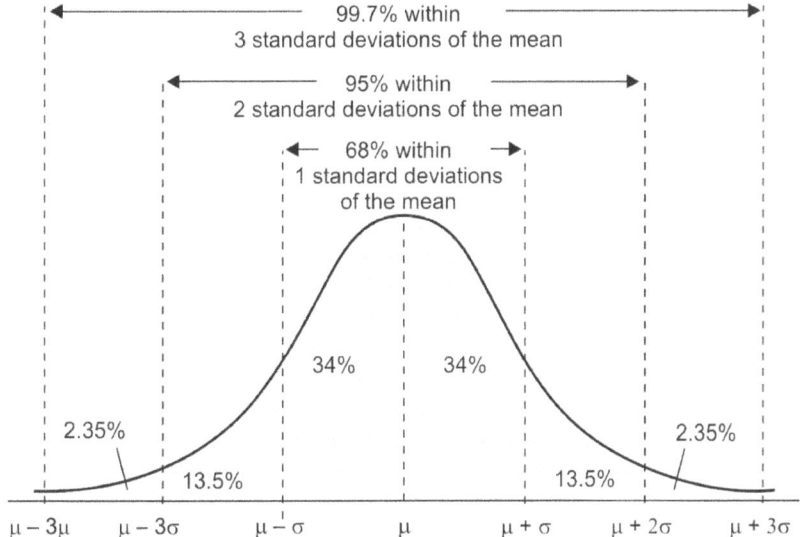

Fig. 12.13: Shape of normal distribution curve.

Skewness and Kurtosis

Skewness

The positions of the mean, median, and mode are affected by whether a distribution is normally distributed or skewed. The data are normally distributed when Mean = Median = Mode, any deviation in symmetry of data called skewness. It may be negative or positive in nature.

Positive skewness: In a positive skewed distribution, the tail of distribution larger towards higher value of the variables and right hand side and hump is to the left side (Fig. 12.14).

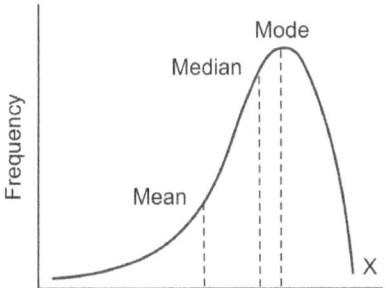
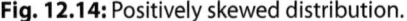
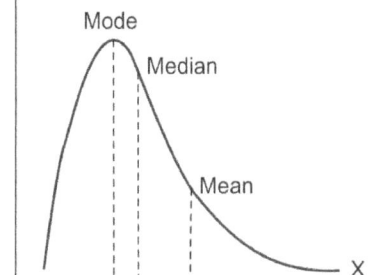

Fig. 12.14: Positively skewed distribution.　　Fig. 12.15: Negatively skewed distribution.

Negative skewness: In a negative skewed distribution, the tail of the distribution longer towards lower values of the variables and left hand side and hump is to the right side (Fig. 12.15).

Measures of Skewness

The following measures are used to compute skewness in the distribution of data.

a. Karl-Pearson's coefficient of skewness

$$= \frac{\text{Mean} - \text{Mode}}{2}$$

b. Bowley's coefficient of skewness

$$= \frac{Q_3 + Q_1 - \text{Median}}{Q_3 - Q_1}$$

Kurtosis

The expressions 'kurtosis' is used to describe the peakness or flatness of normal distribution curve. Usually, all the frequency curves expose different degree of flatness or peakness. It is called Kurtosis (Fig. 12.16).

Measures of Kurtosis

It is based on frequency distribution and denoted by β_2.

$$\beta_2 = \frac{\mu_3}{\mu_2}$$

If,

$\beta_2 = 3$ = Mesokurtic curve
$\beta_2 > 3$ = Leptokurtic curve
$\beta_2 < 3$ = Platykurtic curve

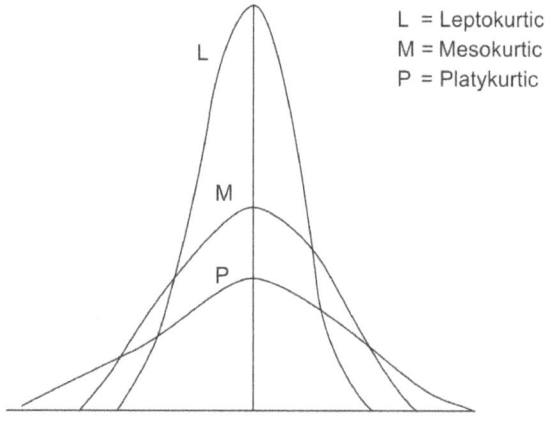

Fig. 12.16: Kurtosis.

INFERENTIAL STATISTICS

Inferential statistics involves techniques for making inferences about the whole population on the basis of observations obtained from a random sample. It use a random sample from selected population to draw conclusion or inference about the whole population. Inferential statistics helps a researcher to answer or test the hypothesis.

The findings of inferential statistics are usually expressed in term of probability. Probability is the measure of the likelihood that an event will occur. Probability value quantified between 0 to 1 (0- no event, 1- true event). Examples, student t-test, z-test, one way ANOVA, and regression, etc.

HYPOTHESIS TESTING

Statistical hypothesis testing provides objective criteria for deciding whether hypotheses are accepted or rejected. To test a hypothesis, a researcher need three basic information. The first is type of information or data or level of measurement. The second is sample size and this is whether sample are paired or unpaired or in other words dependent or independent to each others. Hypothesis testing need to devise of two opposite hypotheses.

A researcher should ensure that enough evidence is available to reject or accept null (statistical) hypothesis. By rejecting null hypothesis the researcher can 'accept' research or alternate hypothesis. A researcher has to state both null and research hypothesis to test the significance. For example, impact of 0.5 mL normal saline instillation on blood pressure variation during suctioning. Here, a researcher has to answer whether the change in blood pressure is by chance or because of intervention (0.5 mil normal saline) by comparing the group with other group (control). Statistical hypothesis testing allow a researcher to make objective conclusion about the study findings.

a. The null hypothesis (H_0): The null hypothesis state no significant group difference between experimental and control group on assertiveness skill score:
$$H_0 = \mu_E = \mu_C$$
b. The research hypothesis (H_1): The research hypothesis state a significant group difference between experimental and control group on assertiveness skill score.
$$H_1 = \mu_E \neq \mu_C$$

Level of Significance

To test the hypothesis, a cutoff point is selected before data collection. The cutoff point referred to as alpha (α) or the level of statistical significance. It is a point at which the level of statistical analysis judged to indicate a statistical significant difference between the groups. The two most preferred level of significance are (known as alpha or α) are 0.01 and 0.05. With a 0.01 significant level, we accept the risk that out of 100 sample, a true hypothesis wrongly rejected one time. In 99 out of 100 cases, however, a true null hypothesis would be correctly accepted. With 0.05 significant level, the risk of making type I error is higher than 0.01 level of significance. It indicates that in 5 sample out of 100 would be wrongly reject the null hypothesis. However, 0.05 is the most preferred level of significance in nursing studies. The level of significance is dichotomous, which means that difference is either significant or nonsignificant: there is no 'degrees' of significance.

Type I and Type II Errors

Statistical inference about accepting or rejecting a hypothesis based on incomplete information, so there is always risk. While testing hypothesis, a researcher can make following two types of errors.
- Type I error
- Type II error

Type I Error

Researcher can make a type I error by rejecting the null hypothesis when it is actually true. Type I error also called as level of significance and denoted by alpha (α). Type I error is usually fixed in advance by choosing the level of significance employed on the test, i.e. 5% or 1%, etc. In medical studies, type I error is more serious than type II and may allow a bad intervention or unsafe drug to come into the market.

Type II Error

Researcher can make type II error by rejecting a research hypothesis when it is actually true. Type II error denoted by beta (β). Higher the type II error prevent a good intervention/drug to come into the market. Although, the chances of type II error is still unknown.
- *Beta (β):* The probability of failing to reject the null hypothesis when it is actually false
- *Power (or statistical power):* The probability of rejecting the null hypothesis when it is actually false.

Both beta and power are calculated for specific possible values of the alternatives hypothesis.

Table 12.12: Type I and type II errors.

Inference	Accept it	Reject it
H_0 is true	Correct decision (√)	Type I error
H_0 is false	Type II error	Correct decision (√)

To minimize the errors of chance, we should take a large and random sample as possible and interpret the result at 5% level of significance. In one tailed test, if the result is interpreted at 10% (equivalent to 5% in two tailed test) level, the risk of minimizing type I error is reduced. Normally, a researcher want to reduce the risk of committing both types of errors, but unfortunately lowering the risk of type I error increase the risk of committing type II error.

PARAMETRIC AND NONPARAMETRIC TESTS

Parametric Tests

Parametric tests involve estimation of parameter which are at interval or ratio level. Parametric test involves several assumptions like normal distribution of data and large sample size, etc. Parametric tests application is lengthy and laborious process. Parametric test includes t-test, one way ANOVA, simple and linear regression, and Pearson's correlation coefficient, etc.

Nonparametric Test

Generally, nonparametric tests are easy and simple to apply. They do not require any assumptions to be followed like distribution of population in normal fashion and large sample size. For this reason, nonparametric test sometimes called as *distribution free test*. These tests are appropriate choice for data distributed on nominal and ordinal scale. Usually, nonparametric tests can be applied to small sample size and therefore is a good alternatives for study a rare phenomenon or disease. Nonparametric test includes sign test, Kruskal-Wallis test, Spearman's rho correlation and Mann Whitney test, etc. A comparison of parametric and nonparametric test is discussed in Table 12.13.

Table 12.13: Parametric and nonparametric tests: A comparison.

Basis	Parametric tests	Nonparametric tests
Data distribution	Normal	Any distribution
Assumed variance	Homogenous	Any
Type of data	Interval or ratio level	Nominal or ordinal
Measure of central tendency used	Mean	Median
Data set relationships	Independent	Any
Types of tests	T-test (paired and unpaired), Pearson correlation coefficient (r) ANOVA (one way and two way)	Sign test, Friedman test, Median test, Mann Whitney U test, Kruskal-Wallis test

Degree of Freedom (df)

The goal of statistical analysis is to understood how the variables (or parameter to be studied) and observations are linked to each others. Degree of freedom is an abstract and difficult statistical concept. Many elementary statistics textbook introduces this concept in terms of the number that are 'free or vary'. It is index number for identifying which distribution is used.

Hence, degree of freedom is function of both sample size (N) and the number of independent observation (N) or the number of the subjects in the data, minus number of parameter (k) estimated. A researcher may estimate parameters using different amount and pieces of information and the number of independent pieces of information he or she uses to estimate a statistics or a parameter called degree of freedom and denoted by df. The procedure of calculation df is vary from test to test.

TESTS OF SIGNIFICANCE

Chi-Square Test

The chi-square (χ^2) test used to test hypothesis to find out group differences in proportion. It was developed by Karl Pearson called chi-square denoted with the Greek letter (χ) and read as 'kye'. The chi-square has following three important applications:
- Tests of independence or association
- Test of homogeneity
- Test of goodness of fit.

Assumptions of the Chi-square Test Application

The basic assumptions underlying the application of the chi-square test are as follows:
1. The observation are independent to each other and should not have any influence of one observation over other.
2. The expected cell frequency should be large enough to apply chi-square test. A frequency of more than 5 is considered large enough. However, a frequency smaller than five necessitate the application of Yate's correction.

Chi-Square Test of Association/Independence

A test of independence tests the null hypothesis that there is no association between two variables in the contingency table where the data is collected from a single population.
- H_0: The two categorical variables are independent, (i.e. there is no relationship between them)
- H_A: The two categorical variables are dependent, (i.e. there is a relationship between them).

Steps of Chi-Square Calculation

a. Make the contingency table: The frequency observed (O) in class of one event, row wise, i.e. horizontally and then the number in each group of the other events, column wise, i.e. vertically.

Groups	Result outcomes		Total
	Died	Survived	
Experimental	15	25	40
Control	5	40	45
	20	65	85

b. Determine the expected frequencies (E) in each cell: Expected frequency in contingency table calculated by using the following formula:

$$\text{Expected frequency (E)} = \frac{\text{Raw Total} \times \text{Column Total}}{\text{Grand Total}}$$

c. Find the difference between the observed and expected frequencies in each cell of table (O - E)
d. Sum up all values and substitute in following formula to compute χ^2 value

$$\chi^2 = \Sigma \frac{(O-E)^2}{E}$$

e. Calculate degree of freedom (df)

$$df = \text{row} - 1 \times \text{column} - 1$$

In an experiment of immunization of cattle from tuberculosis, the following results are obtained.

Immunization status	Affected	Not affected
Inoculated	12	26
Not inoculated	16	6

	Affected	Not affected	Total
Inoculated (O)	12	26	38
E	17.73	20.27	
Not inoculated (O)	16	6	22
E	10.27	11.73	
Total	28	32	06

Calculate (O–E), (O–E)² and $\frac{(O-E)^2}{E}$

(O – E)	(O – E)²	$\frac{(O-E)^2}{E}$
–5.73	32.83	1.85
5.73	32.83	3.19
5.73	32.83	1.62
–5.73	32.83	2.79
		$\sum \frac{(O-E)^2}{E} = 9.45$

So, chi-square value is 9.45.

Direct Method of Chi-Square Calculation (2 × 2 table)

In case of 2 × 2 contingency table, Chi-square can also be calculated by using following formula

A	B
C	D

$$\chi^2 = \frac{(ad - bc)^2 (a+b+c+d)}{(a+b)(c+d)(a+c)(b+d)}$$

Chi-Square Test for Homogeneity

Test of homogeneity test the null hypothesis that different groups have the similar characteristics on a given variables. Usually, in experimental study, chi-square test is used to test homogeneity between experimental and control group. In case the calculated p value s more than 0.05, then the groups are considered homogeneous on a particular variable. A example of homogeneity testing is given as follows.

Variables	Exp group	Control group	χ^2, df and p-value
Age (Years)			
20–25	10	10	9.87
26–30	15	12	2
31–35	05	08	0.09
Gender			5.98
Male	20	10	1
Female	10	20	.08

Chi-Square Test of Goodness of Fit (Normality Test)

In hypothesis testing, it is difficult to find out the distribution pattern of data collected from a large dispersed population. The Goodness of fit test examine the validity of data distribution before actual statistic application. It is the mean of the differences between the observed and expected frequencies, each squared and divided by the expectations. The formula is given as follows:

$$Q^2 = \sum_{i=1}^{k} \frac{(O_i - E_i)^2}{E_i}$$

Here,
O_i = Observed outcome frequency
E_i = Expected (theoretical frequency)
$i = 1, 2, 3, \ldots\ldots\ldots k$ is the class number

Limitations of Chi-Square Application
- Chi-square test only convey the presence and absence of an association but does not measure the strength of association
- Chi-square statistical findings does not indicate the cause and effect relationship.

THE t-TEST

Theoretical work on t-distribution was done by WS Gossett (1876–1937). He has given this test and thereafter, this 't' distribution is named on his pet name 'student' and thereafter, called student 't' test. It is applied to find out the significant difference between two means or means of two groups. This test can be applied in following conditions:

Assumptions of t-Test Application

t-test application based on assumption of parametric test. A few important assumption are as follow:
- Sample drawn from a population should show normal distribution
- The two samples of comparison must be independently sample from a same population
- The two sample of comparison should be of equal variance and drawn randomly from a same population.

Types of t-Tests

The t-test is further divided in following ways:
1. Unpaired/Independent sample t-test
2. Paired/Dependent sample t-test
3. t-test for one sample.

Paired/Dependent Sample t-Test

This test is used when there are two different interventions and all subjects exposed to both experimental conditions. This is also called as paired sample t-test. For example, a researcher interested to look the effect of relaxation therapy on the anxiety level in geriatric population.

$$H_0 = \mu_A = \mu_B$$

$$t = \frac{\bar{d} - 0}{SD} \times \sqrt{n} \text{ or } \frac{\bar{d}\sqrt{n}}{SD}$$

Where,
$$SD = \sqrt{\frac{(d - \bar{d}^2)}{n - 1}}$$

For example, to verify the effect of a class on performance in a test on 12 students before and after the class.

Before class	After class	Difference (d)	d²
44	53	+9	81
40	38	−2	44
61	69	+8	64
52	57	+5	25
32	46	+14	196
44	39	−5	25
70	73	+3	9
41	48	+7	49
67	73	+6	36
		$\Sigma d = 45$	$\Sigma d^2 = 489$

$$\bar{d} = \frac{\Sigma d}{n} = \frac{45}{9} = 5$$

$$SD = \sqrt{\frac{\Sigma d^2 - n(\bar{d})^2}{n-1}}$$

Substitute the value in given formula to compute t-value.

So, t-value is 5.74.

Since the calculated t-value is greater than table value (1.45, at 5% level, 8 df) we reject the null hypothesis and accept alternative hypothesis.

Unpaired/Independent Sample t-Test

This test is used where there are two interventions and different group or subjects are exposed to different intervention. It is called *independent sample test*.

$$\tau = \frac{\bar{X}_1 - \bar{X}_2}{SD} \times \frac{n_1 n_2}{n_1 + n_2}$$

for

$$SD = \sqrt{\frac{\Sigma(X_1 - \bar{X}_1)^2 + \Sigma(X_2 - \bar{X}_2)^2}{n_1 + n_2 - 2}}$$

Where,

$\bar{X}_1$ = Mean of first sample
$\bar{X}_2$ = Mean of the second sample
n_1 = Number of observation of first sample
n_2 = Number of observation of second sample
SD = Combined standard deviation

For example, two types of drugs were used on five patients and seven patients for reducing their weight.

Drug A	10	12	13	11	14		
Drug B	8	9	12	14	15	10	9

Apply independent sample t-test

$$\tau = \frac{\bar{X}_1 - \bar{X}_2}{SD} \times \frac{n_1 n_2}{n_1 + n_2}$$

X_1	$(X_1 - \bar{X}_1)$	$(X_1 - \bar{X}_1)^2$	X_2	$(X_1 - \bar{X}_2)$	$(X_1 - \bar{X}_2)^2$
10	−2	4	8	−2	4
12	0	0	9	−1	1
13	1	1	12	2	4
11	−1	1	14	4	16
14	2	4	15	5	25
			10	0	0
			9	−1	1
$\Sigma X_1 = 60$		$\Sigma(X_1 - \bar{X}_1)^2 = 10$	$\Sigma X_2 = 77$		$\Sigma(X_2 - \bar{X}_2)^2 = 44$

Now, substitute the values in above given formula

$$\bar{X}_1 = \frac{\Sigma X_1}{N_1} = \frac{60}{5} = 12$$

$$\bar{X}_2 = \frac{\Sigma X_2}{N_2} = \frac{77}{11} = 7$$

Calculate value of

$$SD = \sqrt{\frac{\Sigma(X_1 - \bar{X}_1)^2 + \Sigma(X_2 - \bar{X}_2)^2}{n_1 + n_2 - 2}} = \sqrt{\frac{10 + 44}{5 + 7 - 2}} = 2.32$$

Substitute the value of SD and mean to compute t-value. So, t-value = 6.28.

To Test the Significance of the Mean of a Random Sample

The one sample t-test is to determine the difference between a mean value in a sample compared to the population.

$$t = \frac{X - \mu}{SD} \times \sqrt{n}$$

$$SD = \sqrt{\frac{(X - \bar{X})^2}{n - 1}} \text{ (for deviation from mean)}$$

$$= \sqrt{\frac{\Sigma d^2 - n(d)^2}{n - 1}} \text{ (for assumed mean method)}$$

Where,

$\bar{X}$ = The mean of the sample
μ = The actual or hypothetical mean of the population
n = Sample size
SD = Standard deviation
d = Deviation from assumed mean

Degree of Freedom for t-test

Degree of freedom for independent and dependent sample test will be calculated as follows.
Independent sample *t*-test = Number of observation–2 (n–2)
Dependent (paired) sample *t*-test = Number of observation–1 (n–1).

THE Z-TEST

When the sample size large enough (>30), and a researcher want to compare the difference in population mean or the difference between two sample means, use of Z-test has advantage over t-test. A researcher should follow following assumptions before applying Z-test:
a. The selected sample or samples should be random in nature
b. The data must be quantitative and on interval or ratio level
c. The ample should be normally distributed
d. The sample size should be large enough (>30)

Application of Z-test

Z-test for mean had two applications as given below:
- To test the mean difference between a sample mean and a known value of the population mean. It can be used by using following formula:

$$Z = \frac{\text{Mean (X)} - \text{Population } (\mu)}{\text{SE of sample mean}}$$

- To test the mean difference of two sample means or between one experimental and control means. Use of following formula will help to find it:

$$Z = \frac{\text{Observed difference between two sample means}}{\text{SE of difference between two sample means}}$$

However, calculation of standard error of mean (SE) and mean difference is calculation is similar to the t-test.

Interpretation of Z-Test

In Z-test df is not computed to determine the significance of Z-value in comparison of p-value. The interpretation will be done by taking the help of computed table on the basis of normal distribution. If the calculates Z-value is greater than tabulated Z-value, the result is significant and we reject the null hypothesis. In other side, if calculated Z-value is less than tabulated Z-value, the result is not significant and we accept the null hypothesis.

ANALYSIS OF VARIANCE (ANOVA)

Analysis of variance technique is developed by RA Fisher in 1920s. Analysis of variance frequently referred as ANOVA. It is a statistical technique specially designed to test the significant difference in sample means of more than two quantitative population means. Basically, it consists of classifying and cross classifying statistical results and testing the significant differences in means of population. Although, t-test is also useful to detect the significant difference in means of more than two populations but application of t-test will be laborious process and increase the chances of type I error. These limitations can be overcome by use of ANOVA in place of t-test. Therefore, it is understood that ANOVA is used to compare the means of more than two samples drawn from normally distributed population.

For example, a researcher wants to see the effect of 0.5 mL, 01 mL, 1.5 mL and 2.0 mL normal saline instillation on change in vital parameters like blood pressure, respiration, and heart rate. To test whether changes in vital parameters differ significantly to instillation of amount of normal saline or not, F-test or analysis of variance test (ANOVA) has to apply. Here, application of ANOVA gives precise results than t-test.

Assumptions of ANOVA Applications

ANOVA is a parametric test used to measure difference between means of more than two groups. A researcher has to follow certain assumptions before application of one way ANOVA. The following assumptions should be followed before application of ANOVA.
- *Variability:* The variability of each group must be approximately equal to the variability of every other group in the analysis.
- *Normal distribution of data:* Score of the independent must be normally distributed.
- *Data on ratio and interval scale:* The data for dependent variable must be on interval and ratio level.
- *Large sample size:* For better statistical inference, a large sample size is needed for ANOVA applications.

Steps of ANOVA Calculation

For example, whiteness reading made in 17 cloths with four types of detergents A, B, C, D is given below,

A	B	C	D
77	74	73	76
81	66	78	85
61	58	57	77
76		69	64
69		63	
$\Sigma A = 364$	$\Sigma B = 198$	$\Sigma C = 340$	$\Sigma D = 302$

Steps of Computation of ANOVA
- Calculate the total sum of the observations of the group under study by suing following formula
$$= (\Sigma A)^2 + (\Sigma B)^2 + (\Sigma C)^2 + (\Sigma D)^2$$
- Calculate the correction factors (C) by using the following formula
$$C = \frac{(\Sigma A + \Sigma B + \Sigma C + \Sigma D)^2}{n_A + n_B + n_C + n_D}$$

$$C = \frac{(\text{Total Sum of Observation})^2}{\text{Total number of observation}(n)}$$

- Calculate total sum of the squares of all the observations by using following formula
$$= (\Sigma A)^2 + (\Sigma B)^2 + (\Sigma C)^2 + (\Sigma D)^2 - C$$
- Calculate total sum of squares between the groups by using following formula
$$SS_B = (\Sigma A)^2 + (\Sigma B)^2 + (\Sigma C)^2 + (\Sigma D)^2 - C$$
- Calculate sum of the squares with in groups by using following formula
$$SS_W = SS_T - SS_B$$
- Calculate the df for between and within groups
  - For between groups = number of groups −1
  - For with in groups = number of subjects in all groups−number of groups
  - df total = number of subjects in all groups −1
- Finally, calculate the F-ratio by using the given formula:

$$\text{F-ratio} = \frac{\text{Mean of the sum of the squares between the groups}}{\text{Mean of the sum of the squares within the groups}}$$

Preparation of ANOVA Table

The ANOVA table is looks as given below:

Sources of variation	Sum of squares	df	Mean square	F- ratio
Between subjects	216.67	k − 1 = 4 − 1 = 3	72.22	1.07
Within subjects	873.80	N − k = 17 − 4 = 13	67.22	

$$\text{F-ratio} = \frac{\text{Sum of Square between groups}}{\text{Sum of Square with in groups}} = \frac{SS_B}{SS_W} = \frac{72.22}{67.22} = 1.07$$

Interpretation of ANOVA Value

Acceptance or rejection of null hypothesis is decided from the column labeled as variance Ratio (F-Ratio), if calculated F-value is greater than F-tabulated critical value for given degrees of freedom at 5% (or selected level of significance) level then reject the null hypothesis or if the calculated F-value is less than F-tabulated critical value for a given degrees of freedom at 5% level than accept the null hypothesis.

In given example, The F-Ratio does not fall in critical region between four types of detergents. So, null hypothesis got rejected and alternate hypothesis got accepted.

STATISTICAL PACKAGES AND ANALYSIS

Computer-based statistical packages are an important tool for researcher in the social sciences. The mathematics behind statistical analysis can be daunting for those who have little formal training in either mathematics or in the use of statistics. The development of specialist statistical packages has greatly reduced the mathematical challenges of undertaking many analyses. The packages have however reduced the need for researchers to be able to undertake many of the calculation that are required for statistical analysis.

Statistical software packages are same like other software packages; changed greatly since the advent of the personal computer a little over 20 years ago.

Selection of Statistical Packages

Selection of statistical package for personal and professional use depends upon many factors. These factors are as follows:
- The availability of a package
- Cost of the package
- Types of functions software can perform
- Familiarity with software.

A number of statistical packages are available for statistical analysis. The commonly used packages are described here:

- *Statistical Packages for Social Sciences (SPSS):* The SPSS Corporation first produced the SPSS software package in 1980s and has recently released version 16. It is one of the most commonly used statistical packages throughout world. The advantages of the SPSS are its ease of use, familiarity to many statistical experts, and its functionality. The disadvantage is it cost. The different packages have licenses that also differ. In most case the license are set up to expire automatically after a limited period after which the package can no longer be used.
- *Excel:* Microsoft excel is a very popular and useful program that can be used for data analysis. Excel can be used for computation of many descriptive and inferential test application like t-test, chi-square test, mean, median and mode and standard deviation, etc. Excel also helpful for constructing graph, chart, pie diagram, histogram and Ogive.
- *R:* The R system for statistical computing is an environment for data analysis and graphics. The root of the R is the S language, developed by John Chambers and colleagues at Bell Laboratories in 1960s. R system helpful to perform different tests for descriptive and inferential statistics.
- *SAS:* The Statistical Analysis System (SAS) is very comprehensive software developed by North Caroline State University in 1966s. The SAS institute for advanced analytics, business intelligence, data management and predictive analytics. The SAS software suite has more than 200 components.
- *SYSTAT:* SYSTAT is a comprehensive desktop statistical package that is simple enough for beginners, yet powerful enough for experts. SYSTAT is a powerful statistics and statistical graphics software package developed by Leland Wilkinson in late 1970s. It employs a staggering range of powerful techniques to help conduct many types of research. SYSTAT has recently released version 13.0. SYSTAT also offers a huge data worksheet for powerful data handling. SYSTAT handle most of the format like Excel, SPSS, SAS, and MINITAB, etc. All matrix and computations are menu driven in SYSTAT. The advantages of SYSTAT are high speed and ease of use.
- *Stata*: Stata is statistical software designed in 1985 by StataCorp. It is used by researcher in economics, sociology, biomedicine and epidemiology. Stata is offered in many licenses; for students to professional use. Stata helpful for descriptive and inferential statistical analysis.

REVIEW QUESTIONS AND ANSWER

Long and Short Answer Questions

1. What is a statistical average? Describe the characteristics of a good statistical average.
   (TNMGRMU, MSc N-2017)
2. What is meant by analysis of variance?
   (RGUHS, MSc N-2011)

3. What is a statistical average? Describe the characteristics of a good statistical average.
   (BFUHS, MSc N-2004)
4. Explain the procedure of test of significance. (AIIMS, MSc N-2006)
5. Discuss testing of hypothesis procedure. (RGUHS, MSc N-2009)
6. Discuss assumptions of Karl Pearson correlation, coefficient methods. (PGI, MSc N-2014)
7. Explain the different types of diagrammatic presentation and mention the advantages.
   (PGI, MSc N-2002)
8. Role of statistics in nursing research. (RGUHS, MSc N-2005)

Multiple Choice Questions

1. Linear relationship between weight (in kg) and height (in cm) of nursing students can be calculated by:
   a. One-way ANOVA
   b. Chi-square test
   c. Correlation coefficient
   d. Independent sample t-test

2. In a data distribution you noticed that mean is lesser than median, then the data is said to be:
   a. Negatively skewed
   b. Positively skewed
   c. Normal distribution
   d. Unequitable distribution

3. Which of the following is NOT a feature of normal distribution curve?
   a. Breast shaped
   b. Symmetrical
   c. Mean = Median = Mode
   d. Positive skewness

4. Identify the mode of the following given observation.
   2, 3, 3, 5, 3, 4, 3, 3, 3, 4, 2, 2
   a. 2
   b. 3
   c. 4
   d. 5

5. It is a measure of central tendency that depict the exact middle of a set of a score is:
   a. Mean
   b. Median
   c. Mode
   d. Standard deviation

6. Which of the following observation fall above the median is?
   a. 60%
   b. 50%
   c. 75%
   d. 95%

7. In a normally distributed data set, what percentage of population fall within two standard deviation of the mean?
   a. 34%
   b. 95.4%
   c. 68%
   d. 99.6%

8. Which of the following formula is used to calculate degree of freedom in chi-square statistics?
   a. Row total × Column total
   b. Column total – Row total -1
   c. Row total × Column total +1
   d. Row total × Column total -1

9. Which of the following measure of central tendency is appropriate in case of data has significant variability?
   a. The mean
   b. The median
   c. The mode
   d. Variance

10. Probability value fall on a scale between:
    a. 0 and 1
    b. −1 to +1
    c. 0.001 to 1
    d. 0.05 to 0.01

Answer Key

1.	2.	3.	4.	5.	6.	7.	8.	9.	10
c.	a.	d.	b.	b.	b.	b.	d.	d.	a.

SUGGESTED READING

1. Ali Z, Bhaskar SB. Basic statistical tools in research and data analysis. Indian Journal of Anaesthesia. 2016; 60(9), 662-69.
2. Altman DG, Bland JM. Statistics notes: the normal distribution. BMJ. 1995;310(6975). 298.
3. Burn N, Grove SK. Understanding nursing research–building an evidence based practice, 4th edition. St Louis: Saunders Elsevier; 2007.
4. Garrett HE. Statistics in psychology and education, New Delhi: Paragon International Publishers; 2007.
5. Guilford JP. Fundamental statistics in psychology and education. New York: McGraw Hill; 1956.
6. Gupta SK. Statistical methods. New Delhi:Sultan Chand and Sons; 2008.
7. Hinkle DE, Wiersma W, Jurs SG. Applied statistics for the behavioral sciences, 5th edition. Boston: Houghton Mifflin; 2003.
8. Holgado–Tello P, et al. Polychoric versus Pearson correlations in exploratory and confirmatory factor analysis of ordinal variables. Quantity and Quality. 2011; 44.
9. Jothikumar J. Statistics, Chennai: Tamil Nadu Textbook Corporation; 2004.
10. Kim TK. T-test as a parametric statistics. Korean Journal of Anesthesiology. 2015; 68(6): 540-6.
11. Mahajan BK. Methods in biostatistics, 7th edition. New Delhi: Jaypee Brothers Medical Publishers;2010.
12. Manikandan S. Measures of central tendency: median and mode. J Pharmacol Pharmcother. 2011;2(3):214-5.
13. Manikandan S. Measures of central tendency: the mean. Journal of Pharmacology & Pharmacotherapeutics.2011; 2(2): 140-2.
14. Mukaka M. A guide to appropriate use of Correlation coefficient in medical research. Malawi Medical Journal : The Journal of Medical Association of Malawi. 2012 24(3), 69–71.
15. Negi KS. Biostatistics. New Delhi: AITBS. 2010.
16. Pillai RSN. Statistics (Theory and practical). S. Chand Publishing; 2008.
17. Polit D, Beck C. Essential of nursing research: methods, appraisal and utilization, 6th edition. Philadelphia: Lippincott William Wilkins; 2006.
18. Polit D, Beck C. Nursing research—principle and methods, 7th edition. Philadelphia: Lippincott William Wilkins; 2004.
19. Singh AK. Tests measurement and research methods in behaviorals: Bharti Bhawan (P & D); (2013).
20. Stevens SS. On the Theory of Scales of Measurement. Science. 1946; 103: 677-80.
21. Talbot LA. Principles and practice of nursing research, 1st edition. St Louis: Mosby Year Book Inc.; 1995.
22. Thompson CB. Descriptive data analysis. Air Medical Journal. 2009;28(2):56-9.

Appendices

Appendix I: Distribution of Chi-Square (χ^2)—Probability levels.

d.f.	.995	.99	.975	.95	.9	.1	.05	.025	.01
1	0.00	0.00	0.00	0.00	0.02	2.71	3.84	5.02	6.63
2	0.01	0.02	0.05	0.10	0.21	4.61	5.99	7.38	9.21
3	0.07	0.11	0.22	0.35	0.58	6.25	7.81	9.35	11.34
4	0.21	0.30	0.48	0.71	1.06	7.78	9.49	11.14	13.28
5	0.41	0.55	0.83	1.15	1.61	9.24	11.07	12.83	15.09
6	0.68	0.87	1.24	1.64	2.20	10.64	12.59	14.45	16.81
7	0.99	1.24	1.69	2.17	2.83	12.02	14.07	16.01	18.48
8	1.34	1.65	2.18	2.73	3.49	13.36	15.51	17.53	20.09
9	1.73	2.09	2.70	3.33	4.17	14.68	16.92	19.02	21.67
10	2.16	2.56	3.25	3.94	4.87	15.99	18.31	20.48	23.21
11	2.60	3.05	3.82	4.57	5.58	17.28	19.68	21.92	24.72
12	3.07	3.57	4.40	5.23	6.30	18.55	21.03	23.34	26.22
13	3.57	4.11	5.01	5.89	7.04	19.81	22.36	24.74	27.69
14	4.07	4.66	5.63	6.57	7.79	21.06	23.68	26.12	29.14
15	4.60	5.23	6.26	7.26	8.55	22.31	25.00	27.49	30.58
16	5.14	5.81	6.91	7.96	9.31	23.54	26.30	28.85	32.00
17	5.70	6.41	7.56	8.67	10.09	24.77	27.59	30.19	33.41
18	6.26	7.01	8.23	9.39	10.86	25.99	28.87	31.53	34.81
19	6.84	7.63	8.91	10.12	11.65	27.20	30.14	32.85	36.19
20	7.43	8.26	9.59	10.85	12.44	28.41	31.41	34.17	37.57
22	8.64	9.54	10.98	12.34	14.04	30.81	33.92	36.78	40.29
24	9.89	10.86	12.40	13.85	15.66	33.20	36.42	39.36	42.98
26	11.16	12.20	13.84	15.38	17.29	35.56	38.89	41.92	45.64
28	12.46	13.56	15.31	16.93	18.94	37.92	41.34	44.46	48.28

Contd...

Contd...

d.f.	.995	.99	.975	.95	.9	.1	.05	.025	.01
30	13.79	14.95	16.79	18.49	20.60	40.26	43.77	46.98	50.89
32	15.13	16.36	18.29	20.07	22.27	42.58	46.19	49.48	53.49
34	16.50	17.79	19.81	21.66	23.95	44.90	48.60	51.97	56.06
38	19.29	20.69	22.88	24.88	27.34	49.51	53.38	56.90	61.16
42	22.14	23.65	26.00	28.14	30.77	54.09	58.12	61.78	66.21
46	25.04	26.66	29.16	31.44	34.22	58.64	62.83	66.62	71.20
50	27.99	29.71	32.36	34.76	37.69	63.17	67.50	71.42	76.15
55	31.73	33.57	36.40	38.96	42.06	68.80	73.31	77.38	82.29
60	35.53	37.48	40.48	43.19	46.46	74.40	79.08	83.30	88.38
65	39.38	41.44	44.60	47.45	50.88	79.97	84.82	89.18	94.42
70	43.28	45.44	48.76	51.74	55.33	85.53	90.53	95.02	100.43
75	47.21	49.48	52.94	56.05	59.79	91.06	96.22	100.84	106.39
80	51.17	53.54	57.15	60.39	64.28	96.58	101.88	106.63	112.33
85	55.17	57.63	61.39	64.75	68.78	102.08	107.52	112.39	118.24
90	59.20	61.75	65.65	69.13	73.29	107.57	113.15	118.14	124.12
95	63.25	65.90	69.92	73.52	77.82	113.04	118.75	123.86	129.97
100	67.33	70.06	74.22	77.93	82.36	118.50	124.34	129.56	135.81

Appendix II: Distribution of *t*-Probability values.

cum. prob	$t_{.50}$	$t_{.75}$	$t_{.80}$	$t_{.85}$	$t_{.90}$	$t_{.95}$	$t_{.975}$	$t_{.99}$	$t_{.995}$	$t_{.999}$	$t_{.9995}$
one-tail	0.50	0.25	0.20	0.15	0.10	0.05	0.025	0.01	0.005	0.001	0.0005
two-tails	1.00	0.50	0.40	0.30	0.20	0.10	0.05	0.02	0.01	0.002	0.001
df											
1	0.000	1.000	1.376	1.963	3.078	6.314	12.71	31.82	63.66	318.31	636.62
2	0.000	0.816	1.061	1.386	1.886	2.920	4.303	6.965	9.925	22.327	31.599
3	0.000	0.765	0.978	1.250	1.638	2.353	3.182	4.541	5.841	10.215	12.924
4	0.000	0.741	0.941	1.190	1.533	2.132	2.776	3.747	4.604	7.173	8.610
5	0.000	0.727	0.920	1.156	1.476	2.015	2.571	3.365	4.032	5.893	6.869
6	0.000	0.718	0.906	1.134	1.440	1.943	2.447	3.143	3.707	5.208	5.959
7	0.000	0.711	0.896	1.119	1.415	1.895	2.365	2.998	3.499	4.785	5.408
8	0.000	0.706	0.889	1.108	1.397	1.860	2.306	2.896	3.355	4.501	5.041
9	0.000	0.703	0.883	1.100	1.383	1.833	2.262	2.821	3.250	4.297	4.781
10	0.000	0.700	0.879	1.093	1.372	1.812	2.228	2.764	3.169	4.144	4.587
11	0.000	0.697	0.876	1.088	1.363	1.796	2.201	2.718	3.106	4.025	4.437
12	0.000	0.695	0.873	1.083	1.356	1.782	2.179	2.681	3.055	3.930	4.318
13	0.000	0.694	0.870	1.079	1.350	1.771	2.160	2.650	3.012	3.852	4.221
14	0.000	0.692	0.868	1.076	1.345	1.761	2.145	2.624	2.977	3.787	4.140
15	0.000	0.691	0.866	1.074	1.341	1.753	2.131	2.602	2.947	3.733	4.073
16	0.000	0.690	0.865	1.071	1.337	1.746	2.120	2.583	2.921	3.686	4.015
17	0.000	0.689	0.863	1.069	1.333	1.740	2.110	2.567	2.898	3.646	3.965
18	0.000	0.688	0.862	1.067	1.330	1.734	2.101	2.552	2.878	3.610	3.922
19	0.000	0.688	0.861	1.066	1.328	1.729	2.093	2.539	2.861	3.579	3.883
20	0.000	0.687	0.860	1.064	1.325	1.725	2.086	2.528	2.845	3.552	3.850
21	0.000	0.686	0.859	1.063	1.323	1.721	2.080	2.518	2.831	3.527	3.819
22	0.000	0.686	0.858	1.061	1.321	1.717	2.074	2.508	2.819	3.505	3.792
23	0.000	0.685	0.858	1.060	1.319	1.714	2.069	2.500	2.807	3.485	3.768
24	0.000	0.685	0.857	1.059	1.318	1.711	2.064	2.492	2.797	3.467	3.745
25	0.000	0.684	0.856	1.058	1.316	1.708	2.060	2.485	2.787	3.450	3.725
26	0.000	0.684	0.856	1.058	1.315	1.706	2.056	2.479	2.779	3.435	3.707
27	0.000	0.684	0.855	1.057	1.314	1.703	2.052	2.473	2.771	3.421	3.690
28	0.000	0.683	0.855	1.056	1.313	1.701	2.048	2.467	2.763	3.408	3.674
29	0.000	0.683	0.854	1.055	1.311	1.699	2.045	2.462	2.756	3.396	3.659

Contd...

Contd...

cum. prob	$t_{.50}$	$t_{.75}$	$t_{.80}$	$t_{.85}$	$t_{.90}$	$t_{.95}$	$t_{.975}$	$t_{.99}$	$t_{.995}$	$t_{.999}$	$t_{.9995}$
one-tail	0.50	0.25	0.20	0.15	0.10	0.05	0.025	0.01	0.005	0.001	0.0005
two-tails	1.00	0.50	0.40	0.30	0.20	0.10	0.05	0.02	0.01	0.002	0.001
30	0.000	0.683	0.854	1.055	1.310	1.697	2.042	2.457	2.750	3.385	3.646
40	0.000	0.681	0.851	1.050	1.303	1.684	2.021	2.423	2.704	3.307	3.551
60	0.000	0.679	0.848	1.045	1.296	1.671	2.000	2.390	2.660	3.232	3.460
80	0.000	0.678	0.846	1.043	1.292	1.664	1.990	2.374	2.639	3.195	3.416
100	0.000	0.677	0.845	1.042	1.290	1.660	1.984	2.364	2.626	3.174	3.390
1000	0.000	0.675	0.842	1.037	1.282	1.646	1.962	2.330	2.581	3.098	3.300
z	0.000	0.674	0.842	1.036	1.282	1.645	1.960	2.326	2.576	3.090	3.291
	0%	50%	60%	70%	80%	90%	95%	98%	99%	99.8%	99.9%
Confidence Level											

Appendix III: Z-Distribution table (area under the standard normal curve from 0 to Z).

z	.00	.01	.02	.03	.04	.05	.06	.07	.08	.09
−3.4	.0003	.0003	.0003	.0003	.0003	.0003	.0003	.0003	.0003	.0002
−3.3	.0005	.0005	.0005	.0004	.0004	.0004	.0004	.0004	.0004	.0003
−3.2	.0007	.0007	.0006	.0006	.0006	.0006	.0006	.0005	.0005	.0005
−3.1	.0010	.0009	.0009	.0009	.0008	.0008	.0008	.0008	.0007	.0007
−3.0	.0013	.0013	.0013	.0012	.0012	.0011	.0011	.0011	.0010	.0010
−2.9	.0019	.0018	.0018	.0017	.0016	.0016	.0015	.0015	.0014	.0014
−2.8	.0026	.0025	.0024	.0023	.0023	.0022	.0021	.0021	.0020	.0019
−2.7	.0035	.0034	.0033	.0032	.0031	.0030	.0029	.0028	.0027	.0026
−2.6	.0047	.0045	.0044	.0043	.0041	.0040	.0039	.0038	.0037	.0036
−2.5	.0062	.0060	.0059	.0057	.0055	.0054	.0052	.0051	.0049	.0048
−2.4	.0082	.0080	.0078	.0075	.0073	.0071	.0069	.0068	.0066	.0064
−2.3	.0107	.0104	.0102	.0099	.0096	.0094	.0091	.0089	.0087	.0084
−2.2	.0139	.0136	.0132	.0129	.0125	.0122	.0119	.0116	.0113	.0110
−2.1	.0179	.0174	.0170	.0166	.0162	.0158	.0154	.0150	.0146	.0143
−2.0	.0228	.0222	.0217	.0212	.0207	.0202	.0197	.0192	.0188	.0183
−1.9	.0287	.0281	.0274	.0268	.0262	.0256	.0250	.0244	.0239	.0233
−1.8	.0359	.0351	.0344	.0336	.0329	.0322	.0314	.0307	.0301	.0294
−1.7	.0446	.0436	.0427	.0418	.0409	.0401	.0392	.0384	.0375	.0367
−1.6	.0548	.0537	.0526	.0516	.0505	.0495	.0485	.0475	.0465	.0455
−1.5	.0668	.0655	.0643	.0630	.0618	.0606	.0594	.0582	.0571	.0559
−1.4	.0808	.0793	.0778	.0764	.0749	.0735	.0721	.0708	.0694	.0681
−1.3	.0968	.0951	.0934	.0918	.0901	.0885	.0869	.0853	.0838	.0823
−1.2	.1151	.1131	.1112	.1093	.1075	.1056	.1038	.1020	.1003	.0985
−1.1	.1357	.1335	.1314	.1292	.1271	.1251	.1230	.1210	.1190	.1170
−1.0	.1587	.1562	.1539	.1515	.1492	.1469	.1446	.1423	.1401	.1379
−0.9	.1841	.1814	.1788	.1762	.1736	.1711	.1685	.1660	.1635	.1611
−0.8	.2119	.2090	.2061	.2033	.2005	.1977	.1949	.1922	.1894	.1867
−0.7	.2420	.2389	.2358	.2327	.2296	.2266	.2236	.2206	.2177	.2148
−0.6	.2743	.2709	.2676	.2643	.2611	.2578	.2546	.2514	.2483	.2451
−0.5	.3085	.3050	.3015	.2981	.2946	.2912	.2877	.2843	.2810	.2776
−0.4	.3446	.3409	.3372	.3336	.3300	.3264	.3228	.3192	.3156	.3121
−0.3	.3821	.3783	.3745	.3707	.3669	.3632	.3594	.3557	.3520	.3483
−0.2	.4207	.4168	.4129	.4090	.4052	.4013	.3974	.3936	.3897	.3859
−0.1	.4602	.4562	.4522	.4483	.4443	.4404	.4364	.4325	.4286	.4247
−0.0	.5000	.4960	.4920	.4880	.4840	.4801	.4761	.4721	.4681	.4641

Appendix IV: Z-Distribution table with level of significance.

z	.00	.01	.02	.03	.04	.05	.06	.07	.08	.09
0.0	.5000	.5040	.5080	.5120	.5160	.5199	.5239	.5279	.5319	.5359
0.1	.5398	.5438	.5478	.5517	.5557	.5596	.5636	.5675	.5714	.5753
0.2	.5793	.5832	.5871	.5910	.5948	.5987	.6026	.6064	.6103	.6141
0.3	.6179	.6217	.6255	.6293	.6331	.6368	.6406	.6443	.6480	.6517
0.4	.6554	.6591	.6628	.6664	.6700	.6736	.6772	.6808	.6844	.6879
0.5	.6915	.6950	.6985	.7019	.7054	.7088	.7123	.7157	.7190	.7224
0.6	.7257	.7291	.7324	.7357	.7389	.7422	.7454	.7486	.7517	.7549
0.7	.7580	.7611	.7642	.7673	.7704	.7734	.7764	.7794	.7823	.7852
0.8	.7881	.7910	.7939	.7967	.7995	.8023	.8051	.8078	.8106	.8133
0.9	.8159	.8186	.8212	.8238	.8264	.8289	.8315	.8340	.8365	.8389
1.0	.8413	.8438	.8461	.8485	.8508	.8531	.8554	.8577	.8599	.8621
1.1	.8643	.8665	.8686	.8708	.8729	.8749	.8770	.8790	.8810	.8830
1.2	.8849	.8869	.8888	.8907	.8925	.8944	.8962	.8980	.8997	.9015
1.3	.9032	.9049	.9066	.9082	.9099	.9115	.9131	.9147	.9162	.9177
1.4	.9192	.9207	.9222	.9236	.9251	.9265	.9279	.9292	.9306	.9319
1.5	.9332	.9345	.9357	.9370	.9382	.9394	.9406	.9418	.9429	.9441
1.6	.9452	.9463	.9474	.9484	.9495	.9505	.9515	.9525	.9535	.9545
1.7	.9554	.9564	.9573	.9582	.9591	.9599	.9608	.9616	.9625	.9633
1.8	.9641	.9649	.9656	.9664	.9671	.9678	.9686	.9693	.9699	.9706
1.9	.9713	.9719	.9726	.9732	.9738	.9744	.9750	.9756	.9761	.9767
2.0	.9772	.9778	.9783	.9788	.9793	.9798	.9803	.9808	.9812	.9817
2.1	.9821	.9826	.9830	.9834	.9838	.9842	.9846	.9850	.9854	.9857
2.2	.9861	.9864	.9868	.9871	.9875	.9878	.9881	.9884	.9887	.9890
2.3	.9893	.9896	.9898	.9901	.9904	.9906	.9909	.9911	.9913	.9916
2.4	.9918	.9920	.9922	.9925	.9927	.9929	.9931	.9932	.9934	.9936
2.5	.9938	.9940	.9941	.9943	.9945	.9946	.9948	.9949	.9951	.9952
2.6	.9953	.9955	.9956	.9957	.9959	.9960	.9961	.9962	.9963	.9964
2.7	.9965	.9966	.9967	.9968	.9969	.9970	.9971	.9972	.9973	.9974
2.8	.9974	.9975	.9976	.9977	.9977	.9978	.9979	.9979	.9980	.9981
2.9	.9981	.9982	.9982	.9983	.9984	.9984	.9985	.9985	.9986	.9986
3.0	.9987	.9987	.9987	.9988	.9988	.9989	.9989	.9989	.9990	.9990
3.1	.9990	.9991	.9991	.9991	.9992	.9992	.9992	.9992	.9993	.9993
3.2	.9993	.9993	.9994	.9994	.9994	.9994	.9994	.9995	.9995	.9995
3.3	.9995	.9995	.9995	.9996	.9996	.9996	.9996	.9996	.9996	.9997
3.4	.9997	.9997	.9997	.9997	.9997	.9997	.9997	.9997	.9997	.9998

Appendix V: The correlation coefficient at 5% and 1% level of significance.

n	2-tailed testing			1-tailed testing		
	α = .1	α = .05	α = .01	α = .1	α = .05	α = .01
5	0.805	0.878	0.959	0.687	0.805	0.934
6	0.729	0.811	0.917	0.608	0.729	0.882
7	0.669	0.754	0.875	0.551	0.669	0.833
8	0.621	0.707	0.834	0.507	0.621	0.789
9	0.582	0.666	0.798	0.472	0.582	0.750
10	0.549	0.632	0.765	0.443	0.549	0.715
11	0.521	0.602	0.735	0.419	0.521	0.685
12	0.497	0.576	0.708	0.398	0.497	0.658
13	0.476	0.553	0.684	0.380	0.476	0.634
14	0.458	0.532	0.661	0.365	0.458	0.612
15	0.441	0.514	0.641	0.351	0.441	0.592
16	0.426	0.497	0.623	0.338	0.426	0.574
17	0.412	0.482	0.606	0.327	0.412	0.558
18	0.400	0.468	0.590	0.317	0.400	0.543
19	0.389	0.456	0.575	0.308	0.389	0.529
20	0.378	0.444	0.561	0.299	0.378	0.516
21	0.369	0.433	0.549	0.291	0.369	0.503
22	0.360	0.423	0.537	0.284	0.360	0.492
23	0.352	0.413	0.526	0.277	0.352	0.482
24	0.344	0.404	0.515	0.271	0.344	0.472
25	0.337	0.396	0.505	0.265	0.337	0.462
26	0.330	0.388	0.496	0.260	0.330	0.453
27	0.323	0.381	0.487	0.255	0.323	0.445
28	0.317	0.374	0.479	0.250	0.317	0.437
29	0.311	0.367	0.471	0.245	0.311	0.430
30	0.306	0.361	0.463	0.241	0.306	0.423
40	0.264	0.312	0.403	0.207	0.264	0.367
50	0.235	0.279	0.361	0.184	0.235	0.328
60	0.214	0.254	0.330	0.168	0.214	0.300
80	0.185	0.220	0.286	0.145	0.185	0.260
100	0.165	0.197	0.256	0.129	0.165	0.232
120	0.151	0.179	0.234	0.118	0.151	0.212
140	0.140	0.166	0.217	0.109	0.140	0.196

Contd...

Contd...

	2-tailed testing			1-tailed testing		
n	$\alpha = .1$	$\alpha = .05$	$\alpha = .01$	$\alpha = .1$	$\alpha = .05$	$\alpha = .01$
160	0.130	0.155	0.203	0.102	0.130	0.184
180	0.123	0.146	0.192	0.096	0.123	0.173
200	0.117	0.139	0.182	0.091	0.117	0.164
300	0.095	0.113	0.149	0.074	0.095	0.134
400	0.082	0.098	0.129	0.064	0.082	0.116
500	0.074	0.088	0.115	0.057	0.074	0.104

Appendix VI: Critical values for Spearman's rank correlation coefficient.
Use this table to determine the significance of your result for this test. For example, if you had 20 pairs of data and a value of 0.53 then there would be a probability of between 0.01 and 0.005 that it had occurred by chance. In other words, you might expect to get this result occurring **by chance** once every 100–200 times. This, therefore, indicates a very significant correlation between the two sets of data.

n (number of pairs)	Probability that your result occurred by chance				
	0.1	0.05	0.025	0.01	0.005
4	1.0000	1.0000	1.0000	1.0000	1.0000
5	0.7000	0.9000	0.9000	1.0000	1.0000
6	0.6571	0.7714	0.8286	0.9429	0.9429
7	0.5714	0.6786	0.7857	0.8571	0.8929
8	0.5476	0.6429	0.7381	0.8095	0.8571
9	0.4833	0.6000	0.6833	0.7667	0.8167
10	0.4424	0.5636	0.6485	0.7333	0.7818
11	0.4182	0.5273	0.6091	0.7000	0.7545
12	0.3986	0.5035	0.5874	0.6713	0.7273
13	0.3791	0.4780	0.5604	0.6484	0.6978
14	0.3670	0.4593	0.5385	0.6220	0.6747
15	0.3500	0.4429	0.5179	0.6000	0.6536
16	0.3382	0.4265	0.5029	0.5824	0.6324
17	0.3271	0.4124	0.4821	0.5577	0.6055
18	0.3170	0.4000	0.4683	0.5425	0.5897
19	0.3077	0.3887	0.4555	0.5285	0.5751
20	0.2992	0.3783	0.4438	0.5155	0.5614
21	0.2914	0.3687	0.4329	0.5034	0.5487
22	0.2841	0.3598	0.4227	0.4921	0.5368
23	0.2774	0.3515	0.4132	0.4815	0.5256
24	0.2711	0.3438	0.4044	0.4716	0.5151
25	0.2653	0.3365	0.3961	0.4622	0.5052
26	0.2598	0.3297	0.3882	0.4534	0.4958
27	0.2546	0.3233	0.3809	0.4451	0.4869
28	0.2497	0.3172	0.3739	0.4372	0.4785
29	0.2451	0.3115	0.3673	0.4297	0.4705
30	0.2407	0.3061	0.3610	0.4226	0.4629

Appendix VII: Table of critical values for the F-distribution (for use with ANOVA). Critical values of F for the 0.05 significance level.

	1	2	3	4	5	6	7	8	9	10
1	161.45	199.50	215.71	224.58	230.16	233.99	236.77	238.88	240.54	241.88
2	18.51	19.00	19.16	19.25	19.30	19.33	19.35	19.37	19.39	19.40
3	10.13	9.55	9.28	9.12	9.01	8.94	8.89	8.85	8.81	8.79
4	7.71	6.94	6.59	6.39	6.26	6.16	6.09	6.04	6.00	5.96
5	6.61	5.79	5.41	5.19	5.05	4.95	4.88	4.82	4.77	4.74
6	5.99	5.14	4.76	4.53	4.39	4.28	4.21	4.15	4.10	4.06
7	5.59	4.74	4.35	4.12	3.97	3.87	3.79	3.73	3.68	3.64
8	5.32	4.46	4.07	3.84	3.69	3.58	3.50	3.44	3.39	3.35
9	5.12	4.26	3.86	3.63	3.48	3.37	3.29	3.23	3.18	3.14
10	4.97	4.10	3.71	3.48	3.33	3.22	3.14	3.07	3.02	2.98
11	4.84	3.98	3.59	3.36	3.20	3.10	3.01	2.95	2.90	2.85
12	4.75	3.89	3.49	3.26	3.11	3.00	2.91	2.85	2.80	2.75
13	4.67	3.81	3.41	3.18	3.03	2.92	2.83	2.77	2.71	2.67
14	4.60	3.74	3.34	3.11	2.96	2.85	2.76	2.70	2.65	2.60
15	4.54	3.68	3.29	3.06	2.90	2.79	2.71	2.64	2.59	2.54
16	4.49	3.63	3.24	3.01	2.85	2.74	2.66	2.59	2.54	2.49
17	4.45	3.59	3.20	2.97	2.81	2.70	2.61	2.55	2.49	2.45
18	4.41	3.56	3.16	2.93	2.77	2.66	2.58	2.51	2.46	2.41
19	4.38	3.52	3.13	2.90	2.74	2.63	2.54	2.48	2.42	2.38
20	4.35	3.49	3.10	2.87	2.71	2.60	2.51	2.45	2.39	2.35
21	4.33	3.47	3.07	2.84	2.69	2.57	2.49	2.42	2.37	2.32
22	4.30	3.44	3.05	2.82	2.66	2.55	2.46	2.40	2.34	2.30
23	4.28	3.42	3.03	2.80	2.64	2.53	2.44	2.38	2.32	2.28
24	4.26	3.40	3.01	2.78	2.62	2.51	2.42	2.36	2.30	2.26
25	4.24	3.39	2.99	2.76	2.60	2.49	2.41	2.34	2.28	2.24
26	4.23	3.37	2.98	2.74	2.59	2.47	2.39	2.32	2.27	2.22
27	4.21	3.35	2.96	2.73	2.57	2.46	2.37	2.31	2.25	2.20
28	4.20	3.34	2.95	2.71	2.56	2.45	2.36	2.29	2.24	2.19
29	4.18	3.33	2.93	2.70	2.55	2.43	2.35	2.28	2.22	2.18
30	4.17	3.32	2.92	2.69	2.53	2.42	2.33	2.27	2.21	2.17
31	4.16	3.31	2.91	2.68	2.52	2.41	2.32	2.26	2.20	2.15
32	4.15	3.30	2.90	2.67	2.51	2.40	2.31	2.24	2.19	2.14

Contd...

Contd...

	1	2	3	4	5	6	7	8	9	10
33	4.14	3.29	2.89	2.66	2.50	2.39	2.30	2.24	2.18	2.13
34	4.13	3.28	2.88	2.65	2.49	2.38	2.29	2.23	2.17	2.12
35	4.12	3.27	2.87	2.64	2.49	2.37	2.29	2.22	2.16	2.11
36	4.11	3.26	2.87	2.63	2.48	2.36	2.28	2.21	2.15	2.11
37	4.11	3.25	2.86	2.63	2.47	2.36	2.27	2.20	2.15	2.10
38	4.10	3.25	2.85	2.62	2.46	2.35	2.26	2.19	2.14	2.09
39	4.09	3.24	2.85	2.61	2.46	2.34	2.26	2.19	2.13	2.08
40	4.09	3.23	2.84	2.61	2.45	2.34	2.25	2.18	2.12	2.08
41	4.08	3.23	2.83	2.60	2.44	2.33	2.24	2.17	2.12	2.07
42	4.07	3.22	2.83	2.59	2.44	2.32	2.24	2.17	2.11	2.07
43	4.07	3.21	2.82	2.59	2.43	2.32	2.23	2.16	2.11	2.06
44	4.06	3.21	2.82	2.58	2.43	2.31	2.23	2.16	2.10	2.05
45	4.06	3.20	2.81	2.58	2.42	2.31	2.22	2.15	2.10	2.05
46	4.05	3.20	2.81	2.57	2.42	2.30	2.22	2.15	2.09	2.04
47	4.05	3.20	2.80	2.57	2.41	2.30	2.21	2.14	2.09	2.04
48	4.04	3.19	2.80	2.57	2.41	2.30	2.21	2.14	2.08	2.04
49	4.04	3.19	2.79	2.56	2.40	2.29	2.20	2.13	2.08	2.03
50	4.03	3.18	2.79	2.56	2.40	2.29	2.20	2.13	2.07	2.03
51	4.03	3.18	2.79	2.55	2.40	2.28	2.20	2.13	2.07	2.02
52	4.03	3.18	2.78	2.55	2.39	2.28	2.19	2.12	2.07	2.02
53	4.02	3.17	2.78	2.55	2.39	2.28	2.19	2.12	2.06	2.02
54	4.02	3.17	2.78	2.54	2.39	2.27	2.19	2.12	2.06	2.01
55	4.02	3.17	2.77	2.54	2.38	2.27	2.18	2.11	2.06	2.01
56	4.01	3.16	2.77	2.54	2.38	2.27	2.18	2.11	2.05	2.01
57	4.01	3.16	2.77	2.53	2.38	2.26	2.18	2.11	2.05	2.00
58	4.01	3.16	2.76	2.53	2.37	2.26	2.17	2.10	2.05	2.00
59	4.00	3.15	2.76	2.53	2.37	2.26	2.17	2.10	2.04	2.00
60	4.00	3.15	2.76	2.53	2.37	2.25	2.17	2.10	2.04	1.99
61	4.00	3.15	2.76	2.52	2.37	2.25	2.16	2.09	2.04	1.99
62	4.00	3.15	2.75	2.52	2.36	2.25	2.16	2.09	2.04	1.99
63	3.99	3.14	2.75	2.52	2.36	2.25	2.16	2.09	2.03	1.99
64	3.99	3.14	2.75	2.52	2.36	2.24	2.16	2.09	2.03	1.98
65	3.99	3.14	2.75	2.51	2.36	2.24	2.15	2.08	2.03	1.98

Contd...

Contd...

	1	2	3	4	5	6	7	8	9	10
66	3.99	3.14	2.74	2.51	2.35	2.24	2.15	2.08	2.03	1.98
67	3.98	3.13	2.74	2.51	2.35	2.24	2.15	2.08	2.02	1.98
68	3.98	3.13	2.74	2.51	2.35	2.24	2.15	2.08	2.02	1.97
69	3.98	3.13	2.74	2.51	2.35	2.23	2.15	2.08	2.02	1.97
70	3.98	3.13	2.74	2.50	2.35	2.23	2.14	2.07	2.02	1.97
71	3.98	3.13	2.73	2.50	2.34	2.23	2.14	2.07	2.02	1.97
72	3.97	3.12	2.73	2.50	2.34	2.23	2.14	2.07	2.01	1.97
73	3.97	3.12	2.73	2.50	2.34	2.23	2.14	2.07	2.01	1.96
74	3.97	3.12	2.73	2.50	2.34	2.22	2.14	2.07	2.01	1.96
75	3.97	3.12	2.73	2.49	2.34	2.22	2.13	2.06	2.01	1.96
76	3.97	3.12	2.73	2.49	2.34	2.22	2.13	2.06	2.01	1.96
77	3.97	3.12	2.72	2.49	2.33	2.22	2.13	2.06	2.00	1.96
78	3.96	3.11	2.72	2.49	2.33	2.22	2.13	2.06	2.00	1.95
79	3.96	3.11	2.72	2.49	2.33	2.22	2.13	2.06	2.00	1.95
80	3.96	3.11	2.72	2.49	2.33	2.21	2.13	2.06	2.00	1.95
81	3.96	3.11	2.72	2.48	2.33	2.21	2.13	2.06	2.00	1.95
82	3.96	3.11	2.72	2.48	2.33	2.21	2.12	2.05	2.00	1.95
83	3.96	3.11	2.72	2.48	2.32	2.21	2.12	2.05	2.00	1.95
84	3.96	3.11	2.71	2.48	2.32	2.21	2.12	2.05	1.99	1.95
85	3.95	3.10	2.71	2.48	2.32	2.21	2.12	2.05	1.99	1.94
86	3.95	3.10	2.71	2.48	2.32	2.21	2.12	2.05	1.99	1.94
87	3.95	3.10	2.71	2.48	2.32	2.21	2.12	2.05	1.99	1.94
88	3.95	3.10	2.71	2.48	2.32	2.20	2.12	2.05	1.99	1.94
89	3.95	3.10	2.71	2.47	2.32	2.20	2.11	2.04	1.99	1.94
90	3.95	3.10	2.71	2.47	2.32	2.20	2.11	2.04	1.99	1.94
91	3.95	3.10	2.71	2.47	2.32	2.20	2.11	2.04	1.98	1.94
92	3.95	3.10	2.70	2.47	2.31	2.20	2.11	2.04	1.98	1.94
93	3.94	3.09	2.70	2.47	2.31	2.20	2.11	2.04	1.98	1.93
94	3.94	3.09	2.70	2.47	2.31	2.20	2.11	2.04	1.98	1.93
95	3.94	3.09	2.70	2.47	2.31	2.20	2.11	2.04	1.98	1.93
96	3.94	3.09	2.70	2.47	2.31	2.20	2.11	2.04	1.98	1.93
97	3.94	3.09	2.70	2.47	2.31	2.19	2.11	2.04	1.98	1.93
98	3.94	3.09	2.70	2.47	2.31	2.19	2.10	2.03	1.98	1.93
99	3.94	3.09	2.70	2.46	2.31	2.19	2.10	2.03	1.98	1.93
100	3.94	3.09	2.70	2.46	2.31	2.19	2.10	2.03	1.98	1.93

Appendix VIII: Critical values of F for the 0.01 significance level.

	1	2	3	4	5	6	7	8	9	10
1	4052.19	4999.52	5403.34	5624.62	5763.65	5858.97	5928.33	5981.10	6022.50	6055.85
2	98.50	99.00	99.17	99.25	99.30	99.33	99.36	99.37	99.39	99.40
3	34.12	30.82	29.46	28.71	28.24	27.91	27.67	27.49	27.35	27.23
4	21.20	18.00	16.69	15.98	15.52	15.21	14.98	14.80	14.66	14.55
5	16.26	13.27	12.06	11.39	10.97	10.67	10.46	10.29	10.16	10.05
6	13.75	10.93	9.78	9.15	8.75	8.47	8.26	8.10	7.98	7.87
7	12.25	9.55	8.45	7.85	7.46	7.19	6.99	6.84	6.72	6.62
8	11.26	8.65	7.59	7.01	6.63	6.37	6.18	6.03	5.91	5.81
9	10.56	8.02	6.99	6.42	6.06	5.80	5.61	5.47	5.35	5.26
10	10.04	7.56	6.55	5.99	5.64	5.39	5.20	5.06	4.94	4.85
11	9.65	7.21	6.22	5.67	5.32	5.07	4.89	4.74	4.63	4.54
12	9.33	6.93	5.95	5.41	5.06	4.82	4.64	4.50	4.39	4.30
13	9.07	6.70	5.74	5.21	4.86	4.62	4.44	4.30	4.19	4.10
14	8.86	6.52	5.56	5.04	4.70	4.46	4.28	4.14	4.03	3.94
15	8.68	6.36	5.42	4.89	4.56	4.32	4.14	4.00	3.90	3.81
16	8.53	6.23	5.29	4.77	4.44	4.20	4.03	3.89	3.78	3.69
17	8.40	6.11	5.19	4.67	4.34	4.10	3.93	3.79	3.68	3.59
18	8.29	6.01	5.09	4.58	4.25	4.02	3.84	3.71	3.60	3.51
19	8.19	5.93	5.01	4.50	4.17	3.94	3.77	3.63	3.52	3.43
20	8.10	5.85	4.94	4.43	4.10	3.87	3.70	3.56	3.46	3.37
21	8.02	5.78	4.87	4.37	4.04	3.81	3.64	3.51	3.40	3.31
22	7.95	5.72	4.82	4.31	3.99	3.76	3.59	3.45	3.35	3.26
23	7.88	5.66	4.77	4.26	3.94	3.71	3.54	3.41	3.30	3.21
24	7.82	5.61	4.72	4.22	3.90	3.67	3.50	3.36	3.26	3.17
25	7.77	5.57	4.68	4.18	3.86	3.63	3.46	3.32	3.22	3.13
26	7.72	5.53	4.64	4.14	3.82	3.59	3.42	3.29	3.18	3.09
27	7.68	5.49	4.60	4.11	3.79	3.56	3.39	3.26	3.15	3.06
28	7.64	5.45	4.57	4.07	3.75	3.53	3.36	3.23	3.12	3.03
29	7.60	5.42	4.54	4.05	3.73	3.50	3.33	3.20	3.09	3.01
30	7.56	5.39	4.51	4.02	3.70	3.47	3.31	3.17	3.07	2.98
31	7.53	5.36	4.48	3.99	3.68	3.45	3.28	3.15	3.04	2.96
32	7.50	5.34	4.46	3.97	3.65	3.43	3.26	3.13	3.02	2.93
33	7.47	5.31	4.44	3.95	3.63	3.41	3.24	3.11	3.00	2.91
34	7.44	5.29	4.42	3.93	3.61	3.39	3.22	3.09	2.98	2.89

Contd...

Contd...

	1	2	3	4	5	6	7	8	9	10
35	7.42	5.27	4.40	3.91	3.59	3.37	3.20	3.07	2.96	2.88
36	7.40	5.25	4.38	3.89	3.57	3.35	3.18	3.05	2.95	2.86
37	7.37	5.23	4.36	3.87	3.56	3.33	3.17	3.04	2.93	2.84
38	7.35	5.21	4.34	3.86	3.54	3.32	3.15	3.02	2.92	2.83
39	7.33	5.19	4.33	3.84	3.53	3.31	3.14	3.01	2.90	2.81
40	7.31	5.18	4.31	3.83	3.51	3.29	3.12	2.99	2.89	2.80
41	7.30	5.16	4.30	3.82	3.50	3.28	3.11	2.98	2.88	2.79
42	7.28	5.15	4.29	3.80	3.49	3.27	3.10	2.97	2.86	2.78
43	7.26	5.14	4.27	3.79	3.48	3.25	3.09	2.96	2.85	2.76
44	7.25	5.12	4.26	3.78	3.47	3.24	3.08	2.95	2.84	2.75
45	7.23	5.11	4.25	3.77	3.45	3.23	3.07	2.94	2.83	2.74
46	7.22	5.10	4.24	3.76	3.44	3.22	3.06	2.93	2.82	2.73
47	7.21	5.09	4.23	3.75	3.43	3.21	3.05	2.92	2.81	2.72
48	7.19	5.08	4.22	3.74	3.43	3.20	3.04	2.91	2.80	2.72
49	7.18	5.07	4.21	3.73	3.42	3.20	3.03	2.90	2.79	2.71
50	7.17	5.06	4.20	3.72	3.41	3.19	3.02	2.89	2.79	2.70
51	7.16	5.05	4.19	3.71	3.40	3.18	3.01	2.88	2.78	2.69
52	7.15	5.04	4.18	3.70	3.39	3.17	3.01	2.87	2.77	2.68
53	7.14	5.03	4.17	3.70	3.38	3.16	3.00	2.87	2.76	2.68
54	7.13	5.02	4.17	3.69	3.38	3.16	2.99	2.86	2.76	2.67
55	7.12	5.01	4.16	3.68	3.37	3.15	2.98	2.85	2.75	2.66
56	7.11	5.01	4.15	3.67	3.36	3.14	2.98	2.85	2.74	2.66
57	7.10	5.00	4.15	3.67	3.36	3.14	2.97	2.84	2.74	2.65
58	7.09	4.99	4.14	3.66	3.35	3.13	2.97	2.84	2.73	2.64
59	7.09	4.98	4.13	3.66	3.35	3.12	2.96	2.83	2.72	2.64
60	7.08	4.98	4.13	3.65	3.34	3.12	2.95	2.82	2.72	2.63
61	7.07	4.97	4.12	3.64	3.33	3.11	2.95	2.82	2.71	2.63
62	7.06	4.97	4.11	3.64	3.33	3.11	2.94	2.81	2.71	2.62
63	7.06	4.96	4.11	3.63	3.32	3.10	2.94	2.81	2.70	2.62
64	7.05	4.95	4.10	3.63	3.32	3.10	2.93	2.80	2.70	2.61
65	7.04	4.95	4.10	3.62	3.31	3.09	2.93	2.80	2.69	2.61
66	7.04	4.94	4.09	3.62	3.31	3.09	2.92	2.79	2.69	2.60
67	7.03	4.94	4.09	3.61	3.30	3.08	2.92	2.79	2.68	2.60
68	7.02	4.93	4.08	3.61	3.30	3.08	2.91	2.79	2.68	2.59

Contd...

Contd...

	1	2	3	4	5	6	7	8	9	10
69	7.02	4.93	4.08	3.60	3.30	3.08	2.91	2.78	2.68	2.59
70	7.01	4.92	4.07	3.60	3.29	3.07	2.91	2.78	2.67	2.59
71	7.01	4.92	4.07	3.60	3.29	3.07	2.90	2.77	2.67	2.58
72	7.00	4.91	4.07	3.59	3.28	3.06	2.90	2.77	2.66	2.58
73	7.00	4.91	4.06	3.59	3.28	3.06	2.90	2.77	2.66	2.57
74	6.99	4.90	4.06	3.58	3.28	3.06	2.89	2.76	2.66	2.57
75	6.99	4.90	4.05	3.58	3.27	3.05	2.89	2.76	2.65	2.57
76	6.98	4.90	4.05	3.58	3.27	3.05	2.88	2.76	2.65	2.56
77	6.98	4.89	4.05	3.57	3.27	3.05	2.88	2.75	2.65	2.56
78	6.97	4.89	4.04	3.57	3.26	3.04	2.88	2.75	2.64	2.56
79	6.97	4.88	4.04	3.57	3.26	3.04	2.87	2.75	2.64	2.55
80	6.96	4.88	4.04	3.56	3.26	3.04	2.87	2.74	2.64	2.55
81	6.96	4.88	4.03	3.56	3.25	3.03	2.87	2.74	2.63	2.55
82	6.95	4.87	4.03	3.56	3.25	3.03	2.87	2.74	2.63	2.55
83	6.95	4.87	4.03	3.55	3.25	3.03	2.86	2.73	2.63	2.54
84	6.95	4.87	4.02	3.55	3.24	3.03	2.86	2.73	2.63	2.54
85	6.94	4.86	4.02	3.55	3.24	3.02	2.86	2.73	2.62	2.54
86	6.94	4.86	4.02	3.55	3.24	3.02	2.85	2.73	2.62	2.53
87	6.94	4.86	4.02	3.54	3.24	3.02	2.85	2.72	2.62	2.53
88	6.93	4.86	4.01	3.54	3.23	3.01	2.85	2.72	2.62	2.53
89	6.93	4.85	4.01	3.54	3.23	3.01	2.85	2.72	2.61	2.53
90	6.93	4.85	4.01	3.54	3.23	3.01	2.85	2.72	2.61	2.52
91	6.92	4.85	4.00	3.53	3.23	3.01	2.84	2.71	2.61	2.52
92	6.92	4.84	4.00	3.53	3.22	3.00	2.84	2.71	2.61	2.52
93	6.92	4.84	4.00	3.53	3.22	3.00	2.84	2.71	2.60	2.52
94	6.91	4.84	4.00	3.53	3.22	3.00	2.84	2.71	2.60	2.52
95	6.91	4.84	4.00	3.52	3.22	3.00	2.83	2.70	2.60	2.51
96	6.91	4.83	3.99	3.52	3.21	3.00	2.83	2.70	2.60	2.51
97	6.90	4.83	3.99	3.52	3.21	2.99	2.83	2.70	2.60	2.51
98	6.90	4.83	3.99	3.52	3.21	2.99	2.83	2.70	2.59	2.51
99	6.90	4.83	3.99	3.52	3.21	2.99	2.83	2.70	2.59	2.51
100	6.90	4.82	3.98	3.51	3.21	2.99	2.82	2.69	2.59	2.50

Glossary

A

Abstract: An brief and concise summary of a research paper, usually placed at the beginning of the paper.

Accessible population: Portion of the population to which researcher has reasonable access.

Accidental sampling: Selection of most readily available person as participants in a study; sometimes called *convenience sampling*.

Adherence to treatment: The degree to which experimental group shows compliance to treatment in experimental research.

Analysis: The process of organizing and synthesizing data so as to answer research questions and test hypotheses.

Alternative hypothesis: In hypothesis testing, a hypothesis different from the one actually being tested-usually different the null hypothesis.

Analysis of covariance (ANCOVA): A statistical procedure used to test mean group differences on a dependent variable, while controlling for one or more covariate.

Analysis of variance (ANOVA): A statistical procedure for testing mean differences among three or more groups by comparing variability between groups to variability within groups, yielding an *F-Ratio* statistics.

Analytic triangulation: The use of two or more analytic approaches to analyze the same set of data.

Ancestory approach: It is a literature search techniques where a researcher use citation of existing relevant studies to track down the research.

Anonymity: Protection of participants' confidentiality in such a manner that even researcher cannot link individuals with information provided.

Applied research: Research designed to find a solution to an immediate practical problem.

Assent: The affirmative agreement of a subject (e.g. a child) to participate in a study, typically supplemented formal consent by a parent and guardian.

Associate relationship: A relationship between two or more than two variables that cannot be described as casual.

Assumption: A principle that is accepted being true based on logic or custom, without proof.

Asymmetric distribution: A skewed distribution of data in a measurement, with two halves that are not mirror images of each others.

Assignment: The process in experiment research where the researcher allocates subjects into two or more groups to achieve having groups as identical as possible.

Attrition: The loss of participants over a course the course of a study, which can create bias by changing the composition of the sample initially drawn.

Axial coding: The second level of coding in grounded theory research using the Strauss and Corbin approach, involves the process of categorizing, recategorizing and condensing first level of codes by connecting a category and its subcategories.

B

Back translation: The translation of translated text back into original language, so that original and back translated version can be compared as a means of enhancing semantic equivalence.

Basic risk: An expression of the likelihood that a particular event will occur within a particular population.

Basic research: Research designed to extend the base of knowledge in a discipline for the sake of knowledge production or theory construction, rather than for solving an immediate problem.

Before-after study: A method of control in which results from experimental subjects are compared with outcomes from patients before the new intervention was available.

Bell shaped curve: The characteristic shape of the curve of a normal distribution, where the data are equally distributed around the mean.

Beneficence: An ethical principal implying that every effort should be made to maximize the benefits to the subjects in health research.

Beta (β): In statistical testing, the probability of a type II error.

Between subject design: A type of research design in which separate groups of people are compare (e.g. alcoholics and non-alcoholics).

Bias: It is under representation and over representation of study results.

Bimodal distribution: A distribution of data values with two peaks.

Bivariate statistics: Statistics derived from analyzing two variables simultaneously to assess the empirical relationship between them.

Blind review: The review of manuscript or proposal in such a manner that neither the author nor the reviewers are identified by other party.

Blinding: A way of making sure that people involved in a research study—participants, clinicians and researcher-do not know each other's. It is also known as *'masking'.*

Bonferroni correction: An adjustment made to establish a more conservative alpha level when multiple statistical test are being run from the same data set; the correction is computed by dividing the desired α β the number of tests.

Bracketing: In phenomenological study, a process of identifying and holding in abeyance any preconceived belief and opinions about the underlying phenomena.

C

Carry over effect: The influence that one treatment can have on subsequent treatment, notably in cross over design.

Case control study: A type of observational analytical longitudinal retrospective study in which a group of subjects with a specified condition or disease and a healthy group are compared to identify risk factors, and treatment effectiveness.

Case study: A research method involving a through, in-depth analysis of an individual, group, or other social unit.

Categorical variables: Data where each individual variable is one of a member of mutually exclusive classes.

Cause and effect relationship: A relationship between two variable where presence or absence of one variable (the "cause") determine presence and absence of another variable (the "effect").

Central (core) category: The main category or pattern of behavior in grounded theory analysis using the Strauss and Corbin approach.

Central tendency: A statistical index of what is "typical" in a set of score, derived from the center of the score distribution; the mean, median or mode for numerical data in a frequency distribution.

Chi-square: A statistical test used for categorical data. It is based on comparison of the frequencies observed and the frequencies expected in the various categories.

Cluster sampling: A type of random sampling, based on random selection of certain subgroups, from which the sample can be taken.

Clinical research: Research designed to generate knowledge to guide practice in nursing and health care fields.

Close ended question: A question that offers respondents a set of specific response options.

Cluster randomization: The random assignment of intact groups or sites—rather than individual subjects—no treatment conditions.

Cluster sampling: A form of sampling in which a large grouping (clusters) are selected first and proceeds to successive subsampling of smaller units.

Code of ethics: The fundamental ethical principles to guide researchers conduct in research with human (or animal) subjects.

Code book: A record documenting categorization and coding decisions.

Coding: A process of labeling and classification of data by giving some numerical meaning.

Coefficient alpha (Cronbach's alpha): A reliability index that estimate the internal consistency or homogeneity of a composite measure composed of several items or subjects.

Coercion: The use of implicit or explicit threat to gain cooperation of people in research.

Cohort design: A non-experimental design in which a group of people is followed over a period of time to study outcomes for subsets of the cohort.

Comparison group: A group of subjects whose scores on dependent variables are used to evaluate the outcomes of the group of primary interest.

Concealment: A method involving collection of research data without participant's knowledge and or consent. Usually data are collected to obtain an accurate view of natural phenomena when the known presence of an investigator would change the phenomena of interest.

Concept: An abstraction inferred from observation of behaviors, situations, or circumstances.

Concurrent validity: The degree to which scores on an instrument are correlated with an external criterion, measured at the same time.

Confidence interval: The range of values within which a population parameter is estimated to lie, at a specified probability (e.g. 95% CI).

Confidentiality: The measures used by researcher to protect the sensitive and other private information of participants to expose publically.

Conformability: A criterion for integrity in a qualitative inquiry, referring to the objectivity or neutrality of the data and interpretations.

Confounding variables: A variable that is not a part of research study and extraneous to study but may confound the relationship between independent and dependent variables.

Conflict of interest: Investigators may have vested interest in the research. These may be intellectual property interest as well as commercial interest. Such interest should be explicitly declared.

Consecutive sampling: A sampling procedure in which subjects available in a defined period of time are enrolled in study.

Consent form: A written agreement signed by a study participant and a researcher concerning the term and condition of voluntary participation in a study.

Consistency check: A procedure performed in cleaning a set of data to ensure that the data are internally consistent.

CONSORT guidelines: Consolidated Standards of Reporting Trails, a widely adopted guideline for reporting information of a randomized controlled trails.

Constant comparison: A procedure used in grounded theory analysis wherein newly collected data are compared in an ongoing fashion with data obtained earlier, to refine theoretically relevant categories.

Construct: An abstraction or concept that is deliberately invented by researcher for a scientific purpose (e.g. interpersonal relationship).

Construct validity: The validity of inferences from observed person, settings, and interventions in a study to the construct that these instances might represent; with an instrument, the degree to which it measure the construct under investigation.

Contamination: The inadvertent, undesirable influence of one treatment condition on another treatment condition, as when member of the control group receive the intervention; sometimes called *treatment diffusion*.

Content analysis: The process of organizing and integrating material from documents, often narrative information from a qualitative study, according to key concept and themes.

Content validity: The degree to which an instrument represent all possible items for the concept being measured.

Content validity index (CVI): An index of degree of agreement for an instrument based on aggregated rating of a panel of experts.

Contingency table: A two-dimensional table in which the frequencies of two categorical variables are cross tabulated.
Continuous variables: Data which are measured on a continuous scale and can take infinite range of value along a specified continuum (e.g. all physical parameters).
Control: The process of holding constant extraneous influences on the dependent variable under study.
Control group: Subjects in an experimental study who do not receive intervention and whose performance is evaluated against experimental group.
Controlled trails: A clinical trials that has a control, with or without randomization.
Convenience sampling: Selection of most readily and feasible subjects in a study.
Convergent validity: An approach to measure constructs validity which measures the degree of similarity of two methods measuring a construct.
Correlation: The strength and direction of the association between two variables. Correlation does not mean causation.
Correlation coefficient: A statistics designed to measure size and direction of the association between two variables. The value varies between 0 and +1.
Correlational research: Research that explore relationship between two or more than two variables.
Cost-benefit analysis: A type of economic study design in which both cost and benefits of intervention are expressed in monetary terms.
Counterbalancing: The process of systematically changing the order of administration of intervention to control for ordering effects, especially in cross over design.
Covert data collection: The collection of data in a study without knowledge of participants.
Critical region: The area in the sampling distribution representing value that are "improbable" if the null hypothesis is true.
Cross over study: An experimental design in which one group of subject is exposed to more than one conditions of treatment.
Cross sectional study: An observational study design in which measurement are made on a single occasion.
Cross-tabulation tables: Frequency distribution tables that examines the relationship between several variables at one time to look for differences and relevant association.

D

Data: The piece of information obtained in a study (singular is *datum*).
Data cleaning: The process of preparing data for analysis by checking certain points like consistency and accuracy.
Data collection: The process of gathering information for research purpose.
Data saturation: See *saturation*.
Data set: The total collection of data on all variables for all study participants.
Data transformation: A process to make the data organized and in order to proceed for data analysis.

Data triangulation: The use of multiple methods to collect information on an underlying phenomenon.

Debriefing: A sort of communication with study subjects once the data collection is over.

Deception: The deliberate effort to withhold information or providing false and incomplete information to study subjects.

Degree of freedom (*df*): The number of sample values free to vary (e.g. with a given sample mean, all but one value would be free to vary).

Delphi survey: A technique for obtaining judgment from experts about an issue under study: experts are asked to give suggestions in several rounds to achieve some consensus.

Dependability: Its referring to the stability of the qualitative data over time and condition; analogues to reliability in quantitative research.

Dependent variables: The variable hypothesized to depend on or be caused by another variable name independent variable; the outcome variable of interest.

Descriptive research: Research that typically has its main objective to describe the characteristics of underlying phenomena.

Descriptive statistics: Statistics designed to summarizes and describe characteristics of the data. Descriptive statistics help us to make sense of a large volume of data.

Descriptive study: An observational study that simply describe the distribution of a characteristic.

Dichotomous variable: A variable having only two values or categories (e.g. gender).

Directional hypothesis: A hypothesis that makes a specific prediction about the direction of the relationship between two variables.

Discourse analysis: A qualitative tradition, from the discipline of sociolinguistics, that seeks to understand the rules, mechanism, and structure of conversation.

Discrete variable: Numerical variables that have definite value and cannot be measured on a continuous scale.

Discriminate validity: An aspect of construct validity that involves assessing the degree to which a single method for measuring two construct yield different results.

Disproportionate sampling: A type of sampling in which researcher select the sample disproportionally from different population.

Domain analysis: One of the Spradley's levels of ethnographic analysis, focusing on the identification of domains, or unit of cultural knowledge.

Double blind study: A experimental study, often a situation in which neither the subjects not those who administer the intervention know who is in experimental or control group.

Duplicate or redundant publication: Publication of a paper that overlaps substantially with one already published paper by the same authors.

E

Effect size: A statistical expression of the magnitude of relationship between two variables.

Eligibility criteria: The criteria designating the specific attributes of the target population, by which people are selected for inclusion in the study.

Emergent design: A design that emerge in the course of qualitative study as the researcher makes ongoing designs decisions reflecting what has already been learned.
Emic perspective: A ethnographic term indicating how the member of a culture themselves view their culture; the insider view.
Empirical evidence: Evidence which are rooted in reality and collected through one's senses (e.g. seeing, testing, or hearing).
Equivalence: The degree of similarity between alternate forms of a measuring instrument.
Ethics: A system of moral values that is concerned with the degree to which research procedures adhere to professional, legal and social obligation of the study.
Ethnography: A branch of human inquiry that focuses on the culture of a group of people.
Ethic perspective: A ethnographic term indicating experience of the outsiders towards a culture; the outside view.
Evaluation research: A research that focus on evaluation of program, policy or a programme.
Event sampling: A sampling plan that involves selection of integral behavior or events to be observed.
Evidence-based practice: A clinical problem-solving approach that emphasizes the integration of best evidences, with clinical expertise and patient preferences.
Exclusion criteria: Sampling criteria specifying characteristics that population does not have.
Experimental group: The subjects who are exposed or receive intervention.
Exploratory research: A study that explores the dimensions of a phenomenon or that develops or refines hypotheses about relationship between phenomena.
External criticism: In historical research, the systematic evaluation of the authenticity and genuineness of data.
Extraneous variable: A variable that confound the relationship between independent and dependent variables and that needs to be controlled either in the research design.

F

F-ratio: The statistics obtained in several statistical tests (e.g. ANOVA) in which variation attributable to different sources.
Face validity: The extent to which a measuring instrument looks as though it is measuring what it purport to measure.
Factorial design: Experimental designs in which two or more independent variable are simultaneously manipulated, permitting separate analysis of main effect of the independent variables and their interaction.
Feasibility study: A small scale rehearsal or trial run of main study to test feasibility of research methodology; also called *pilot study*.
Filed diary: A daily record of events and conversations in the field; also called a *log book*.
Field notes: The notes collected by researcher while conducting unstructured interview in the field.
Fisher's exact test: A statistical test used to test the significant difference in proportion when sample size small or cells in the contingency table have no observations.

Fit: In grounded theory analysis, the process of identifying one piece of data and comparing them with the characteristics of another data to determine similarity.

Focus group interview: An interview with a group of people who have similar problems of disease conditions.

Follow up study: A study conducted to ascertain the outcomes of individuals who have specified conditions or who have received a specified treatment.

Frequency distribution: A systematic arrangement of numeric values from lowest to the highest, together with a count of the number of times each values was obtained.

Frequency polygon: Graphic display of a frequency distribution, in which dots connected by a straight line indicate the number of times score values occur in a data set.

Friedman test: A nonparametric analogue of ANOVA, used with paired groups or repeated measures situations.

Full disclosure: The communication of complete information about a study to potential study participants.

Functional relationship: A relationship between two variables in which it cannot be assumed that one variable caused others.

G

Gaining entry: The process of getting access to study participants through the cooperation of key gatekeepers in the selected community or site.

Grand theory: A broad theory aimed at describing large segment of the physical, social, or behavioral world; also called *macro theory*.

Graphic rating scale: A scale in which respondents are asked to rate a concept along an ordered, numbered continuum, typically on a bipolar dimensions (e.g. "excellent" to "very poor").

Grounded theory: An approach to collecting and analyzing qualitative data that aims to develop theories grounded in real world observations.

H

Hawthorne effect: The effect on the dependent variable resulting from subjects awareness that they are participating under study.

Hermeneutics: A phenomenological study design, drawing on interpretive phenomenology, which focuses on the lived experience of human, and how they interpret those experiences.

Heterogeneity: The degree to which one object is dissimilar to another on an attribute.

Histogram: A graphic presentation of frequency distribution data.

Historical research: Systematic studies designed to discover facts and relationship about past events.

History threat: The occurrence of events external to an intervention that can affect the dependent variable and threaten the study's internal validity.

Homogeneity: (1) In term of reliability of an instrument, the degree to which its subparts are internally consistent. (2) More generally, the degree to which objects are similar (i.e. characterized by low variability).

Hypothesis: A statement predicted population parameter or relationship between two variables.

I

Impact factor: An annual measure of citation frequency for an average article in a given journal, that is, the ratio between citations and citable items published in the journal in a specified period.

Implied consent: Consent to participate in a study that a researcher assumes has been given based on participants' action, such as returning a complete questionnaire.

IMRaD format: The organization of research report into four sections: the Introduction, Method, Results and Discussion sections.

Incidence rate: The rate of new cases with a specified condition over a given period of time.

Independent variable: The variable that is believed to cause or influence the dependent variable; in experimental research, the manipulated (treatment) variable.

Inference: In research, conclusion drawn from the study evidence, taking into account the methods used to generate that evidence.

Inferential statistics: Statistics that permit inferences about whether results observed in a sample are likely to be found in the larger populations.

Informant: An individual who provides information to researchers about a phenomena under study, usually in qualitative study.

Informed consent: An ethical principle that requires researchers to obtain the voluntary participation of subjects, after informing them of a possible risks and benefits.

Inquiry audit: An independent scrutiny of qualitative data and relevant supporting documents by an external reviewer, to evaluate the dependability and conformability of qualitative data.

Institutional Review Board (IRB): A group of experts to review proposal and ongoing studies with respect to ethical considerations.

Instrument: A device used to collect information from research participants, e.g. questionnaire, rating scale and checklist, etc.

Interaction effect: The effect of two or more independent variables acting in combination on a dependent variable.

Intercoder reliability: The degree of agreement decision of two coders coding an construct.

Internal consistency: The degree to which subparts of an instrument are all measuring the same construct or attribute.

Internal criticism: In historical research or record analysis, evaluation of worth of evidences.

Internal validity: The degree of strength of relationship between independent and dependent variable.

Interpretation: The process of drawing conclusion and sense of study results and examining their implications.

Interquartile range: A measure of variability show the difference between Q_3 (75th percentile) and Q_1 (25th percentile).

Interrater (interobserver) reliability: The degree to which two rater of observer, operating independently, assign the same rating or category for a construct or attribute.

Interval measurement: A level of measurement in which an attribute of a variable is rank ordered on a scale that has an equal distance between two points.

Intervention: In experiment, the treatment being used.

Intervention fidelity: The degree of faithfulness of implementation of intervention on subjects in a study.

Intervention protocol: A detailed description of intervention and its related aspects in experimental research.

Intervention research: Research focused on development, implementation and testing of an intervention.

Interview: A data collection method in which researcher and participants sit face to face to collect information on underlying issue.

Intuiting: The second step in descriptive phenomenology, when researcher use to remain open to the meaning attributed to the phenomena by those who experienced it.

Investigator triangulation: The use of two or more researchers to analyze and interpret the data to enhance rigor.

Item: A single question on an instrument, or a single statement on a scale.

Item analysis: A type of analysis used to assess whether items on a scale are tapping the dame construct and are sufficiently discriminating.

Item difficulty: The amount of an attribute (such as knowledge) that a respondent must possess in order to "pass" the item.

J

Joint interview: An interview where two or more people are interviewed simultaneously or collect information on underlying attribute in a study.

Journal club: A group that meet in clinical setting to discuss and critique research report publishing in a journal.

K

Kappa: An index, used to measure the degree of an agreement between two or more than two raters.

Kendall's tau: A correlation coefficient used to measure the degree of strength between ordinal levels of data.

Key informant: A participant, usually in qualitative study, who agree to provide information on an attribute.

Keyword: An important term used to search for references on a topic in a bibliographic databases, used by other researcher to enhance the likelihood that their report will be found.

Known group technique: A technique for estimating the construct validity of an instrument through an analysis of the degree to which the instrument separates groups predicted to differ based on known characteristics or theory.

Kruskal-Wallis test: A nonparametric test used to test the difference between three and more independent groups, based on ranked scores.

L

Level of measurement: A system of classifying measurement according to the nature of the measurement and the type of permissible mathematical operations; the levels of measurement are nominal, ordinal, interval, and ratio.

Level of significance: The risk of making a type I error in a statistical analysis. With the criterion (alpha) established by the researcher beforehand (e.g. $\alpha = 0.05$ or 0.01).

Life history: A narrative self-report about a person's life experiences, e.g. a theme of interest.

Likert scale: A composite measure of attribute involving the summation of score on a set of item that respondent rate for their degree of agreement or disagreement.

Literature review: A critical summary of research on a topic of interest, often prepared to put a research problem.

Longitudinal study: A study designed to collect data at more than one point in time, in contrast to a cross-sectional study.

M

Macro theory: A broad theory aimed at describing large segment of the physical, social, and behavioral world; also called *grand theory*.

Manipulation: An intervention introduced by researcher to assess the impact on the dependent variable.

Manipulation check: In experimental studies, a test used to assess whether the manipulation was implemented or experienced as intended.

Mann-Whitney U test: A nonparametric test used to test difference between two independent groups, based on ranked scores.

Matching: It is process of paring two groups on the basis of certain characteristics, to enhance the overall comparability of groups.

Maturation threat: A threat to the internal validity of a study that results when changes to the outcomes measure result from the passage of time.

McNemar test: A statistical test for comparing differences in proportions when values are derived from paired groups.

Mean: A measure of central tendency, computed by summing all scores and dividing by the total number of cases.

Median test: A nonparametric test involving the comparison of median values of two independent groups to test whether the groups are from population with different medians.

Members check: A method of validating the credibility of qualitative data through debriefings and discussions with informants.

Meta-analysis: A statistical technique for quantitatively integrating the result of multiple similar studies addressing the same research question.

Meta-synthesis: It is a non-statistical technique used to integrate, evaluate and interpret the findings of multiple qualitative research studies.

Method triangulation: The use of multiple methods of data collection about the same phenomena, to enhance rigor or validity.

Methodologic research: Research designed to develop or refine methods of obtaining, organizing, or analyzing data.

Middle-range theory: A theory that focuses on only a portion of reality or human experience, involving selected number of concepts (e.g. theory of caregiver burden).

Minimal risk: Anticipated risks that are no greater than those ordinarily encountered in daily life or during the performance of routine tests of procedure.

Mixed design: A design that lends itself to comparisons both within groups overtime and between different groups of participants.

Mode: A measure of central tendency, the score value that occur most frequently in a distribution of scores.

Model: A symbolic representation of concepts or variables, and interrelationships among them.

Moderator variable: A variable that affects the strength or direction of a relationship between the independent and dependent variable.

MOOSE guidelines: Guidelines used to report meta-analysis of observational studies.

Mortality threat: A threat to the internal validity of a study, referring to loss of participants from different groups.

Multistage sampling: A sampling strategy that proceeds through a set of stages from large to smaller sampling unit.

Multivariate analysis of variance (MANOVA): A parametric statistics used to find the difference between the means of two or more groups on two or more independent variables.

N

Narrative analysis: A qualitative approach that focuses on stories as the object of the inquiry.

Negative relationship: A relationship between two variables in which there is a tendency for high values on one variable to be associated with low values on the other.

Negative skewed distribution: An asymmetric distribution of data values with a disproportionally high number of cases at the upper end; when displayed graphically, the tail points to the left.

Network sampling: The selection of participants based on referral from others already in the sample; also called *chain* or *snowball sampling*.

Nominal measurement: The lowest level of measurement involving the assignment of characteristics into categories (male, category 1; females, category 2).

Non-directional sampling: A research hypothesis that does not stipulate the expected direction of the relationship between variables.

Nonequivalent control group design: A quasi experimental design involving a comparison group that was not created through random assignment.

Non-experimental research: Studies in which researcher collects data without introducing an intervention; also called *observational study*.

Nonparametric test: A test statistics that does not follow assumption of distribution of data, also called *distribution free test*.

Nonprobability sampling: The selection of sample from population using nonrandom procedures.

Nonsignificant result: The relationship or association between groups indicating that observed difference or association have occurred by chance, at a given probability level.

Normal distribution: A distribution of data in a measurement in bell shaped and symmetrical curve; also called *normal distribution* or a *Gaussian distribution*.

Novelty effect: A threat to construct validity that can occur when participants change their behavior because of new intervention of instrument.

Null hypothesis: A hypothesis predicting no relationship between the variables under study; used for statistical testing.

Nursing research: Systematic inquiry designed to develop knowledge about issues of importance to the nursing professions.

O

Objectivity: The extent to which independent researchers would arrive at similar judgment or conclusions.

Observational research: An observer's in-depth description about events and conversation observed in naturalistic settings.

One tailed test: A statistical test in which only values in one tail of a distribution are considered in determine significance; sometimes used when researcher use directional hypothesis in study.

Open ended question: A type of question in questionnaire or interview that does not restrict respondents' answer to underlying construct.

Open coding: The first level of coding in a grounded theory study, referring to the basic descriptive coding of the content of the narrative materials.

Operational definition: The definition of concept or variable in term of the procedure by which it is to be measured.

Ordinal measurement: A measurement level that rank orders phenomena along some dimension.

Outcome measure: A term often used to refer to the dependent variable, that is, the measure that captures the outcomes of an intervention.

Outcome research: Research study deigned to documents the effectiveness of healthcare services and the end results of patient care.

Outliers: Value that lie outside the normal range of values for other cases in a data set.

P

P value: In statistical testing, the probability value to accept or reject statistical hypothesis.

Panel study: A longitudinal study in which data are collected from the same people over a period of time.

Parameter: A characteristics of a population (e.g. the mean age of Indian population).

Parametric tests: A type of statistical tests that involves assumptions about the distribution of variables and the estimation of a parameter.

Participant observation: A observation method of collecting data through the participation in and observation of a group.

Pearson's r: A correlation coefficient designating the magnitude of relationship between two variables measured at least an interval scale; also known as *product-moment correlation*.

Peer debriefing: Session with peers to review and explore various aspects of a study, sometimes used to enhance the trustworthiness in a qualitative study.

Perfect relationship: A correlation between two variables in which change in one variable permit perfect prediction of another variable.

Person triangulation: The collection of data from different levels of persons to validate the data through multiple perspectives on the phenomena.

Personal notes: In field studies, written comments about the observer's own feelings during the research process.

Phenomenon: The abstract concept under study, often used by qualitative researchers in lieu of the term variable.

Phenomenology: A qualitative research based on live experience of the person.

Phi coefficient: A statistical index describing the magnitude of relationship between two dichotomous variables.

Pilot study: A small scale rehearsal or trial run of main study to test feasibility of research methodology.

Placebo: A pseudo intervention, often used as a control group condition.

Placebo effect: A change in the dependent variable attributable to the placebo condition.

Point estimation: A statistical procedure in which information from a sample is used to estimate the single value that best represent the population parameter.

Population: A group of people or objects having some common characteristics.

Positive relationship: A relationship between two variable in which high value of one variable is related to high value of another variable.

Positively skewed distribution: An asymmetric distribution of values with a disproportionally high number of cases at the lower end; when displayed graphically, the tail points to the right.

Poster session: A session at professional conference in which several researcher simultaneously present visual displays of their studies and have question answer session with conference participants.

Post-test: The collection of information or data after administration of intervention.

Post-test only design: An experimental design in which data are collected after administration of an intervention.

Power: The ability of a design or analysis strategy to detect true relationships that exist among variables.

Power analysis: A procedure used to determine the sample size in experimental study or the likelihood of committing a type II error.

Predictive validity: The degree to which an instrument can predict a criterion observed at a future time.

Pretest: The collection of baseline information prior to administering intervention from the subjects.

Pretest post-test design: An experimental research in which data are collected before and after giving intervention.

Prevalence study: An epidemiological cross-sectional study designed to identify the number of old as well news cases of a disease or condition at a given time.

Primary sources: The first hand sources which are written or developed by the investigator who conduct the study or work.

Principal investigator (PI): The individual who is lead researcher and who will have primary responsibility for overseeing a study.

PRISMA guidelines: Guidelines used to report findings of true experimental studies.

Probability sampling: The selection of sample on the basis of random procedures.

Problem statement: An expression of a perplexing and puzzling situation that need investigation.

Process consent: In qualitative study, an ongoing transactional process of negotiating consent with study participants to take part in research study to perform their role.

Prolonged engagement: It is process of investing sufficient time to collect data in qualitative study.

Propensity score: A score that captures the conditional probability of exposure to a treatment, given various pre-intervention characteristics; can be used to match comparison groups or as a statistical control variable to enhance internal validity.

Proposal: A well written document communicate research problem, its significance, procedure for collecting information, and when funding is sought, how much the study will cost.

Prospective design: A study that begin with a presumed causes and then goes forward in time to observe presumed effects.

Purposive sampling: A nonprobability sampling method in which the researcher selects participants based on personal judgment about which ones will be most informative; sometimes called *judgmental sampling.*

Q

Q-sort: A data collection method in which participants sort statements into a number of piles (usually 9 or 11) according to some bipolar dimension.

Qualitative data: Information collected in the form of narrative description such as dialogues from transcript of an unstructured interview.

Qualitative research: The investigation of an phenomena, typically in an in-depth and holistic fashion, through the collection of rich narrative materials using a flexible research design.

Quantitative data: Information collected in numeric form; usually in quantitative research.

Questionnaire: A document contains series of questions to gather information on a particular attribute or phenomenon.

Quota sampling: A nonrandom sampling technique in which quota for certain sample characteristic are fixed to improve representativeness.

R

Random assignment: A process of assigning the subjects in experimental and control group in a random manner; sometimes called *randomization*.

Random sampling: The sampling technique in which each sample has equal and independent chance of selection in study.

Randomization: A process of assigning the subjects in experimental and control group in a random manner; sometimes called *random assignment*.

Randomized block design: An experimental design involving two or more factors (independent variables), with one or more factors experimentally manipulated and one or more factors not manipulated.

Randomized control trials (RCT): An ideal intervention procedure involving random assignment to treatment group; sometimes, phase III of a full clinical trials.

Range: A measure of variability, computed by subtracting the lowest value from highest values in a distribution of scores.

Rating scale: A scale that require rating of an object or concept along a continuum.

Ratio measurement: A measurement level with equal distances between score and true meaningful zero point (e.g. height).

Raw data: Data in the form in which they are collected, before proceeding to coding, organizing and analysis process.

Reflexive notes: Notes that document a qualitative researcher's personal experience, reflections and progress in the field.

Relationship: A connection between two or more variables.

Reliability: The degree of consistency and accuracy of an instrument to measure a construct on different occasions.

Reliability coefficient: A index, usually range from 0.00 to 1.00, that provides an estimate of how reliable an instrument is. (e.g. KR_{20}, Crohnback lapha).

Repeated measure ANOVA: An analysis of variance used when there are multiple measures of the dependent variable over time.

Replication study: The deliberate repetition of research procedures in a second investigation for the purpose of determining or checking the authenticity of earlier results.

Representative sample: A sample whose characteristics are comparable to population from which it is taken.

Research: It is systematic, controlled, empirical and critical investigation in an attempt to discover of conform the findings.

Research design: The overall plan for addressing a research question, including specifications for enhancing the study's integrity.

Research hypothesis: The statement which state relationship between two or more than two variables.

Research method: The techniques used to structure a study and to gather and analyze information in a systematic fashion.

Research misconduct: Fabrication, falsification and plagiarism, or other deliberate ways to change the study methods, and reported results.

Research problem: An enigmatic or perplexing condition that can be studied through disciplined inquiry.
Research question: A statement of the specific query the researcher wants to answer to address a research problem.
Research report: A well written concise document summarizing the main features of a study, including the research question, methods, findings and the interpretation of the findings.
Research utilization: The use of some aspect of a study in an anticipation unrelated to the original research.
Researcher credibility: It is faith of a researcher based on his training, qualifications, and experience.
Respondents: In self-report method, the study participants who respond to self report method.
Response set bias: The measurement errors resulting from the tendency of some individuals to respond to items in either always positive or vice versa.
Results: The answer to research question, obtained through an analysis of the collected data.
Retrospective design: A study design that begin with effect or outcome and go back to search for presumed cause of the event.
Risk/benefit ratio: The relative cost and benefit, to an individual subject to society at large, of participation in a study; also the relative cost and benefits of implementing an innovation.
Rival hypothesis: An alternative explanation, competing with the researcher's hypothesis, for interpreting the results of a study.

S

Sample: A subset of population, enrolled for study.
Sampling: The process of drawing a desired number of sample size from accessible population.
Sampling bias: A over-representation or under-representation of sample to the characteristics of population.
Sampling error: The variation in value from one sample to another drawn from the same sample.
Sampling frame: A list of all the elements in the population, from which the sample is drawn.
Sampling plan: A formal plan that specify sampling method, size and procedure to collect sample.
Saturation: The collection of qualitative data to the point where new data yield duplicate or redundant information from the subjects.
Scale: A composite measure of an attribute, involving the combination of several items that have a logical and empirical relationship to each other, resulting in the assignment of a score to place people on a continuum with respect to the attribute.
Scatter plot: A graphic representation of magnitude of relationship between two variables.
Scientific method: A set of orderly, systematic, controlled procedure for acquiring authentic information on underlying construct.
Screening instrument: An instrument used to determine whether potential subjects for a study meet eligibility criteria, or for determining whether a person tests positive for a specified condition.

Secondary analysis: A form of research which are based on the data collected by other researcher to answer new questions or test rival hypothesis. Secondary source: It is second hand account of information. A description of information prepared by someone else than original researcher.

Selective coding: A level of coding in grounded theory that involves selection of the core category and integrating relationship between core categories and other categories.

Selection threat: A threat to external validity of the study resulting from preexisting group differences between groups under study.

Self-determination: A person's ability to voluntarily decide whether or not to participate in a research study.

Self-report: A method of data collection involving collection of information from the person who are being studied (e.g. questionnaire or interview).

Semantic differential: A technique used to measure attitudes in which respondents rate underlying concept on a series of bipolar rating scale.

Semi-structured interview: A type of interview in which a researcher has a list of all possible questions related to concepts in a study.

Sensitivity: The ability of an instrument to correctly identify a "case", that is, to correctly diagnose a condition.

Setting: The venue or location in which data collection takes place in a study.

Significance level: The probability that an observed relationship could be caused y chance; significance at 0.05 level indicates the probability that a relationship of the observed magnitude would be found by chance only 5 times out of 100.

Sign test: A nonparametric test used to compare two paired groups based on the relative ranking of values between the pairs.

Simple random sampling: It is basic probability sampling technique involve selection of sample members through random procedure (e.g. lottery method, table of random number).

Site: The overall location where a study is undertaken.

Skewed distribution: The asymmetric distribution of a set of data values around a central point.

Snowball sampling: The selection of samples through referral from earlier participants; also called as *network* or *chain sampling*.

Spearman's rank correlation (Spearman's rho): A correlation coefficient indicate the magnitude of relationship between two variables measured at ordinal level.

Specificity: The ability of a screening instrument to correctly identify noncases.

Standard deviation: The most frequently used statistic for measuring the degree of variability in a set of score.

Standard error: The standard deviation of a sampling distribution, such as sampling distribution of the mean.

Standard scores: Score expressed in terms of standards deviations from the means, with raw scores transformed to have a mean of zero and a standard deviation of one; also called *z scores*.

Statement of purpose: A broad declarative statement of the overall goals of study.

Statistics: An estimate of a parameter, calculated from sample data.

Index

Page numbers followed by *b* refer to box, *f* refer to figure, and *t* refer to table.

A

Abstract 52, 343
Accessing records, problems in 201
Accidental sampling 343
Acquiring knowledge in nursing, methods of 5
Action research 140
    example of 143*b*
    limitation of 143
    strengths of 143
    typology 141*t*
Addressing ethical issues 58
Adolescent Coping Orientation for Problem Experiences 97
Adolescent, height and weight of 289*t*
Aggrement in cohen kappa, level of 209*t*
Alcohol and alcohol problems science databases 78
American Nurses Association 63
American Psychological Association 263
    style 263
    of references 264
Analytic triangulation 343
Analytical studies 123, 123*b*
Animal studies, sample size for 169
Anova applications, assumptions of 322
Anova calculation, steps of 322
Anova table, preparation of 323
Anova value, interpretation of 323
Applied research 14, 343
    example of 14*b*
Arithmetic mean, properties of 291
Assess internal consistency, measures to 210
Assignment 344
Associate relationship 343
Associative hypothesis, example of 44*b*
Assumptions 40, 343
    hypotheses 41
    in research, importance of 42
    types of 41
Asymmetric distribution 344
Attributes of reliability 210*t*
Attrition 344
    effects 105
    rate 169
Authority 5
Authorship abuses 269
Authorship order 270
Axial coding 250, 344

B

Back translation 344
Background data 182
Back-translation 214
Bar diagram 283
    subdivided 285*f*
Bar graphs 229, 230
Basic and applied research 13, 13*t*
Basic research 13, 344
    example of 14*b*
Basic risk 344
Before-after study 344
Behavior/phenomenon, selection of 197
Bell shaped curve 344
Beneficence 344
    principle of 63
Benner's model 93
Best research evidence 21
Bias 344
    and barriers identification 173
Bibliographic trail 75
Bimodal distribution 344
Biophysiological measurement, purposes of 199
Biophysiological methods 198
    limitations of 200
    strengths of 199
    types of 198
Biostatistics 277

Bivariate statistics 344
Blind review 344
Blinding 344
Body 281
Bonferroni correction 344
Book 263, 264
Borrowing 6
Bowley's coefficient of skewness 312
Bracketing 344
Brainstorming 5
British Nursing Index 78
Budget estimation 269

C

Cafeteria question 180
  example of 180b
Calculate sampling interval, example to 158b
Cancer literature (CanerLit) 78
Caption heading 281
Carry over effect 345
Case control study 345
  sample size for 168
Case study 139, 345
  example of 140b
  limitations of 140
  strengths of 140
Case-control designs 123
  limitation of 124
  strengths of 123
Case-control study, example of 124b
Casual hypotheses 44
  example of 45b
Categorical variables 52, 345
Category system 197
Cause-effect relationship 345
Central category 345
Central tendency 345
  measures of 221, 290
Cerebrovascular accident 151
Charts 229, 237
Checklist
  limitations of 189
  strengths of 189
Children in Indian families, number of 290t
Chi-square 345
  calculation
    direct method of 317
    steps of 316
  distribution of 327

Chi-square test 240, 315
  application, assumptions of 315
  for homogeneity 317
  of association/independence 316
  of goodness of fit 317
Chronological analysis 249
Circular systematic sampling 159
Classical experimental design 110
Classical measurement theory 208b
Client system 95
Clinical data and history 22
Clinical expertise 21
Clinical research 345
Close ended question 345
  example of 179b
Cluster randomization 107, 345
Cluster sampling 159, 345
  example of 160b
  limitations of 160
  steps of 159
  strengths of 160
Cochrane library 79
Code book 345
Code notes 246
Code of ethics 61, 345
  for nurses 62b
Code, type of 246, 250
Coding 345
Coding data 223
Coding in qualitative data analysis, types of 246t
Coding qualitative data 245
Coding sheet 223
Coefficient alpha 211, 345
Coefficient correlation
  (r)-direct method, calculation of 306
  calculation of 308
  interpretation of 306b
  significance of 306
Coercion 345
Coercive authorship 270
Cohort design 124, 345
Cohort study
  example of 124b
  process of 124f
Colaizzi approach 252f
Colaizzi method 251
Collect data from subjects 4
Collecting data 55
Column heading 281
Combined health information databases 78
Common statistical methods, list of 222b

Common statistical terms 279
Communicating findings 56
Communication
   and dissemination of research 257
   barriers related to 273
   of research findings 257
   select method of 258
Comparative and relative figures 226
Comparative designs 121
Comparative study, examples of 121b
Comparative survey 127
Comparison group 345
Completion techniques 205
Complex hypothesis 43
   example of 43b
Complex table, example of 226
Componential analysis 248, 249
Computation of anova, steps of 322
Computer generated random numbers 107
Computer software application in data analysis 243
Computer table 156
Computer-assisted
   interviews 193
   method 182
Computing coefficient correlation, steps of 209
Concealment 346
   and non-participant 196
   and participant 196
Concept mapping 247
Conceptual equivalence 213
Conceptual framework 43, 88, 91
   basic elements of 91
   development, process of 97
   purposes of 90
Conceptual model 91
Conclusion and interpretation 138
Concurrent validity 346
Conducting interviews
   guidelines for 192
   tips for 192b
Conference proceeding 263
Confidence interval 346
Confidentiality 346
Confirmability 131, 244
Conflict of interest 346
Conformability 346
Confounding variables, example of 37b
Consecutive sampling 346
   example of 164b
   limitations of 164
   strengths of 164

Consent form 346
Consent, types of 66
Consistency check 346
Consort guidelines 346
Constant comparative analysis 249
Constant comparison 346
Construct 346
Construct validity 206, 207, 346
Construct/concept, selection of 181
Constructing good checklist, guidelines of 189
Constructing vignettes, steps of 203
Construction of self-report methods, steps of 181
Construction projective techniques 204
Contact information 66
Contains instrument 45
Contamination 346
Content analysis 346
   limitations of 247
   strengths of 247
Content equivalence 213
Content validity 206, 207, 346
   coefficient, interpretation of 207
   index 346
   measurement of 207
Contingency question 180
   example of 180b
Contingency table 347
Continuous data 279
Continuous frequency distribution table 227
Continuous variables 52, 347
Control group 347
   interrupted time series design 116
   use of 108
Control in experimental research 108
Control problem 4
Controlled trails 347
Convenience sampling 160, 347
   limitations of 161
   strengths of 161
Convenient to select sample 154
Convergent validity 206, 347
Cooperation of colleagues and others 35
Copyright issue 270
Corbin's method 250t
Core category 345
Correlation coefficient 305, 333, 347
   types of 306, 307f
Correlational research 122, 347
   limitations of 123
   strengths of 123
   types of 122

Correlational survey 127
Cost 35
Cost effectiveness in nursing practice, improve 19
Cost-benefit analysis 347
Council of Science Editors 263
Counterbalanced design 117
    example of 117b
Counterbalancing 109, 347
Covariance, analysis of 343
Cover letter 183
Covert data collection 347
Creativity 243
Credibility (internal validity) 130, 244
Criterion equivalence 213
Criterion validity 206, 207
Critical appraisal
    of research report 264
    of review 83, 83b
Critical assessment of plan 176
Critical region 347
Critique whole report 265
Critiquing quantitative research, guidelines for 267t
Cronbach's alpha 211, 345
Cross over study 347
Cross-sectional design 125
    example of 126b
Cross-sectional study 347
    limitations of 126
    strengths of 126
Cross-sectional survey 127
    designs, sample size for 167
Cross-tabulation tables 347
Cultural equivalence of instrument 213
Cumulative frequency 228
    curve 229,235, 283, 288
    table 229t
Current issues of profession 8

D

Data 347
    analysis of 4
    cleaning 224, 347
    coding 223
    collectors, training to 176
    determine quantum of 138
    editing 223
    for analysis, preparing 56
    fraction of 242
    input 224
    interpretation of 4, 242
    into categories, classification of 251
    precision of 154
    saturation 58, 347
    set 347
    sources of 174, 282
        evaluate strengths of 138
        specify types of 138
    transformation 347
    triangulation 348
    types of 15, 65, 174
    verification 224
Data analysis 138, 219
    and interpretation 219
    duration of 15
    plan for 269
    process, description of 243
Data collection 133, 138, 347
    duration of 15
    essential of 175, 175b
    methods 176, 176f, 177
    in research 173
    selection of 177
    plan 175, 269
        development of 175
    purposes of 173
    selecting tools for 58
    techniques of 177
    tool for 177, 177t
Data presentation 225
    methods of 281
Data processing 223
    steps of 225
Data-oriented reflection 243
Debriefing 348
Degree of freedom 315, 348
    for T-test 321
Delimitations 46, 47
    example of 47b
    in research, purposes of 47
Delphi survey 348
Delphi technique 143
    advantages and limitations of 144t
    crux of 144b
Democratic impulse 142
Dependability (reliability) 131, 244, 348
Dependent and independent variables,
    example of 36b
Dependent sample t-test 318
Description and exploration 241
Descriptive question 34
Descriptive research 120, 348

Descriptive statistics 219, 281, 348
Descriptive study 122, 348
	example of 122b
Descriptive survey 126
Develop model and framework for nursing practice 19
Develop reward system for nurses 273
Developing category scheme 245
Developing coding frame 223
Developing conceptual framework 54
Developing intervention protocol 55
Developing research design 58
Developmental research 124
Dichotomous
	question 178
	variable 52, 348
Difficulty index of scale 213
Directional hypothesis 44, 348
	example of 44b
Discourse analysis 348
Discovery and explanation 241
Discrete data 279
Discrete frequency distribution table 227
Discriminate validity 348
Disease pattern, distribution of 173
Disproportionate sampling 348
Disproportionate stratified random sampling 157
Disseminating research, steps of 258
Dissemination of research findings, purposes of 257
Dissertation and thesis 264
Distribution free test 314, 354
Divergent validity 206
Domain analysis 248, 249, 348
Dot diagram 229, 236, 283, 289
Double blind study 348
Draw-a-person test 204
Duplicate publication 270, 348

E

Easy language 183
EBP in nursing, significance of 24
Educational research, sampling in 151
E-journals 264
Electronic databases 77
	list of 78b
Electronic sources 77
Element 152
	elimination 251
Eligibility criteria 153, 348
	specify 165

Email questionnaire 182
Emergent design 16, 349
Emersion in data 242
Emphasis 227
Empirical evidence 349
Empirical phase 55
End questionnaire in proper way 183
Ensure credibility of nursing profession 19
Entry in research setting 58
Environment, preparation of 192
Environmental characteristics/attributes 195
Epidemiological research 122
Equivalence 209, 349
E-thesis 264
Ethic 349
	in research, importance of 63
	perspective 349
Ethical consideration 4, 35, 55, 269
Ethical dimension 266
Ethical issues 102
	in animal research 68
	in research 61
Ethical principles 64f
Ethical violations in research 61
Ethnographic analysis 248
Ethnographic study 135b
	example of 135b
	limitations of 136
Ethnography 134, 349
	strengths of 136
Evaluate outcomes and revise 2
Evaluation criteria for research problem 34
Evaluation research 349
Evaluative study 128
	example of 128b
Evaluative survey 127
Even observations, median for 294
Event sampling 197, 349
Evidence
	analyze 2, 24
	levels of 22b
Evidence-based practice 20, 22, 271, 272, 349
	components of 21
	five A's of 24b
	history of 20
	model 21f
	steps of 22, 23f
Exclusion criteria, example of 154b
Exclusive class interval 228, 228t
Experimental designs, symbols in 111b
Experimental group 349

Experimental research 106
   characteristics of 106
   limitations of 114
   steps in 109
   strengths of 114
   types of 106
Experimental studies, sample size for 168
Experimenter effects 105
Explanatory survey 127
Exploitation in elderly 72
Exploratory designs 121
Exploratory research 349
   example of 121b
Exploratory survey 127
Exponential discriminative snowball sampling 162
Exponential nondiscriminative snowball sampling 161
Expressive techniques 205
External criticism 201, 349
Extraneous variable 37, 52, 349
   example of 37b
Extrapersonal stressors 95
Extreme climate condition 213

F

Fabrication 271
Face pain scale for infant 187f
Face to face
   interviews 193
   method 182
Face validity 349
Facilitate comparison 229
Facilitate statistical processing 229
Facilitating research utilization 273
Factorial design 112, 349
   example of 112b
Factors affecting
   external validity 105
   internal validity 104
   literature review 72
   reliability 212
   sampling/sample size 164
   selection of study design 102
Feasibility study 214, 349
Field notes 349
Filed diary 349
Final draft, preparation of 182
Fisher's exact test 240, 349
Fittingness 131
Flexible line of defense 95

Flipping coin 107
Flowcharts 229, 239
Focus group interview 350
Focused group discussion 191
Footnotes 282
Formulate research question 138
Formulating hypothesis 54
Formulating research problem 53
F-ratio 349
Frequency curve 229, 233, 233f, 283, 286, 287f
Frequency distribution 221, 350
   table 227t
Frequency polygon 229, 234, 235f, 236f, 283, 287, 288f, 350
Friedman test 350
F-test 322
Functional relationship 350
Fundamental research terms 52

G

Gaussian distribution 355
Geared towards evidences development 8
General and specific objectives, example of 39b
General nursing and midwifery 11
Ghost author 270
Giorgi method 252
Glaser and Strauss method 249, 250t
Good chart 237b
Good hypothesis, characteristics of 45
Good measure of dispersion, characteristics of 297
Good questionnaire, essentials of 182
Good research
   characteristics of 8
   design, characteristics of 102
   question, elements of 33
   report 260
Good sample, characteristics of 154
Good table
   construction of 281
   essentials of 282
Goodness of fit, test of 315
Grand theory 92, 350
Graph presentation 225, 229, 282
   principles of 230, 282
Graphic rating scale 184, 188, 350
   example of 188b
   limitation of 188
   strengths of 188
Graphical presentation
   methods of 283
   significance of 282

Grounded theory 136, 350
  analysis 249
  limitations of 137
  strengths of 137
Group homogeneity 213

H

Hawthorne effect 105, 196, 350
Health Insurance and Portability and Accountability Act 65
Health STAR 78
Heideggerian hermeneutics school of phenomenology 253
HELLP syndrome 93
Help references 229
Hermeneutics 350
Heterogeneity 350
Hierarchical statement, development of 98
Histogram 229, 230, 232, 232f, 283, 285f, 350
Historical research 137, 350
  example of 139b
  limitations of 138
  steps of 138
  strengths of 138
History effects 104
History threat 350
Holistic approach 253
Homogeneity 350
  of population 165
  test of 315
  testing 109
House-tree-person test 204
Human behavior complexity 4
Hypotheses 42, 46, 46b, 91, 350
  alternative 343
  associative 44
  classification of 43
  components of 46
  example of 45b
  in research, purposes of 42
  non-directional 44
  sources of 43
  testing 173, 177, 240, 313
Hypothetical identification 251

I

Identify population 165
Identifying research problem, steps of 32, 32f
Impact factor 351
Implied consent 66, 351

Importance question, example of 181b
IMRaD format 351
In vitro measurement 199
In vivo measurement 199
Incidence rate 121b, 351
Incidence studies 120
Inclusion criteria, example of 153b
Inclusive class interval 227, 228t
Independent sample t-test 319
Independent variable, manipulation of 108
Index medicus 78
Indian Council of Medical Research 63, 68
Indian National Science Academy 68
Indian Nursing Council 18
Individual in provision of care 62
Inductive data analysis 16
Inferential statistics 239, 312, 351
  types of 240
Informant 351
Information, source of 227
Informed consent 65, 351
Informed written consent 66
Initial data analysis 250
Inquiry audit 351
Institutional Animal Ethics Committee 68
Institutional Ethical Committee 67
Institutional Review Board 67, 351
Instrument 46, 177, 351
  length of 212
  translation into new language 213
  validity, types of 207t
Instrumentation effects 105
Integrated and systematic review 75t
Integrated literature review 74
Interaction effect 351
Interactional analysis 249
Intercoder reliability 351
Interest and motivation 102
Internal consistency 210, 351
Internal criticism 201, 351
Internal validity 206, 351
International Nursing Journals 79
International standard
  book numbers 75
  serial numbers 75
Internet and other electronic sources 264
Interpersonal stressors 95
Interpersonal wording of question 183
Interpretation 351
Interpretive dimension 266
Interpretive phenomenology 133

Interquartile range 222, 297, 298, 351
Interrater (interobserver) reliability 351
Interrupted time series design 115
Interval measurement 280, 351
Interval scale 220
Interval-level measurement 220b
   example of 280b
Intervention 352
Intervention protocol 352
   in experimental research 109
Intervention research 352
Interviews 352
   limitations of 194
   method 190
   preparation, guidelines for 192
   strengths of 193
   types of 190
   unstructured 190
Interviewing process 193
Intrapersonal stressors 95
Introduction and instructions 181
Intuiting 352
Intuition 5, 31
Investigate thoroughly 6
Investigator triangulation 131, 352
Item 352
   analysis 352
   difficulty 352
Item-total correlations 212

J

Joint interviews 191, 352
Journal 264
   club 352
   offline 79
   online 79
Judgmental sampling 163
Justice, principle of 63, 65

K

Kappa 352
Karl-Pearson's coefficient of skewness 312
Kendall's tau 352
Key informant 352
Keyword 352
Knowledge and experience of investigator 102
Known group technique 352
Kruskal-Wallis test 352

Kuder-Richardson formula 211
Kurtosis 312, 312f
   measures of 312

L

Language of items in scale 213
Latin square design 117
Levels-by-treatment design 113
Library call number 75
Life history 353
Likert scale 184, 353
   example of 185t
   limitations of 185
   reverse scoring in 185t
   strengths of 185
   uses of 184
Line diagrams 229, 237, 237f, 283, 289, 290f
Linear systematic sampling 159
Literature review 6, 353
   importance of 73
   organization of 82
   purposes of 73
   sources of 75, 76f, 77b
   steps of 80
   types of 74
Literature sources 78f
   obtaining information from 79
Literature, analyzing 80
Logical construct, development of 98
Logical flow 183
Longitudinal design 125
Longitudinal study
   example of 125b
   limitations of 125
Lottery method 156

M

Macro theory 353
Maintain record 176
Manipulation check 353
Mann-Whitney U test 353
   median test 240
Maps 229, 238
Marker variables 152
Matching 107, 353
Maturation effects 104
Maturation threat 353
McNemar test 353

Index

Mean
  by assumed mean method, calculation of 292
  demerits of 293
  for grouped data, calculation of 292
Mean deviation 222, 299, 304, 304t
  demerits of 300
  merits of 300
Meaning units, discrimination of 252
Measure anova, repeated 358
Measurement
  levels of 220, 279, 353
  related problem 4
Median
  demerits of 295
  for grouped data, calculation of 294
  for ungrouped data, calculation of 293
  merits of 295
  test 353
Members check 353
Memoing 246
Meta-analysis 74, 75, 128, 353
  example of 128b,
Meta-synthesis 74, 75, 129, 353
  example of 129b
Metatheory 92
Method triangulation 131, 353
Methodologic dimension 266
Methodologic research 354
  steps in 129b
Methodological limitations 48
Methodological study 129
  example of 130b
Metro map of Delhi 239f
Middle range theory 92, 93, 354
Midwives information and resource service 78
Minimal risk 354
Mixed design 354
Mode
  demerits of 297
  for grouped data, calculation of 296
  for ungrouped data, calculation of 296
  merits of 296
  types of 296t
Model 87, 354
Moderator variable 354
Molar approach 196
Molecular approach 196
Monthly expenditure
  in particular year 284t
  on different items 231t

Monthly wages of families in India 287t
Moose guidelines 354
Moral-ethical problem 3
Mortality effects 105
Mortality threat 354
Multiple bar
  diagram 284f
  graph 230, 231, 231f
Multiple choice question 179
  example of 179b
Multistage sampling 159, 354
Multivariate analysis of variance 354

N

Narrative analysis 248, 354
National Institute of Nursing Education 12
National Nursing Journals 79
Natural setting 16
Nature of relationship 195
Nature of research design 164
Nazi medical experiment 61
Needs identification 173
Negative relationship 354
Negative skewed distribution 354
Negative skewness 311
Negatively skewed distribution 311f
Network sampling 354
Newspaper article 264
Nominal measurement 279, 354
Nominal scale 220
Nominal-level measurement 220b
  example of 279b
Non-directional hypothesis, example of 44b
Non-equivalent control group
  design 354
  post-test design 115
  pretest design 115
Non-equivalent post-test only design,
  example of 115b
Non-experimental designs 119
Non-experimental research 354
  classification of 120t
  types of 119
Nonmaleficence 64
Non-parametric test 240, 314, 354
Nonparametric tests 315t
Non-probability sampling 160, 355
  reason for use of 164b
  types of 160

Non-randomized pretest post-test design,
   example of 115*b*
Nonverbal communication behavior 195
Normal distribution 355
   curve 221, 222*f*, 309, 310*f*
   shape of 311*f*
   significance of 310
Normality test 317
Novelty effect 105, 355
Null hypothesis 44, 241, 355
   example of 44*b*
Nurse
   barriers related to 25, 272
   respect
      individual's right to privacy 62
      uniqueness of 62
Nursing 1
   and managed care database 78
   journals, list of 79*t*
   practice, provide accountability of 19
   process 90*f*
Nursing research 7, 22, 355
   and evidence-based practice 22*t*
   at international level, major milestone of 9
   at national level, major milestone of 11
   scope and areas of 17
Nursing Research Society of India 12
Nursing students
   marks of 288*t*
   score of 288*t*
Nursing studies index 78
Nursing theory
   research and practice 97*f*
   scope of 92*f*

O

Objective information, focus on 176
Objectivity 355
   in scoring 213
Observation method 195
   limitations of 198
   strengths of 198
   types of 196
Observation schedule, development of 197
Observation, elements of 195
Observational research 355
Observational study 354
Observer-observed relationship 195
Odd observations, median for 293
Odd-even reliability 210

Ogive 289*f*
One group pretest post-test design, example of 118*b*
Open coding 250, 355
Open communication channels 273
Open end question 355
Open end table 228*t*
Open ended question, example of 178*b*
Operational definitions
   examples of 38*b*
   significance of 38
Operational notes 246
Oral report 260
Ordinal measurement 279, 355
Ordinal scale 220
Ordinal-level measurement 220*b*
   example of 280*b*
Orem's self-care theory 93
Organization, barriers related to 25, 272
Organize continuing education events 273
Ovid 78

P

P value 355
Page numbers 75
Panel study 355
Parametric and non-parametric statistics,
   application of 240*b*
Parametric test 240, 314, 315*t*, 356
Participant observation 356
Participant perspective 16
Participant status 65
Participant's selection 66
Participatory character 142
Patient value and preferences 21
Peer debriefing 356
Peer-review 53
Perfect negative relationship 306
Perfect positive relationship 306
Performative analysis 249
Person triangulation 356
Personal data 182
Personal notes 356
Personal reflection 243
Personality traits 259
Phenomena 198
   amenable to observation 195
   of interest, study of 133
Phenomenological analysis 250
Phenomenological data analysis 133, 252*f*

Phenomenology 132, 356
   limitations of 134
   strengths of 134
   study
      example of 133b
      steps of 133
      types of 132
Phenomenon 356
Phi coefficient 356
Physical exploitation 72
PICO approach 34b
   use of 23b
PICO(t) format 23b, 32b
Pictograms 229, 234, 234f, 283, 287
Pictographs 234, 283, 287
Pie
   diagram 233f, 286f
   graphs 229, 232, 283, 286
Pilot study 53, 214, 356
Placebo effect 356
Plagiarism 270
Popham's average congruency procedure 207
Population 46, 47, 151, 269, 356
   accessible 343
   characteristics 165
   selecting 55
Positional average 293
Positive relationship 356
Positively skewed distribution 311f, 356
Poster session 356
Post-test
   only design, example of 111b
   two group 118
Power analysis 169, 356
PQRS approach for literature review 81b
Practice theory 93
Pre-code all questions 183
Prediction research, example of 122b
Predictive validity 206, 356
Pre-experimental designs, types of 118
Pre-experimental research 117
   limitations of 119
   strengths of 119
Preparing Likert scale, tips for 185
Preparing qualitative interview, guidelines for 191
Pretest plan 176
Pretest post-test
   control group designs 110
   design 357
      example of 110b
Prevalence rate 120b
Prevalence studies 120, 357

Primary source 76, 77, 83, 174, 357
   example of 76b, 174b
PRISMA guidelines 357
Privacy and confidentiality 66
Probability sampling 357
   techniques 155
   types of 155
Problem analysis 1
Problem focused triggers 23
Problem statement 30b, 160, 357
   components of 32
Problems with interviews 194
Problem-solving 1
   model 2f
   process 1
Process consent 66, 357
Projective techniques 204
   classification of 204
Prolonged engagement 357
Propensity score 357
Proportional bar graph 230, 231, 231f
Proportionate stratified random sampling 157
Proposal 357
Proposed solution 30
Prospective design 124, 357
Prospective time series design, example of 116b
Protecting basic human rights of
      vulnerable groups 67
Protecting human rights, ethical principles for 63
Protecting right of individual in publication 271
Psychological measurement 199
Psychology test scores 235t
Psychometric properties, evaluation of 182
Public health nursing practice model 93
Publication ethics violations 269
Publication information 75
PubMed 78
Purposive sampling 163, 357
   example of 164b

Q

Q-sort 201, 357
   example of 202b
   strengths of 202
Qualitative analysis, processes of 243
Qualitative content analysis 247
Qualitative data 174, 357
   analysis 241, 243, 249t
      approach 242
      element of 242
      procedure 244
      purpose of 241

Qualitative research 14, 357
    characteristics of 16
    design 130
    example of 16b
    overview 134t
    process, steps of 57f
    study, validity of 130
    types of 132
Qualitative study, steps in 56
Qualitative variables 167
Quality review, characteristics of 72
Quantifying observation 198
Quantitative and qualitative research 14, 15t, 103
Quantitative data 174, 357
Quantitative research 14, 103, 104f
    additional types of 128
    example of 14b
    process 53
        steps of 54f
    validity of 103
Quantitative variables 167
Quartile deviation 222, 297, 298
    coefficient of 298
    for grouped data 299
        calculation of 298
    for ungrouped data, calculation of 298
Quasi-experimental designs 115
Quasi-experimental research 114
    limitations of 117
    strength of 117
Question
    cause-effect 34
    introducing 191
Questionnaire
    administration, methods of 182
    limitations of 184
    on pilot project, administration of 182
    organization of 181
    strengths of 183
    types of 178
    wording of 181
Quota sampling 162, 357
    limitations of 163
    strengths of 163

R

Random assignment 107, 358
Random error 212
Random numbers, table of 107, 156, 156t
Random sampling 358

Randomized block design 113, 358
    example of 113b
Randomized control trials 358
Range 222, 297, 358
Rank order question 179
    example of 179b
Rating question 179
    example of 179b
Rating scale 184, 197, 358
    types of 184
Ratio measurement 280, 358
Ratio scale 220, 221
Ratio-level measurement 221b
    example of 280b
Raw data 279, 358
Reactive measurement effect 105, 196
Reading through manuscript 252
Record analysis 200
    example of 201b
Recruit sample 166
Reduction and linguistic transformation of
    statement 251
Redundant publication 270, 348
References and bibliography 263
Reflective remarks 246
Reflexivity 16
Register clinical trials 271
Reliability coefficient 358
    interpretation of 212
Replication study 358
Report writing 133
Representative sample 152, 358
Research 6, 358
    and nursing research 6
    and publication misconduct 269
    approach 101
    barriers related to 273
    in clinical nursing practice 17
    integrity violations 269
    method 358
    methodology, describe 4
    misconduct 358
    project, complexity of 72
    promotes evidenced based nursing care 19
    purposes of 8
    tools 47
    types of 13, 93
    variables, example of 36b
Research critique
    dimensions of 266
    principles of 265
    purposes of 265

Research design 101, 358
　selecting 54
　selection 15
　types of 120
Research hypotheses 41, 44, 241, 358
　example of 44b
Research in nursing
　administration 18
　education 17
　significance of 19
Research instruments 47, 269
　selecting specific 55
Research objectives 39
　characteristics of 39
　example of 40b
　significance of 39
　types of 39
Research problem 29, 52, 359
　defining 29
　determine feasibility of 35
　identifying 57
　research question and hypothesis 29
　selection of 34b
　　area and 4
　　sources of 30, 31f
Research proposal 266
　development 266
　essentials of 268b
　format of 268
　significance of 266
Research question 33, 34, 359
　and problem statement 33
　example of 34b
　need of 33
　types of 34
Research report 260, 359
　format of 262t
　preparation of 261
Research statement 153, 154
　example of 33b
Research study 258
　reporting guidelines for 258t
　type of 177
Research utilization 271, 272, 359
　and evidence-based practice 272t
　barriers to 272
Researchability of problem 35
Researchers
　background 72
　credibility 359
　experience of 35, 178

　interest of 35
　role of 15
Resources
　availability of 72, 102, 165, 178
　lack of 166
Respect for human dignity, principle of 63, 64
Response set bias 359
Retrospective design 123, 359
Review of literature 4, 71
　steps of 80b
Review process 81f
Rice production per year 230t
Right to fair treatment 65
Right to full disclosure 64
Right to privacy 65
Right to protection from exploitation 64
Right to self-determination 64
Right to withdrawn from study 66
Risk-benefit ratio 359
Risk-benefits assessment 67
Rival hypothesis 359
Roger's theory 93
Root mean square deviation 300
Rorschach inkblot technique 204
Roy's adaptation theory 93

S

Salami slicing 270
Sample and sampling techniques 151
Sample characteristics 178
　identification 173
Sample master data sheet 224t
Sample outlines for research report 261t
Sample representativeness 166
Sample size 15, 269
　analysis problem 166
　calculation 166
　　in animal study 170b
Sampling 53, 152, 359
　bias 153, 166, 359
　criteria 153
　error 153, 359
　frame 152, 359
　in research, importance of 154
　method 164
　mortality/attrition 153
Sampling plan 153, 359
　specify 166
Sampling process 165f
　in quantitative research 165
　knowledge of 166

Sampling technique 269
  types of 155, 155f
  use of 47
Sampling terms 151
Sampling, non-directional 354
Sampling, problems in 166
Scale, duration of 213
Scatter diagram 229, 236, 283, 289
Scatter plot 236f, 289f, 359
Science direct 78
Scientific information, availability of 102
Scientific method 359
  limitations of 3
  steps of 4
Scientific research 6
Screening instrument 359
Searching literature 80
Searching relevant literature
  review 53
  search 58
Secondary sources, example of 77b, 175b
Sector graphs 229, 232, 283, 286
Selection threat 360
Selective approach 253
Selective coding 250, 360
Self-administration 182
Self-determination 360
Self-plagiarism 270
Self-report 360
Semantic differential 360
  scale 184, 185
    dimension of 186b
    example of 186b
    limitations of 187
    uses of 186
Semantic equivalence 213
Semiotic 247
Semi-structured interview 190, 360
Sensitivity 360
Sentence completion tests 204
Short questions 183
Shot gunning 270
Sign test 360
Significance level 360
Silence 191
Simple bar diagram 283f
Simple bar graph 230, 230f
Simple hypothesis 43
  example of 43b

Simple random sampling 156, 360
  limitations of 157
  methods of 156
  strengths of 157
  types of 156
  with replacement 156
  without replacement 156
Single group post-test only design,
  example of 118b
Single item indicator question, example of 181b
Skewed distribution 360
Skewness 311
  and kurtosis 311
  measures of 312
Skill attainment and performance 195
Snowball sampling 161, 360
  limitations of 162
  strengths of 162
  types of 161
Social problems 31
Social sciences, statistical packages for 324
Social work abstracts 78
Sociodemographic variables 37
Sociological abstracts 78
Solomon four group design 111
  example of 111b
Sources, types of 76
Spearman's rank correlation 360
  coefficient 308
    critical values for 335
Spearman's rho 360
Spearman-Brown prophecy formula 211
Specifying behavior 198
Split half-method 210
Stability 209
Standard deviation 169, 222, 300, 304, 304t, 360
  by assumed mean method, calculation of 301
  concept of 300
  for combined observation, calculation of 303
  for group data, calculation of 302
  for ungrouped data, calculation of 300
Standard error 360
Standard scores 360
State hypothesis 4, 46
Statement hierarchy 91
Static groups comparison, example of 119b
Statistical packages
  and analysis 323
  selection of 324
Statistical power 314

Statistical procedures 219
Statistical regression effects 105
Statistics 360
   characteristics of 278
   functions of 278
   use of 15
Strata 152
Stratified random sampling 157
   limitations of 158
   strengths of 158
   types of 157
Stratified sampling technique, steps of 158
Strauss and Corbin method 250
Strengths and weaknesses 2
Stress and coping
   among nursing students, study of 90
   strategies 90
Stressors 95
Structural analysis 249
Structured interviews 190
Structured methods 6
Structured observation 196
   methods in 196
   sampling in 197
Students in strata, number and percentage of 163t
Study
   duration 269
   implications of 103
   instruments 15
   purpose of 65, 102
   time frame 73
Subject/key informant 52
Subjects, availability of 35
Suicidal death 2008 and 2012, number of 237t
Support system, availability of 73
Survey
   examples of 127b
   limitations of 127
   research 126
   strengths of 127
   types of 126
Synthesis 75
Synthesized version by experts, evaluation of 214
Synthesizing literature 80
Systematic and orderly process 8
Systematic random sampling 158
   limitations of 159
   steps of 159
   strengths of 159
   types of 159

Systematic review, stage of 82f
Systematic sampling, repeated 159

T

Table number 281
Table presentation 225, 281
Tabulation, principles of 226
Tabulation, significance of 229
Tax difference per year 231t
Taxonomic analysis 248, 249
Technical equivalence 213
Telephonic interviews 193
Telephonic questionnaire 182
Terminology of theory 87
Testing effects 104
Text recycling 270
Thematic analysis 248
Thematic apperception test 204
Theme analysis 248
Theoretical framework 91
   in research, use of 95
Theoretical limitations 48
Theoretical notes 246
Theoretical sampling 163
Theoretical sensitivity 243
Theory 86, 91
   and conceptual models in research 86
   and corresponding research, types of 93t
   classification
      by level 92
      by purpose 93
   generating research 94
   in nursing, importance of 87
   in research, use of 94
   models and framework in research,
      importance of 93
   research and practice, relationship between 97
   testing research 94
   triangulation 131
   types of 92, 93
Thesis and dissertation 263
Thick description 131
Threats effects, interaction of 105
Three-dimensional analysis 249
Time duration 178
Time frame 35
Time sampling 197
Time series design 115
   types of 116

Time series research
   limitations of 116
   strengths of 116
Title 281
   of table 226, 281
Tool 46
Topic for review, selection of 80
Total enumeration sampling 164
T-probability values, distribution of 329
Track title 75
Tradition 5
Training of observer 198, 212
Transcribing recorded data 245
Translated version, synthesis of 214
Triangulation in ethnography 135b
True experimental
   design
      steps of 110f
      types of 110
   research 106
      characteristics of 107
T-test 318
   application, assumptions of 318
   types of 318

U

Ungrouped data, mean for 291
Unit of measurement 227
United Grant Commission 270
Univariate descriptive designs 120
Unstructured methods 5
Unstructured observation 197
   methods in 197
Utrecht school of phenomenology 253

V

Validating and conforming relationship 98
Validity 205
   and reliability 205
   measures of 206
   of statement 251
Vancouver style 263
   references 263

Variability, measures of 222
Variables 36, 46
   classification of 36
   discrete 52, 348
   knowledge of 15
   of interest 33
   under study 177
Variance test, analysis of 322
Variance, analysis of 321, 343
Variation
   coefficient of 222, 304
   sources of 323
Verbal communication and behavior 195
Vignette, example of 202b
Vignettes 202
   limitations of 203
   strength of 203
Visual analog scale 184, 187, 280
   example of 188b
   for pain 187f
   limitations of 188
   uses and strengths of 188

W

Web-based questionnaire 182
Welcome research in practice, change
      attitude to 273
Well-framed delimitation, characteristics of 47
Wilcoxon rank sum test 240
Word association techniques 204
World association test 205
Writing hypothesis, styles of 46b
Writing literature review, tips for 82
Writing research
   objectives, tips for 40
   question 133
Writing review 81

Z

Z-distribution table 331, 332
Z-test 321
   application of 321
   interpretation of 321

EU GSPR Authorised Reprsentative
Logos Europe, 9 rue Nicolas Poussin
1700, La Rochelle, France
Phone: +33 (0) 6 67 93 73 78
E-mail: contact@logoseurope.eu

www.ingramcontent.com/pod-product-compliance
Ingram Content Group UK Ltd.
Pitfield, Milton Keynes, MK11 3LW, UK
UKHW050455150426
5217IPUK00025B/1689